Download Your Included Ebook Today!

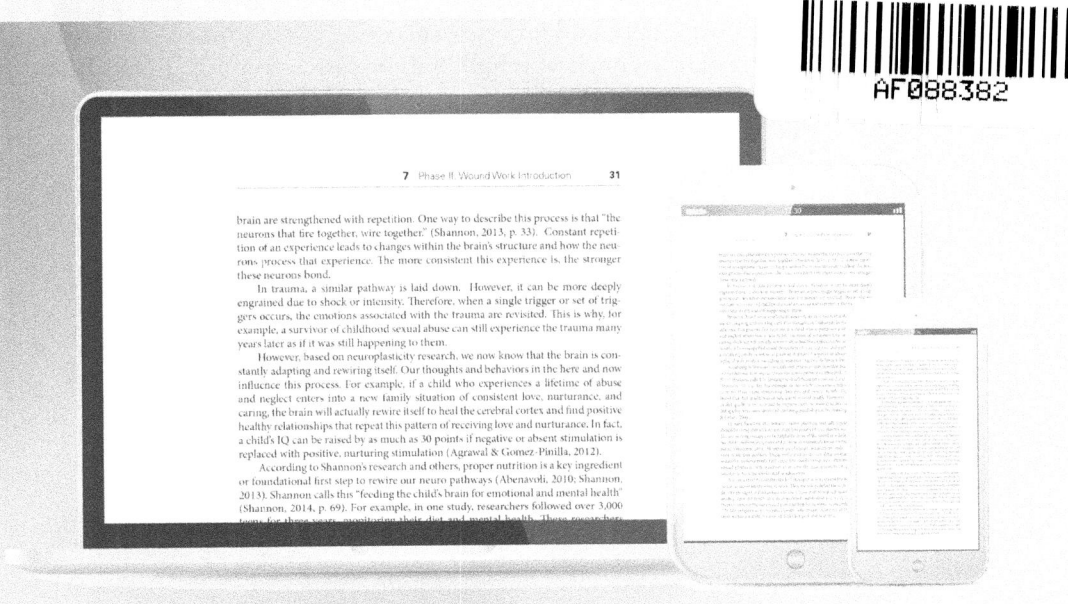

Your print purchase of *Effective Counseling and Psychotherapy* **includes an ebook download** to the device of your choice—increasing accessibility, portability, and searchability!

**Download your ebook today at:
http://spubonline.com/ecp
and enter the access code below:**

1TSHFYC6C

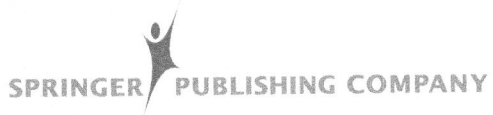

springerpub.com

Bob Bertolino, PhD, is professor of rehabilitation counseling at Maryville University, senior clinical advisor at Youth In Need, Inc., and a senior associate for the International Center for Clinical Excellence. He has taught over 500 workshops throughout the United States and 11 countries and authored or coauthored 14 books. Bob is a licensed marital and family therapist and professional counselor in the state of Missouri, a national certified counselor, a certified rehabilitation counselor, a National Board–certified fellow in hypnotherapy, and a clinical member of the American Association for Marriage and Family Therapy.

Effective Counseling and Psychotherapy

An Evidence-Based Approach

BOB BERTOLINO, PhD

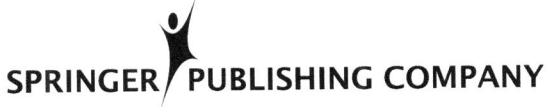

Copyright © 2018 Springer Publishing Company, LLC

All rights reserved.

No part of this publication may be reproduced, stored in a retrieval system, or transmitted in any form or by any means, electronic, mechanical, photocopying, recording, or otherwise, without the prior permission of Springer Publishing Company, LLC, or authorization through payment of the appropriate fees to the Copyright Clearance Center, Inc., 222 Rosewood Drive, Danvers, MA 01923, 978-750-8400, fax 978-646-8600, info@copyright.com or on the Web at www.copyright.com.

Springer Publishing Company, LLC
11 West 42nd Street
New York, NY 10036
www.springerpub.com

Acquisitions Editor: Sheri W. Sussman
Compositor: S4Carlisle Publishing Services

ISBN: 978-0-8261-4112-5
ebook ISBN: 978-0-8261-4113-2

Student Supplements are available from Springerpub.com/bertolino
Student Exercises: 978-0-8261-4118-7

Instructor's Materials: Qualified instructors may request supplements by emailing textbook@springerpub.com:
Instructor's Manual: 978-0-8261-4114-9
Instructor's PowerPoints: 978-0-8261-4116-3
Test Bank: 978-0-8261-4115-6

The author and the publisher of this Work have made every effort to use sources believed to be reliable to provide information that is accurate and compatible with the standards generally accepted at the time of publication. The author and publisher shall not be liable for any special, consequential, or exemplary damages resulting, in whole or in part, from the readers' use of, or reliance on, the information contained in this book. The publisher has no responsibility for the persistence or accuracy of URLs for external or third-party Internet websites referred to in this publication and does not guarantee that any content on such websites is, or will remain, accurate or appropriate.

Library of Congress Cataloging-in-Publication Data
Names: Bertolino, Bob, 1965- author.
Title: Effective counseling and psychotherapy : an evidence-based approach / Bob Bertolino, PhD.
Description: New York : Springer Publishing Company, [2018] | Includes bibliographical references and index.
Identifiers: LCCN 2018001601 | ISBN 9780826141125
Subjects: LCSH: Psychotherapy. | Counseling. | Evidence-based medicine.
Classification: LCC RC480 .B47 2018 | DDC 616.89/14--dc23 LC record available at https://lccn.loc.gov/2018001601

Contact us to receive discount rates on bulk purchases.
We can also customize our books to meet your needs.
For more information please contact: sales@springerpub.com

Printed in the United States of America.

*To my dad, Anthony Bertolino (1939–2015):
Thank you for teaching me to be curious about the world and to understand the value of hard work. I learned as much from your humility as I did from your intellect. I miss you every day.*

Contents

Preface   ix
Acknowledgments   xiii

1. **The Influence of the Therapist   1**
   An Evolution in Psychotherapy?   2
   The Good News, Bad News Conundrum   3
   An Evolution in Context   5
   Methods, Models, and Techniques   5
   Training and Supervision   8
   Exploring Therapist Performance   10
   Therapist Effects   13

2. **Principles and Core Strategies of Effective Therapy   25**
   Evidence-Based Practice and Empirically Supported Treatments:
      One and the Same?   25
   Defining Evidence-Based Practice   27
   Common Factors: A Brief History and Conundrum   30
   Evolving From the Common Factors   34
   The Third Wave: A Strengths-Based Perspective   36
   Strengths-Based Principles: From Evidence to Practice   40
   Putting the Pieces Together: Qualities and Actions of Effective
      Therapists   54

3. **Early Client Engagement   63**
   The Alliance–Outcome Correlation   63
   A Few Words About Words: Strengths-Based Language
      and Conversations   64
   Strengthening the Alliance Through Collaboration Keys   68

4. **Active Client Engagement (ACE): Information-Gathering
      Processes   89**
   The 80/20 Rule in Action: Preparing for Change   90
   Strengths-Based Information Gathering   92

vii

Process 1: ROM in Practice: Partners for Change Outcome Management System   93
Process 2: Interviewing for Strengths   110

5. **Therapeutic Conversations for Achieving Structure and Direction**   135
   Funneling: Bringing Focus to Therapeutic Conversations   135
   Advanced Listening and Attending Skills: Using Language to Strengthen the Alliance and Create Possibilities   153

6. **Matching and Classes of Intervention**   175
   The I-Am Approach to Client Orientations   175
   Matching: Increasing the Factor of Fit   176
   The Path to Models: A Brief Summary   190
   From Philosophy to Theory to Practice   191
   Classes of Problems/Classes of Intervention: Selecting Models   194

7. **Client Progress and the Benefits of Therapy**   201
   The Progression of Therapy in Future Sessions   201
   Category 1: Unimprovement or Deterioration   203
   Responses to Unimprovement and Deterioration   211
   Category 2: Improvement   226
   Revisiting Goals and Outcomes: The Meaning of Progress   235
   Transition From Therapy   239

8. **Professional Development and Clinical Excellence**   247
   Understanding Therapist Effectiveness   247
   The Road to Excellence: Natural and Talented?   248
   Cycle of Excellence   258
   Strategies for Practice to Improve Therapeutic Effectiveness   264
   Deliberate Practice in Context   270
   Future-Forward: Supervision Revisited   272
   The Path to Excellence   277

Appendix: Outcome Measures and Forms   283
Index   295

Preface

In 1862, just prior to signing the Emancipation Proclamation, Abraham Lincoln gave his second annual address to Congress. He urged Congress to use fresh eyes as they considered the situation. Lincoln stated, "The dogmas of the quiet past are inadequate in the stormy present. The occasion is piled high with difficulty. As our case is new, so we must think anew and act anew. We must disenthrall ourselves and then we shall save our country." What did Lincoln mean by disenthrall? He meant that we move through life with ideas that we remain captivated with but are no longer relevant or true (Robinson, 2011). Like most fields, over the last 100 years, the field of psychotherapy has undergone major changes. Unfortunately, available evidence reveals that while there has been a substantial increase in the number of treatment models, outcomes have not improved accordingly. In fact, since the first meta-analytic studies in the 1970s, psychotherapy outcomes have remained flat. Psychotherapy unequivocally works, but its delivery has not improved. As such, a new direction is necessary. However, a new direction does not mean "out with the old and in with the new." Instead, it requires us to shift our attention to those factors that most account for the success of psychotherapy.

This is not a book about treatment models. There are over 55,000 how-to books and a virtual cacophony of articles and chapters on psychotherapy treatment models, methods, and techniques. Rather, the purpose of this book is to direct the therapist toward principles, processes, and practices that underscore effective therapy, regardless of the clinician's theoretical persuasion. To this end, this book is founded on a growing body of research about "what works in therapy," providing specific, evidence-based ways for therapists to improve the benefit of therapy and their individual performance.

TERMINOLOGY

It is important to address terminology from the outset. Throughout this volume, various terms will be used interchangeably, except when examples require specific nomenclature. Because this is a book about psychotherapy, the term *psychotherapy* will primarily be used, with *counseling*, *therapy*, *treatment*, and *behavioral health* periodically substituted. The term *client* will be used when referring to those who are seeking or are already involved in therapy. It is acknowledged that the language used to describe those who receive psychotherapy is largely determined by the contexts in which services are provided, and that the terms *patient* and *consumer* will be more fitting in some settings. To describe persons in support of clients in therapy, *parent*, *guardian*, and *caregiver* will be used.

Four terms—*therapist*, *clinician*, *provider*, and *practitioner*—will primarily be used to refer to those who provide psychotherapy. These terms are inclusive of persons who provide psychotherapy including *counselors*, *psychologists*, *marriage and family therapists*, *social workers*, *substance abuse counselors*, *students*, *case managers*, and other *helping professionals*. Lastly, terms such as *interactions*, *sessions*, *meetings*, *appointments*, *assessments*, and *intakes* appear when referring to interactions between clients and therapists.

HOW THIS BOOK IS ARRANGED

This book is divided into eight chapters. While every chapter has a distinct focus, the chapters are inextricably linked, with each building on previous ones. Collectively, the chapters form a volume that provides both new and experienced therapists guidance for increasing the benefit of services and their individual baseline rates of performance.

Chapter 1, *The Influence of the Therapist*, begins our journey with an exploration of how the field of psychotherapy has evolved. The chapter includes a discussion of promising developments and challenges to improving treatment outcomes and the individual performance of clinicians. The opening chapter also delves into topics such as the effectiveness of treatment models, training and supervision, and therapists' personal philosophies (worldviews). The purpose of this chapter is to orient readers to the current state of the field and offer direction for improving the benefits of psychotherapy.

The second chapter, *Principles and Core Strategies of Effective Therapy*, involves examination of concepts and directions in research and practice that are important to all psychotherapists. The chapter also includes discussion of key movements that represent the field's evolvement, along with corresponding research findings. Included in this examination is a discussion of what it means to be *strengths-based* and principles that define a strengths-based perspective.

Chapter 3, *Early Client Engagement*, focuses on ways to engage clients during initial interactions. Essential to this chapter is examination of specific collaborative processes that help to form and strengthen the therapeutic alliance.

In Chapter 4, *Active Client Engagement (ACE): Information-Gathering Processes*, readers are introduced to the ACE model, which includes *acquiring* information, *creating* a context for collaboration, and *evocation* of clients' strengths and resources. In this detailed chapter, methods for gathering client information and using routine outcome monitoring (ROM) are introduced. An additional part of this chapter involves ways to match clients' communication styles.

The primary focus of Chapter 5, *Therapeutic Conversations for Achieving Structure and Direction*, is creating a direction in therapy with clients. Ideas for gaining clear problem descriptions, establishing goals, and identifying progress toward those goals are provided. Chapter 5 also includes a host of ways of using language to both acknowledge and validate clients' experiences while simultaneously opening up possibilities for change.

Chapter 6, *Matching and Classes of Intervention*, covers several key areas critical to improving the outcome of psychotherapy. Readers are offered ways to increase the *fit* (i.e., how well a model aligns with a particular client) and *effect* (i.e., the outcome) of the treatment. This chapter centers around discussion of how to select and match treatment models with clients to increase the likelihood of success.

In Chapter 7, *Client Progress and the Benefits of Therapy*, the process of monitoring client progress is explored in detail. Of particular importance is how therapists respond to clients who are unimproved or deteriorated. Chapter 7 includes strategies for responding to clients' lack of progress as well as how to build on progress by changing the intensity, dosage form, and type of therapy, to prepare clients for transition when maximum benefit has been achieved.

The final chapter, *Professional Development and Clinical Excellence*, considers ways for therapists to determine their baseline rates of effectiveness, obtain feedback, and engage in deliberate practice to improve their performance. Chapter 8 also includes discussion of the role of supervision, and examples of activities and exercises that therapists can use to develop domain-specific knowledge and evolve over the course of their careers.

To give life to the ideas in this book and connect them to practice, case illustrations, stories, sample dialogues, and discussion questions are used. There is also an appendix with outcome measures as well as graphs and charts that are discussed throughout the book. **Qualfied instructors can also request an Instructor's Manual, PowerPoints, and a test bank to assist with performance development; to access these materials, please send an email to textbook@springerpub.com.**

–Bob Bertolino

Reference

Robinson, K. (2011). *Out of our minds: Learning to be creative* (2nd ed.). West Sussex, UK: Capstone.

Acknowledgments

My deepest appreciation and love to my family—Misha, Morgan, and Claire. Thank you for your love, patience, and support. Life would not have the same meaning without you. And to my mom, stepmom, and brothers and sisters for always being there for me. Family is the greatest gift.

Thank you to my colleagues at Maryville University—especially Dr. Michael Kiener, Dr. Kate Kline, Dr. Chuck Gulas, faculty in the College of Health Professions, and to students who teach me something new almost every day.

A very heartfelt thank-you to the staff of Youth In Need, Inc. (YIN), whom I've had the good fortune of working with for over 25 years. I'd like to especially thank Pat Holtermann-Hommes, Tricia Topalbegovic, Michelle Gorman, Mark Solari, Rob Muschany, Amy Putzler, Melissa Chambers, Cara Merritt, Erin Strohbehn, Joel Durham, and the clinical staff who bring the ideas in this book to life with their clients.

To Covenant Technology Partners (CTP), including Doug Meyer, Kevin Newbern, Alan Richardson, Kurt Rolland, and the many others in our CTP–YIN partnership who have brought our Imagine outcomes management system to life.

A big thank-you to colleagues and friends who have provided indelible support over the years: Scott Miller, Bill O'Hanlon, Jason Seidel, Cynthia Maeschalck, Susanne Bargmann, David Prescott, Charlie Appelstein, and colleagues at the International Center for Clinical Excellence (ICCE).

And my heartfelt gratitude to the Springer Publishing Company. Thank you to Sheri W. Sussman, Mindy Chen, and Michael O'Connor for your vision, patience, and support.

CHAPTER 1

The Influence of the Therapist

In December 1985, the first Evolution of Psychotherapy conference was held in Phoenix, Arizona. Sponsored by the Milton H. Erickson Foundation, the conference was hailed as the "Woodstock" of psychotherapy. Many of the world's top theorists and some 7,000 attendees from 29 countries gathered in the midst of the first snowstorm in Phoenix in over 40 years. Carl Rogers, Virginia Satir, Bruno Bettelheim, Aaron Beck, Jay Haley, James Masterson, Rollo May, Murray Bowen, Salvador Minuchin, Carl Whitaker, and R. D. Laing were among the "legends" leading workshops, participating in panel discussions, and conducting live demonstrations.

The Evolution conference provided an opportunity to debate the differences between various schools of psychotherapy both in terms of theory and practice. Disagreement was expected and even welcomed. Director of the Milton H. Erickson Foundation and conference organizer Jeff Zeig observed, "Ten years ago, these people wouldn't even have sat down together" (Leo, 1985, p. 59). And while there was plenty to debate, there was hope that some points of consensus would emerge for the conference attendees already in practice or the over 2,000 graduate students who were about to begin their professional careers. Perhaps, common ground could be found among an ever-growing sea of theorists, theories, and their respective strategies. In the convocation, Zeig (1987) echoed this sentiment:

> We are here to speak to commonalities that underlie successful clinical work. . . . In the evolution of the infant discipline of psychotherapy, the first 100 years have been divergent. It has been a period of growth, consisting of flowers and weeds. Especially in the last 40 years, there has been a proliferation of discrete schools. Perhaps we can begin this second century in a way that is more convergent. (p. xxvii)

As the conference unfolded, the idea that it could serve as a platform for exploring similarities seemed in jeopardy. Some of the presenters thrived on the thrill of debate, whereas others were less enamored, including behaviorist Joseph Wolpe, who referred to the conference as a "babble of conflicting voices" (Leo, 1985, p. 59). Participants seemed to agree. In a review by *Time* magazine, one attendee commented, "All the experts are here, and none of them agree" (p. 59). Others painted a darker image:

> Many of the speakers resorted to innuendo, "in-jokes," ridicule and references to other theories as being the province of the foolish and misguided. In attempting to present their own position in its clearest, least complicated, and most elementary form for the large audience, the speakers created and subsequently demolished caricatures of opposing viewpoints. . . . A sense of arrogance was frequently projected in the style of presentation, in the lack of adequate preparation and in the manner in which registrants' questions were answered. (Shapiro, 1987, p. 66)

In his introduction to *The Evolution of Psychotherapy*, an edited book published after the event, Zeig (1987) concluded that neither the conference nor the book had succeeded in moving the field in the direction of commonalities and convergence, "Here were the reigning experts on psychotherapy and I could see no way they could agree on defining the territory. Can anyone dispute, then, that the field is in disarray?" (pp. xviii–xix).

Since the inaugural event in 1985, the Evolution conferences have been held in 1990, 1995, 2000, 2005, 2009, 2013, and 2017. Each has provided opportunity for debate, the cross-fertilization of ideas, and high-quality professional training to thousands of attendees. So, after 30 years, we ponder the question, "Has psychotherapy really evolved?"

AN EVOLUTION IN PSYCHOTHERAPY?

Let's consider the evidence. First, in addition to conferences such as the Evolution of Psychotherapy, and stand-alone seminars around the world, high-quality training provided by experts is available face to face, online, and in prerecorded courses and continuing education programs. Next, since the 1960s, the number of psychotherapy models has increased from 60 to over 400 with 145 manualized treatments for 51 of the 297 possible diagnostic categories in the *Diagnostic and Statistical Manual of Mental Disorders* (5th ed.; *DSM-5*; American Psychiatric Association, 2013). The widespread availability of training coupled with an explosion in models and specialized methods suggests that psychotherapy has evolved. And yet, these forms of progress fail to answer two overarching questions relevant to those who practice psychotherapy: (a) How effective is psychotherapy? and (b) How have developments in the field contributed to the overall effectiveness of psychotherapy? Next, we explore each of these questions.

THE GOOD NEWS, BAD NEWS CONUNDRUM

In the 1950s, Hans Eysenck (1952) concluded that patients who were diagnosed with neurosis and received psychoanalytic and eclectic therapies were no better off than those who received no treatment at all. The researcher stated, "The figures fail to support the hypothesis that psychotherapy facilitates recovery from neurotic disorder" (p. 323). Eysenck was quick to qualify his point of view, "The figures quoted do not necessarily disprove the *possibility* of therapeutic effectiveness" [emphasis added] (p. 323), but his remarks made it clear that he considered psychotherapy ineffective. Eysenck's research resulted in considerable controversy regarding how studies were designed, conducted, and compared, and most importantly, the effectiveness of psychotherapy (see Eysenck, 1955; Rosenzweig, 1954; Strupp, 1963). A result was the development of two specific research methods to provide empirical evidence for the efficacy of psychotherapy (Schuckard, Miller, & Hubble, 2017). The first was the clinical trial, which involves assigning clients to an active treatment condition, waitlist, or control group (Wampold, 2013). The second, meta-analysis, allows for results of different studies to be combined to determine the overall efficacy, in this case, of psychological methods (Wampold & Imel, 2015).

The Good News

The National Institute of Mental Health (NIMH), concerned about the ever-growing number of psychotherapy treatments, advocated for the use of clinical trials, in the form of randomized controlled trials (RCTs), to determine which therapies ensured the best outcomes and therefore merited reimbursement (Schuckard, Miller, & Hubble, 2017; Segal, 1975). Following in the footsteps of medicine, the RCT became the "gold standard" of research designs. By the early 1970s, hundreds of clinical trials had shown the benefits of psychotherapy regardless of the approach (Bergin, 1971; Schuckard, Miller, & Hubble, 2017).

Similarly, beginning with Smith and Glass's (1977) meta-analysis involving 375 studies, researchers found psychotherapy to be an effective means of helping persons experiencing the wide array of difficulties and challenges. Studies show that those who receive psychotherapy achieve much better outcomes than they would have had they not received psychotherapy (Lambert & Ogles, 2004; Wampold, 2001, 2007). Meta-analyses in settings ranging from community mental health centers to university counseling centers to independent practices have demonstrated that the average person who is psychologically distressed and receives therapy is better off than 80% of persons who do not (Hubble, Duncan, & Miller, 1999; Wampold, 2001; Wampold & Imel, 2015). These results are robust and provide evidence that psychotherapy produces results on par with various medical procedures and practices (e.g., chemotherapy for breast cancer, heart bypass surgery, treatments for asthma, flu vaccines) and are equal to or exceed the effects of psychotropic medications (Forand, DeRubeis, & Amsterdam, 2013; Lipsey &

Wilson, 1993; Wampold, 2007; Wampold & Imel, 2015). The benefits of psychotherapy are also longer lasting than those of medications (i.e., lower relapse rates after treatment is discontinued) and it is less resistant to additional courses of treatment. Lambert and Ogles (2004) remarked:

> Psychotherapy facilitates the remission of symptoms and improves functioning. It not only speeds up the natural healing process but also often provides additional coping strategies and methods for dealing with future problems. Providers as well as patients can be assured that a broad range of therapies, when offered by skillful, wise and stable therapists, are likely to result in appreciable gains for the client. (p. 180)

In clinical trials, psychotherapy has been shown to be effective in treating depression, anxiety, marital dissatisfaction, substance abuse, health problems (including smoking, pain, and eating disorders), and sexual dysfunction. It also helps treat various populations, including children, adolescents, adults, and elders (Chambless et al., 1998). Psychotherapy is also a flexible vehicle for promoting change, growth, and healing. It can be provided to individual or multiple persons as is the case with couples, families, or groups, and in a variety of settings including, but not limited to, private practices, community agencies, hospitals, and schools. Psychotherapy can be adapted or individualized for the particular client and his or her disorder, problem, or complaint (Wampold, 2010). Another significant benefit of psychotherapy is its cost-effectiveness. Referred to as *cost offset research*, psychotherapy has been shown to reduce health and medical expenditures for high utilizer rates of medical and health-related services (Chiles, Lambert, & Hatch, 1999; Crane & Christensen, 2008; Cummings, 2007; Cummings, Cummings, & Johnson, 1997; Cummings, O'Donohue, & Ferguson, 2002; Law, Crane, & Berge, 2003). When combined with fewer debilitating side effects than psychotropic medications and benefits that last longer, the previous findings suggest that the field of psychotherapy has evolved into an effective means of helping people who experience individual and interpersonal distress (Gøtzsche, Young, & Crace, 2015).

The Bad News

The good news is psychotherapy works. And yet, as with any form of treatment, it does not work for everyone. In clinical trials only about 60% of participants reach what is considered the "recovery" range (Lambert, 2013). Another 30% to 50% of clients do not improve from therapy (Lambert, 2010). These clients do not necessarily get worse, they just don't demonstrate any measurable benefit. Further, 5% to 10% of adults and between 12% and 20% of adolescents deteriorate while in therapy (Hansen, Lambert, & Forman, 2002; Lambert, 2013; Warren et al., 2010). In addition, dropout—the unilateral decision by clients to prematurely end therapy—ranges between 20% and 47% and increases with children and adolescents to 28% to 85% (Garcia & Weisz, 2002; Swift, Greenberg,

Whipple, & Kominiak, 2012). These findings, and others to be discussed later in this chapter, suggest that there is much opportunity for improvement and growth in psychotherapy as it is currently practiced (Schuckard, Miller, & Hubble, 2017).

AN EVOLUTION IN CONTEXT

Given the "good news, bad news" conundrum, a central theme of this book is how to use evidence to improve therapeutic outcomes. To do this, we revisit the second overarching question posed earlier in this chapter: How have developments in the field contributed to the overall effectiveness of psychotherapy? We begin with the influence of therapeutic models followed by discussion of training and supervision. We then consider the role of the therapist in psychotherapy outcomes and how to systematically improve over the course of one's career.

METHODS, MODELS, AND TECHNIQUES

Since the advent of psychotherapy over a century ago, there has been much discussion about the role of models in treatment outcomes. Today, the influence of models and specialized techniques on psychotherapy outcomes continues to be a source of fierce debate (Wampold & Imel, 2015). Here we consider two critical questions. First, are some psychotherapy models more effective than others? Second, are there specific ingredients of models that are largely responsible for change? Given that these and other closely related questions have been discussed in great detail elsewhere, I will summarize the findings as they pertain to our aim of becoming more informed, effective clinicians.

Are Some Models More Effective Than Others?

After years of allowing researchers to test their respective models in RCTs against no treatment conditions (i.e., primarily waitlists), a design in which the experimental group receives the intervention and the control group does not, controversy arose. Whereas neither the administrators nor participants in medication trials know who is receiving the active treatment, it is not possible to blind participants in trials to psychotherapy (O'Leary & Borkovec, 1978; Seligman, 1995; Wampold, 2001). Simply, participants in psychotherapy trials know whether or not they are in the treatment or placebo condition and therapists are more often than not aware that they are delivering a sham or incomplete treatment (Wampold, Minami, Tierney, Baskin, & Bhati, 2005).

The response of the American Psychological Association (APA) to criticisms of RCTs was to form a task force to establish criteria for reviewing evidence and ultimately determine which models met its level of excellence and be deemed "empirically validated" (which was later changed to "empirically supported") (Task Force on the Promotion and Dissemination of Psychological Procedures [TFPP], 1995).

The TFPP, later renamed the Committee on Science and Practice, was to "consider methods for educating clinical psychologists, third-party payers, and the public about effective psychotherapies" (p. 3). The result was the creation of a list of empirically supported treatments (ESTs). To date, there are over 80 ESTs for 27 of the 157 diagnoses in the *DSM-5* (APA, 2013). The APA hoped that the creation of a list of ESTs would provide an appropriate competition to the prevailing biological model of mental illness purported by psychiatry. Schuckard, Miller, and Hubble (2017) summed up the effectiveness of this effort, "In the end, the task force's initiative did little to create an advantage for therapists in the mental health care market" (p. 16).

A further, and perhaps unanticipated, ramification was that an effort to create unity among psychotherapists actually led to further divisiveness. One particular point of contention was the favor given to cognitive and behavioral approaches, studies of which were funded at a far greater rate than those involving other approaches. But the most substantive argument could be found with the APA's actual list of ESTs given that there was little to no evidence that these models were superior to others used in everyday practice (Wampold et al., 1997).

With one qualification, differences in the outcomes of various types of psychotherapies are negligible or altogether absent (Wampold & Imel, 2015). These findings come from clinical trials in which one model is compared to another. Referred to as comparative analyses, studies demonstrate that numerous models can have a positive influence on outcome, but no one model can claim superiority, even when it comes to specific disorders and client issues (Wampold & Imel, 2015). The one qualification occurs when researchers choose to compare a "bona fide" (i.e., legitimate) treatment approach to a model for which there is no coherent explanation of the approach, how it might help the client, and/or no treatment plan (e.g., "supportive therapy," "standard community care") (Wampold & Imel 2015). Although some form of intervention is better than doing nothing for clients, it stands to reason that comparing a bona fide model—one that is actually used by therapists—to one that is made up only for the purposes of comparison in a study and not used in any reputable form of treatment is simply not a good way to demonstrate the efficacy of an approach. By definition, bona fide approaches are:

1. intended to be therapeutic (i.e., has a theoretical base and associated techniques);
2. considered viable by the psychotherapeutic community (e.g., through professional books or manuals);
3. delivered by trained therapists; and,
4. contain ingredients common to all legitimate psychotherapies (e.g., therapeutic relationship) (Bertolino, Bargmann, & Miller, 2013).

When comparison studies involve bona fide approaches, no differences are found between treatments for a wide range of diagnostic categories including anxiety, depression, alcohol addiction, posttraumatic stress disorder, bulimia nervosa, and youth disorders (i.e., attention deficit disorder, anxiety, depression, conduct disorder) (Benish, Imel, & Wampold, 2008; Imel, Wampold, Miller, & Fleming, 2008; Miller, Wampold, & Varhely, 2008; Stefini et al., 2017; Wampold, Minami, Baskin, & Tierney, 2002). Ironically, over a half century prior to the first comparative analyses, psychologist Saul Rosenzweig (1936, 1954) made reference to the Dodo Bird in *Alice in Wonderland* in which contestants started and ended when they wanted. The Dodo exclaimed, "*Everybody* has won, *all* must have prizes.*"* Rosenzweig theorized all psychotherapies produce equivalent outcomes which in psychotherapy became known as the *Dodo bird effect*.

In 2012, the APA took a significant step by its acceptance of a growing body of evidence pointing to the general equivalence of the major models of psychotherapy. In its Resolution on the Recognition of Psychotherapy Effectiveness, the APA stated:

> Comparisons of different forms of psychotherapy most often result in relatively nonsignificant difference, and contextual and relationship factors often mediate or moderate outcomes. These findings suggest that (1) most valid and structured psychotherapies are roughly equivalent in effectiveness and (2) patient and therapist characteristics, which are not usually captured by a patient's diagnosis or by the therapist's use of a specific psychotherapy, affect the results. (American Psychological Association [APA], 2012)

Another argument can be found with those who advocate for the veracity of single studies that show differences between approaches, including those with cognitive and behavior therapies. However, such differences are no more than is to be expected by chance and result from methodological factors such as more reactive criteria involving client factors, therapist effects, or the allegiance effect (Lambert & Ogles, 2004; Luborsky et al., 1999; Wampold, 2001). The *allegiance effect* factors in the influence of the researcher's bias to a particular model within a study. The more researchers believe in, practice, and support particular models, the greater the likelihood that those models will show favorable results in studies involving those models (Wampold, 2001). To summarize, 40 years of outcome research has demonstrated that even though most models effect change, no one approach is significantly and consistently more effective than another (Duncan, Miller, Wampold, & Hubble, 2010).

A second and equally critical point regarding the effectiveness of models relates to the amount of variance in outcomes that can be attributed to any approach. Models, such as those debated for nearly three decades at the Evolution of Psychotherapy conferences, are responsible for only about 1% of the overall variance in treatment outcomes (Duncan, Miller, Wampold, & Hubble, 2010). At the center of dispute is the ideology that models act like medications—for example, penicillin—with active ingredients that are responsible for change. In the psychotherapy literature, there is a distinct absence of evidence demonstrating that therapy models contain active ingredients or "active factors" remedial to a particular disorder or problem (Schuckard, Miller, & Hubble,

2017). Neither component strategies, including dismantling (i.e., studies in which specific ingredients of a model are removed to provide evidence of its therapeutic value), nor additive designs (i.e., an ingredient is added to an existing package) have shown that specific model components (e.g., behavioral activation, automatic thoughts modification, the miracle question, etc.) have any substantive effect on therapy outcomes. Wampold and Imel (2015) summarized, "There is no compelling evidence that the specific ingredients of any particular psychotherapy or specific ingredients in general are critical to producing the benefits of psychotherapy" (p. 253).

Clarifying the Role of Methods and Models

Saying that bona fide treatment models produce results that are equivalent and that there is no evidence of active ingredients in psychotherapy is not saying that clinicians should ignore the significance of choosing an approach or subscribe to the idea that "anything goes." In fact, models are essential to effective psychotherapy, just not in ways originally conceived. As we will discover throughout this text, models provide frameworks for understanding client concerns and developing strategies of intervention, which will be discussed in Chapter 6. Models also provide structure to therapy, which is associated with better outcomes, as long as that structure does not override the experiences of clients. Therapy involves a delicate balance of flexibility and attunement to clients while maintaining focus—a sense of direction and purpose in each interaction. For clinicians to continuously elicit and respond to client feedback regarding improvement, lack thereof, and deterioration, they must balance structure and flexibility.

To this point we have explored the role of models as an indicator of the evolvement of the field of psychotherapy. Next, we consider the efficacy of therapist training and supervision.

TRAINING AND SUPERVISION

Continuing education is a requirement for upkeep of licensure, and in some cases, certifications, for most mental health professionals. Consensus is that professional development *provides opportunities* for clinicians to grow and improve. In contrast, there is much disagreement as to *what kinds* of professional development activities are actually beneficial, particularly when it comes to improving client outcomes. At the center of this debate is a paucity of evidence indicating that psychotherapy training and supervision improve the effectiveness of individual clinicians (Laska, Guran, & Wampold, 2014; Rousmaniere, Goodyear, Miller, & Wampold, 2017). In fact, in one study supervision was shown to contribute less than 1% of the variance in outcome (Rousmaniere, Swift, Babins-Wagner, Whipple, & Berzins, 2014). It was actually *.01%*, but was rounded to "less than 1%" because the researchers thought readers would believe it to be a typo! Further, there is some evidence that the more training, the less effective therapists may actually be (Atkins & Christensen, 2001; Christensen & Jacobson, 1994; Lambert & Ogles, 2004).

Proponents of models argue that improved training and supervision will ensure better adherence and competency and, as a result, better outcomes. By *adherence* we mean that a particular treatment is delivered in full with necessary components and void of any extraneous components. *Competence* refers to the treatment components being delivered skillfully. Wampold (2015) summarized:

> It would seem logical that adherence to the protocol and competence would be related to outcome. That is, for cases, where the therapist followed the protocol and did so skillfully, there should be better outcomes. However, this is not the case. . . . If the specific ingredients of a treatment are critical, then adherence should make a difference—actually delivering those ingredients should be related to outcome. (p. 275)

As an example, in a meta-analysis, Webb, DeRubeis, and Barber (2010) found the effects for adherence and competence were small ($d = .04$, $n = 28$ for adherence; $d = .14$, $n = 18$ for competence). Simply, therapists who adhere to what is expected in a treatment do not get better outcomes than therapists who deviate from the manual. Actually, it appears that therapists who, regardless of how the client responds, stick to the treatment have poorer outcomes. Wampold (2015) states, "There is evidence that rigid adherence to a protocol can attenuate the alliance and increase resistance to treatment" (p. 275). As it turns out, therapists who flexibly provide a treatment achieve the best outcomes (Wampold & Imel, 2015).

The benefit of training expenditures used for model-based training is also questionable (Mukuria et al., 2013). Consider, for example, a year-long study that investigated 43 clinicians who participated in a year-long "high-intensity" cognitive behavioral therapy (CBT) training that included more than 300 hours of training, supervision, and practice (Branson, Shafran, & Myles, 2015). The outcomes of 1,247 service users were monitored and tracked using standardized measures administered at regular intervals. Adherence to and competence in delivering CBT improved throughout the training and yet, contrary to expectations, results showed that greater adherence and competence, acquired through specific CBT training, did not result in better outcomes. The therapists were no more effective following the training than they were before. There is clearly a gap between the idea that training and supervision provide opportunities for clinicians to improve their relative effectiveness and prevailing evidence that casts doubt on their efficacy.

Because both training and supervision are considered primary paths to enhancing therapist development and performance, addressing the issue is of critical importance. How pressing is it? Consider studies indicate that therapist effectiveness plateaus relatively early on (Miller, 2013; Schuckard, Miller, & Hubble, 2017) in clinicians' careers, and in some cases therapists even get worse (Clement, 1994, 2008, 2013; Goldberg et al., 2016). For example, in the largest longitudinal study to date, Goldberg and colleagues (2016) followed 75 therapists over 17 years, finding that on average therapists' outcomes declined over time. Continuing to train and supervise therapists in ways that are ineffective and inefficient is an unreasonable proposition.

Although the issue of therapist growth is a complex one, there is reason to be optimistic moving forward. Extensive scientific literature across multiple disciplines including sports, chess, music, medicine, mathematics, and computer programming led by K. Anders Ericsson (Ericsson, 2006, 2009a, 2009b; Ericsson, Charness, Feltovich, & Hoffman, 2006) has provided guidance for therapist training. Ericsson (2006) and colleagues have identified a *universal set of processes* which, according to Schuckard, Miller, and Hubble (2017), account for superior performance and offer direction for cultivating the individual development of clinicians. In accordance, psychotherapy researchers have begun to more actively study how therapists improve, including the role of professional activities in their development (Chow et al., 2015). These studies suggest that therapist outcomes can improve through very specific training activities and processes. We will learn strategies that clinicians not only can immediately use to improve their effectiveness, but continue to use to develop over the course of their careers. In addition, the aforementioned studies provide guidance for supervisors, trainers, and agencies, which will be discussed throughout this book, culminating with Chapter 8.

The available literature demonstrates the importance of revising our curriculums by shifting away from trainings that are largely based on teaching methods and techniques to ones that emphasize the person of the therapist and other factors correlated with successful outcomes. In their study of 56 therapists and over 1,700 clients, Okiishi, Lambert, Nielsen, and Ogles (2003) echoed this sentiment, "Even though graduate school training and managed health care tend to focus on training in specific techniques, something else, perhaps the individual therapists themselves are responsible for the variance in client outcomes" (p. 370). Contrary to the traditional ideology that therapy approaches are critical to the success or failure of treatment, *who* provides the treatment is a far greater determinant in outcome than *what* model the therapist uses. For the remainder of this chapter we will explore the role of the therapist in therapeutic outcomes.

EXPLORING THERAPIST PERFORMANCE

Over a half century ago, psychologist Hans Strupp (1963) pondered the role of the clinician in treatment outcome when he asked, "What variance is introduced by the person of the therapist practicing them—his degree of expertness, his personality, and attitudes?" (pp. 1–2). A decade later, Ricks (1974) examined the differences in outcome in a child guidance clinic between two therapists with nearly identical caseloads (i.e., level of disturbance, gender, IQ, socioeconomic status, age, ethnicity, period seen, and the frequency of psychotic disturbances in their parents) of adolescents identified as "quite disturbed" and at high risk for developing schizophrenia (p. 280). At follow-up, as adults, 27% of the youth of the first therapist fit the diagnostic criteria for schizophrenia whereas a full 84% of the second therapist qualified. The first therapist not only had demonstrably better outcomes than the second, but was referred to as "supershrink" by youth (p. 278). Ricks' study suggested that therapists working with similar populations may achieve very different outcomes. Surprisingly, Ricks' work went largely unnoticed, falling victim to the annals of history, until nearly two decades later when researchers began to more actively explore the therapist's role in psychotherapy outcomes.

This growing interest in therapist outcomes has brought opportunities to study and learn from the most effective therapists, the "supershrinks," and in contrast, those whose outcomes fall into the average or below average ranges. Doing so involves the use of routine outcome monitoring (ROM), which has been shown to reduce rates of client deterioration (Lambert & Shimokawa, 2011). One of the more revealing findings of researchers is that although many clinicians are interested in regular reports of client progress (Bickman, 2000; Hatfield & Ogles, 2004), most do not use ROM on a regular basis, if at all (Gilbody, House, & Sheldon, 2002; Hatfield & Ogles, 2004; Zimmerman & McGlinchey, 2008). Without a baseline rating of one's effectiveness, it is very difficult to evaluate the effectiveness of training, supervision, and other efforts to improve.

Three Risks to Therapist Effectiveness and Outcomes: Overprediction, Failure to Identify, and Bias

The landscape of therapist performance is further muddied when considering that clinicians' lack of knowledge of their outcomes contributes to failure to identify client deterioration, overprediction of client improvement, and self-assessment bias. For example, in a study by Hannan et al. (2005), the researchers asked 48 clinicians (26 trainees and 22 licensed staff) to review 550 clients to predict which of their clients were likely to end treatment worse off than when they started treatment. The group was informed that the baseline rate of deterioration for the clinic was approximately 8%. The clinicians collectively identified just one of the deteriorated clients as compared to the lab-test/actuarial method, which correctly identified 36 of the 40 who deteriorated. The results revealed two crucial findings. First, "Therapists tend to overpredict improvement and fail to recognize clients who worsen during therapy" (p. 161). Next, "Therapists need independent data to alert them that treatment is not having its intended effects and that deterioration may be forthcoming" (p. 162). These results are consistent with previous studies on clinical versus actuarial predictions (Dawes, 1989; Grove & Meehl, 1996).

Beyond the duality of therapists' tendency to overpredict client improvement and failure to recognize client deterioration is self-assessment bias. Not unlike other fields, therapists are poor evaluators of their own performance (Tetlock &

Gardner, 2015). It seems that the least effective therapists view themselves as effective as the most effective therapists (Brown, Dreis, & Nace, 1999). In fact, on average clinicians overrate their effectiveness by 60% to 65%. In a 2012 study of 129 psychiatrists, psychologists, professional counselors, clinical social workers, and marriage and family therapists, researchers found on average that practitioners viewed their skills to be at the 80th percentile (Walfish, McAlister, O'Donnell, & Lambert, 2012). The researchers also found that:

> None of the respondents self-rated their skills below the 50th percentile, with only 8.4% of the respondents rating their skill below the 75th percentile. Twenty-five percent of the sample self-rated their skill at the 90th percentile or above when compared to their peers. (p. 641)

As discussed, therapists are not alone when it comes to overestimating their effectiveness. In a classic study at the General Electric Company by Meyer (1980), the researcher asked engineers to self-assess their performance compared to other engineers with similar jobs and salaries. The findings were that the average engineer rated his performance to be at the 78th percentile compared to peers, while only 2 of the 92 engineers in the study placed themselves below the 50th percentile. Similar results have been found in a range of performance areas from driving skills to medical practice, suggesting that individuals' self-judgments often surpass their abilities (Dunning, Heath, & Suls, 2004; Elaad, 2003; Kruger & Dunning, 1999).

It can be argued that all three issues—overestimation of client improvement, failure to identify client deterioration, and self-assessment bias—present cause for concern. When it comes to the well-being of others, the consequences of underperformance can be steep. An example can be found with Cincinnati Children's Hospital (CCH), considered one of the foremost treatment centers for patients with cystic fibrosis (CF). Many patients who sought medical treatment did so with the belief that CCH was better in the treatment of persons with CF than other facilities. The fact was that CCH was average; their patients were living to be about 30 years old. At the best treatment centers the outcomes were much better with patients living to around 46 years old.

In his article "The Bell Curve: What Happens When Patients Find Out How Good Their Doctors Really Are?" surgeon Dr. Atul Gawande (2004) explained that CCH faced the conundrum of what to do about the knowledge of their outcomes with CF patients. The hospital administration first made the decision to be transparent by informing their patients of how the hospital's outcomes compared to national norms. CCH then vowed to do something about its performance. They consulted with Don Berwick, then CEO of the Institute for Healthcare Improvement (IHI), a small organization with the mission of transforming healthcare. CCH staff also studied those centers with the best outcomes with CF and narrowed its focus to those factors most linked to longevity. In doing so, CCH learned about subtle differences that account for the majority of outcome. For example, a decrease in just .05% in lung functioning can, over time, compound and be the difference between life and death (Gawande, 2004). CCH understood that there were large consequences when it came to "average" treatment of patients with CF. Average meant shorter life span. They committed themselves to doing what it took to improve and extend the lives of their patients.

In behavioral health, it can also be argued that "average" spells more suffering, unnecessary expenditures, and so on. In a study of 91 therapists, Okiishi, Lambert, Nielsen, and Ogles (2003) found that clients of the top 10% of therapists were twice as likely to recover and 50% less likely to deteriorate as compared to the least effective therapists in the study. It is apparent that there is variability between therapists who work both in private settings and at a given agency (Wampold & Brown, 2005). Some therapists consistently achieve better outcomes than others.

Truly, not every therapist will become a supershrink nor should that be the goal. Rather, our aim is to not accept average performance as "the best we can do," nor is it to implement ROM to satisfy funders or accrediting bodies. Even with a commitment to ROM, the impact of feedback can vary significantly depending on who uses the feedback (Schuckard, Miller, & Hubble, 2017). As it turns out, effective therapy involves a commitment to both ROM *and* performance improvement. Improvement requires careful examination of clinicians, their mindsets, and practices, so we can deepen our knowledge of what is commonly referred to as "therapist effects" in the professional literature, which will be discussed next.

THERAPIST EFFECTS

Research indicates that the variability in outcomes attributed to the therapist is between 5% and 9% (Crits-Christoph & Mintz, 1991; Wampold & Brown, 2005; Wampold & Imel, 2015). One study, involving a naturalistic design, found therapist contributions to be even higher, between 8% and 17% (Lutz, Leon, Martinovich, Lyons, & Stiles, 2007). There appear to be differences between naturalistic/effectiveness studies (i.e., real-world settings) and efficacy studies (i.e., clinical trials), with the former revealing therapist effects of around 7% and the latter of about 5% (Baldwin & Imel, 2013). Chow (2017) suggested a possible reason for the differences between the two settings being "higher amounts of training, supervision, and structure, leading to increased homogeneity" in efficacy settings (p. 328). Differences in settings are particularly relevant given that most clinicians practice in naturalistic environments. Regardless of the setting, it is evident that the therapist contributes 5 to 9 times more to the eventual outcome than the model he or she employs.

A central focus of this book is to become as effective a clinician as possible and continue to improve from an established baseline over time. To properly address the concept of therapy effectiveness and better understand the service provider's role in outcomes, we round out this chapter with the exploration of several key therapist effects. These therapist effects serve as building blocks for effective practice.

Personal Philosophy: The Therapist's Worldview

As clinicians, we have an extraordinary amount of influence in the therapeutic milieu. In a state of vulnerability and distress, clients attend therapy in search of understanding, comfort, and relief. As such, it is understandable that therapists, particularly those new to the profession, want to know the "nuts and bolts"—*what to do*—the tried and true methods and techniques to remediate client distress. And yet, what becomes clear is that the most effective therapists have a good understanding of when and how to use their respective methods, which originate from their worldviews.

Our worldviews or *personal philosophies* represent collective experiences and are shaped by influences including, but not limited to, ethnicity, race, gender, education, environment, family history, genetics, physiology, religion/spirituality, sexual orientation, community, politics, economics, disability, and social relationships. Our experiences are filtered through these influences. Although some influences are more meaningful than others, each contributes to the formation of our respective personal philosophies. Our philosophies affect change as they inform therapy choices and practices. For example, some therapists prefer cognitively oriented models while others are more drawn to interactional (i.e., systemic) approaches. These choices are seldom random; rather, they are reflections of therapists' belief systems. To better understand this idea, Madsen (2007) proposed a three-level system, the first of which is the philosophy of the clinician:

Personal Philosophies	➡	Theories/Models	➡	Practices
"How we are"		"How we think"		"What we do"

Our personal philosophies represent foundational belief systems reflective of preestablished ideas about clients, including their capacities to change. Next is *theories/models*, which are higher-level maps and systems that serve as conceptual templates for how we think about the development and amelioration of client concerns and problems. Models do not represent reality. They are ideological frameworks to guide therapists. Finally, *practices* represent the specific means and methods used in therapy—how we work to facilitate change with clients. Because our personal philosophies both precede and inform theory and practice, they can open up pathways with possibilities or close down such avenues. To gain a better understanding of your own philosophy and worldview, please consider the following questions:

- What are my core beliefs, ideas, and assumptions about people and their capacities for change?
- How have I come to believe what I believe and know what I know about people and their capacities?

- What have been the most significant influences on my beliefs, ideas, and assumptions?
- How have my beliefs and assumptions affected my work with people? With my colleagues? With my community?
- How do I believe that change occurs? What does change involve?
- What do I do to promote change?
- Do I believe that some degree of positive change is possible with every person? (If "yes," end here; if "no," proceed to the next question.)
- How do I work with others whom I believe cannot change? What do I do?
- If I do not believe that people with whom I work can change, what keeps me working in the field? (Bertolino, 2010, 2014)

What did you learn about yourself from the previous questions? How do you think your views might impact your work as a clinician? What, if any, new thoughts do you have about how your philosophy might change or grow and perhaps have greater influence in your work in the present or future? Because personal philosophies are constantly evolving, it is necessary to periodically reexamine our beliefs. Doing so does not mean compromising our individual belief systems: Each of us has a right to believe what we believe. The purpose of ongoing exploration is to stay attuned to the impact our individual philosophies have on the therapeutic encounter.

As a blueprint of our belief systems, our philosophies are most often the point from which impossibility originates. Said differently, therapists who tend to see their clients as incapable, resistant, unmotivated, or oppositional, for example, frequently find their clients as "impossible" or "untreatable" (Miller, Duncan, & Hubble, 1997). In contrast, therapists who view their clients through a lens of hope, competency, and capacity tend to see more opportunities to promote growth and change.

In the professional literature, the term *strengths-based* has become synonymous with a focus on perspectives that highlight factors such as hope, client competencies, the therapeutic relationship, and well-being (functioning and outcome; Bertolino, 2010, 2014, 2015; Bertolino & O'Hanlon, 2002), each of which is a robust influence on the psychotherapy outcomes (Duncan, Miller, Wampold, & Hubble, 2010). In the next chapter, we will explore what it means to be strengths-based in detail. At this juncture, it is important to clarify that a belief in others' abilities—an emphasis on strengths—is not the same as believing that every person has every ability he or she needs to solve every problem. Nor does it imply that people should rely on hope and simply learn to think and speak positively and their problems will evaporate. Such a position can leave clients feeling invalidated and perhaps even more entrenched in their distress. It also ignores real-life challenges (health, financial, social, etc.) that can threaten client well-being.

Instead, clinicians with core beliefs that clients have strengths that can be utilized in the service of change are less likely to give up on their clients, remaining open and responsive in each therapeutic encounter. This is, in effect, practicing a "growth mindset"—being flexible, creative, confident, resilient, and finding value in setbacks (Dweck, 2006). The benefits of a strengths-based, growth mindset extend beyond the therapeutic milieu to the person of the therapist and stand in contrast to a worldview mired with negativity, which can lead to decreased job motivation, effectiveness, and increased stress, dissatisfaction, resentment, anxiety, depression, physical illness, burnout, and, ultimately, the loss of hope.

Myths About Therapist Effectiveness

Much has been learned about the reasons that some therapists consistently achieve better outcomes than others. Interestingly, many of the factors *therapists believe* account for these differences are unsupported. In addition to professional training, there remains no evidence that factors such as age, gender, personality traits, years of experience, professional qualifications, time conducting therapy, or therapist involvement in therapy are related to outcomes or therapist effectiveness (Anderson, Ogles, Patterson, Lambert, & Vermeersch, 2009; Beutler et al., 2004; Chow et al., 2015).

Another common myth is that some professional disciplines (i.e., counseling, marriage and family therapy, social work) produce clinicians who achieve better outcomes. Clinicians from each of the primary behavioral health disciplines consistently work in the same contexts, with the same clientele, with psychotherapy being the most common form of service provision. This overlap between fields has perpetuated comparisons. And yet, psychologist Michael Lambert (2004) noted, "On the basis of much research evidence, no one profession can claim a monopoly on superior service" (p. 5). When it comes to actual psychotherapy practice, distinctions between professional degrees and disciplines matter little (Wampold & Brown, 2005).

Toward Continuity

Earlier in the chapter it was mentioned that there is potential for professional training to positively influence therapist outcomes. At the center of the debate is how to provide training, given that the education of students and practitioners can vary greatly, not only according to a person's chosen professional discipline but also with respect to educational programs and practice settings. In terms of educational programs, instructors and trainers from different schools emphasize different principles, practices, and models. Some models, for example, are privileged more than others and included as part of counseling curriculums; others are given less attention or excluded altogether. An implication is that two people who attend separate graduate programs but obtain the same degree are likely to receive training that is markedly different. Again, these variances should give us pause, because irrespective of the educational path or professional discipline, as we know, those who choose careers as therapists will more often than not work in the same settings, performing the same or similar tasks. There are different accrediting bodies for each discipline and therefore considerable variance as to what constitutes acceptable coursework and training when it comes to preparing students to practice as therapists. This means that the bulk of the educational responsibility begins with faculty and trainers, who must commit to keeping up with research and creating learning opportunities for students to become competent and effective practitioners.

A challenge for both current and future therapists is to maintain an openness to, and awareness of, research both in and outside their respective disciplines. As we will learn, there are ideas, processes, and practices that cross all behavioral health disciplines and account for the largest portion of therapeutic effectiveness that are not the province of any professional orientation. Practitioners should be skilled in each of these areas.

A final consideration in the discussion of professional orientation and training is practice settings. Similar to educational programs providing different curriculums, practice settings can vary significantly in terms of post-degree training opportunities, the quality of clinical supervision, and level of support. Many develop and blossom into very effective therapists when well-supported and afforded opportunities to grow. Unfortunately, some become casualties of the field—often the result of poor support, training, and lack of opportunity. Too many clinicians have given up and left the field altogether from "staff infections," which occur when negativity infiltrates an organization or setting (Bertolino, 2011).

The Reflective Practitioner

Therapist effectiveness is suspect to a gap between what clinicians do not know or assume to know, which poses threats to psychotherapy as a viable and effective means of helping others (Boisvert & Faust, 2006). Insufficient or incorrect knowledge can also present conflicts with licensing boards, regulatory bodies, and insurance panels, each of which create, maintain, and monitor standards of care and practice. Law and ethics necessitate personal accountability for every person who works as or is working toward a career as a therapist. Each current therapist or therapist in training is responsible for maintaining an understanding and awareness of legal and ethical factors and how they affect the scope of practice. Professional competency is further reflected in one's knowledge of the best available research and practices related to clientele served.

In terms of psychotherapy outcomes research, let's briefly review a few robust findings that many clinicians, often at no fault of their own (they were or have not been introduced to the available literature in their graduate programs or professional training), have little or no knowledge. Whether you are new to the field or a seasoned veteran, consider which of these findings is part of your current knowledge base.

A first finding is that most clients achieve some form of change early in therapy (Baldwin, Berkeljon, Atkins, Olsen, & Nielsen, 2009; Howard, Kopta, Krause, & Orlinsky, 1986; Kopta, Howard, Lowry, & Beutler, 1994). Second is the longer clients attend therapy without experiencing a positive change, the greater the likelihood that they will experience a negative or null outcome or dropout (Duncan, Miller, Wampold, & Hubble, 2010). A third finding is clinicians routinely fail to identify which clients will not benefit from therapy (Hannan et al., 2005; Hansen, Lambert, & Forman, 2002; Lambert, 2010; Warren et al., 2010). Fourth, therapists struggle to address dropout in services—which is arguably the greatest threat to psychotherapy (Swift et al., 2012; Wierzbicki & Pekarik, 1993). Lastly, as discussed, most therapists do not know how effective they are, having never measured their outcomes (Hansen, Lambert, & Forman, 2002; Sapyta, Riemer, & Bickman, 2005). As a result, there is a tendency to overrate their effectiveness (Hansen et al., 2002; Lambert, 2010; Sapyta et al., 2005; Walfish, McAlister, O'Donnell, & Lambert, 2012). No amount of professional training will help a therapist to improve if they do not know how effective they are to start.

These and other key findings yet to be discussed represent just a few that should be part of every clinician's knowledge base *and* included in professional training endeavors. Although it is not possible for therapists to know everything from a research standpoint, some findings are crucial to all therapists, regardless of their theoretical approach. And while familiarity with research does not guarantee improved outcomes, its absence precludes that possibility (Boisvert & Faust, 2006). To this end, if you are not where you desire to be in terms of your professional knowledge and skills, there is no need to panic. You are not alone. This book will help you to move forward in your journey to improve as a clinician.

One way to begin the path of ongoing professional development relates back to a point raised earlier in this chapter, the settings within which clinicians practice. Just as not all therapists are equally effective, some settings produce better overall outcomes than others. Therefore, it is important that clinicians consider the settings within which they work, including the kind of support needed to grow and evolve. Skovholt and Rønnestad (1995) stated:

> It is important to have an environment supportive of one's search, an environment where the person is connected to other professional searchers. Such an environment is not dogmatic or rigid but is supportive of professional development and increased competence. Such an environment values high standards of performance and a searching process as opposed to the process of total acceptance of a preordained set of ideological principles. Such an environment supports an exploratory, investigative approach. Such an environment values diversity and has an opening up stance versus a simplification of the complex world, i.e., in working with a client case, such an environment will encourage looking for as many associations on a case as possible versus reinforcing only a narrow, prescribed theory or method. (pp. 106–107)

A second way to begin this journey is to commit to being a reflective practitioner. Doing so means taking the time to employ a simple, yet fundamental process referred to as TAR—Think, Act, and Reflect (Bertolino et al., 2013). Bertolino et al. (2013) described the process of TAR:

> To move beyond the realm of reliable performance, the best engage in forethought. This means setting specific goals for improvement and developing a plan to reach those goals. In the act phase, successful experts track their performance: they monitor on an ongoing basis whether they used each of the steps or strategies outlined in the thinking phase and the quality with which each step was executed. The sheer volume of detail gathered in assessing their performance distinguishes the exceptional from their more average counterparts. During the reflection phase, top performers review the details of their performance, identifying specific actions and alternative strategies for reaching their goals. Where unsuccessful learners paint in broad strokes, attributing failure to external factors and uncontrollable events, the best know exactly what they do, most often citing controllable factors. (p. 20)

Each therapist's path to improvement and excellence may vary; however, without a commitment to lifelong improvement, which involves reflection, it is unlikely any clinician will reach his or her potential (Rousmaniere, Goodyear, Miller, & Wampold, 2017). As such, self-reflection has been shown to be a distinguishing factor between therapists who continue to grow and develop professionally and those who face professional stagnation and burnout (Skovholt & Jennings, 2005; Skovholt & Rønnestad, 1995). Reflective practitioners consider both how they influence and how the therapeutic milieu influences them. They develop and maintain ongoing awareness of matters including, but not limited to, personal biases and issues, philosophical worldviews, selection of strategies and methods, and demonstration of interest in their effectiveness as therapists.

If we are to truly evolve as a field, we must set aside our allegiances to ideologies and pursue a commitment to excellence. In this chapter we explored current issues to be included as part of any discussions to improve therapist effectiveness and performance. In Chapter 2 we delve deeper into research to better understand the factors most responsible for successful outcomes. We will also consider a series of research-based principles to guide practice.

REFERENCES

American Psychiatric Association. (2013). *Diagnostic and statistical manual for mental disorders* (5th ed.). Arlington, VA: American Psychiatric Publishing.

American Psychological Association. (2012). Resolution on the recognition of psychotherapy effectiveness. Retrieved from http://www.apa.org/about/policy/resolution-psychotherapy.aspx

Anderson, T., Ogles, B. M., Patterson, C. L., Lambert, M. J., & Vermeersch, D. A. (2009). Therapist effects: Facilitative interpersonal skills as a predictor of therapist effects. *Journal of Clinical Psychology, 65*(7), 755–768. doi:10.1002/jclp.20583

Atkins, D. C., & Christensen, A. (2001). Is professional training worth the bother? A review of the impact of psychotherapy training on client outcome. *Australian Psychologist, 36*(2), 122–131. doi:10.1080/00050060108259644

Baldwin, S. A., Berkeljon, A., Atkins, D. C., Olsen, J. A., & Nielsen, S. L. (2009). Rates of change in naturalistic psychotherapy: Contrasting dose-effect and good-enough level models of change. *Journal of Consulting and Clinical Psychology, 77*, 203–211. doi:10.1037/a0015235

Baldwin, S. A., & Imel, Z. E. (2013). Therapist effects: Findings and methods. In M. J. Lambert (Ed.), *Bergin and Garfield's handbook of psychotherapy and behavior change* (6th ed., pp. 259–297). Hoboken, NJ: Wiley.

Benish, S., Imel, Z. E., & Wampold, B. E. (2008). The relative efficacy of bona fide psychotherapies of post-traumatic stress disorder: A meta-analysis of direct comparisons. *Clinical Psychology Review, 28*, 746–758. doi:10.1016/j.cpr.2007.10.005

Bergin, A. E. (1971). The evaluation of therapeutic outcomes. In S. L. Garfield & A. E. Bergin (Eds.), *The handbook of psychotherapy and behavior change* (pp. 217–270). New York, NY: Wiley.

Bertolino, B. (2010). *Strengths-based engagement and practice: Creating effective helping relationships*. Boston, MA: Allyn & Bacon.

Bertolino, B. (2011). Building a culture of excellence: Anatomy of a community agency that works. *Psychotherapy Networker, 35*(3), 32–39.

Bertolino, B. (2014). *Thriving on the front lines: Strengths-based youth care work*. New York, NY: Routledge.

Bertolino, B. (2015). *Working with children and adolescents in residential care: A strengths-based approach*. New York, NY: Routledge.

Bertolino, B., Bargmann, S., & Miller, S. D. (2013). Manual 1: What works in therapy: A primer. In B. Bertolino & S. D. Miller (Eds.), *The ICCE manuals of feedback informed treatment*. Chicago, IL: International Center for Clinical Excellence.

Bertolino, B., & O'Hanlon, B. (2002). *Collaborative, competency-based counseling and therapy*. Boston, MA: Allyn & Bacon.

Beutler, L. E., Malik, M., Alimohamed, S., Harwood, T. M., Talebi, H., Noble, S., & Wong, E. (2004). Therapist variables. In M. J. Lambert (Ed.), *Bergin and Garfield's handbook of psychotherapy and behavior change* (5th ed., pp. 227–306). Hoboken, NJ: Wiley.

Bickman, L. (2000). Summing up program theory. *New Directions for Evaluation, 87*, 103–112. doi:10.1002/ev.1186

Boisvert, C. M., & Faust, D. (2006). Practicing psychologists' knowledge of general psychotherapy research findings: Implications for science-practice relations. *Professional Psychology: Research and Practice, 37*(6), 708–716. doi:10.1037/0735-7028.37.6.708

Branson, A., Shafran, R., & Myles, P. (2015). Investigating the relationship between competence and patient outcome with CBT highlights. *Behaviour Research and Therapy, 68*, 19–26. doi:10.1016/j.brat.2015.03.002

Brown, J., Dreis, S., & Nace, D. K. (1999). What really makes a difference in psychotherapy outcome? Why does managed care want to know? In M. A. Hubble, B. L. Duncan, & S. D. Miller (Eds.), *The heart and soul of change: What works in therapy* (pp. 389–406). Washington, DC: American Psychological Association.

Chambless, D. L., Baker, M. J., Baucom, D. H., Beutler, L. E., Calhoun, K. S., Daiuto, A., . . . Woody, S. R. (1998). Update on empirically validated therapies, II. *The Clinical Psychologist, 51*, 3–16.

Chiles, J., Lambert, M. J., & Hatch, A. L. (1999). The impact of psychological interventions on medical cost offset: A meta-analytic review. *Clinical Psychology, 6*(2), 204–220. doi:10.1093/clipsy.6.2.204

Chow, D. L. (2017). The practice and the practical: Pushing your clinical performance to the next level. In D. S. Prescott, S. D. Miller, & C. L. Maeschalck (Eds.), *Feedback-informed treatment in clinical practice: Reaching for excellence* (pp. 323–355). Washington, DC: American Psychological Association.

Chow, D. L., Miller, S. D., Seidel, J. A., Kane, R. T., Thornton, J. A., & Andrews, W. P. (2015). The role of deliberate practice in the development of highly effective psychotherapists. *Psychotherapy, 52*(3), 337–345. doi:10.1037/pst0000015

Christensen, A., & Jacobson, N. S. (1994). Who (or what) can do psychotherapy: The status and challenge of nonprofessional therapies. *Psychological Sciences, 5*, 8–14. Retrieved from http://www.jstor.org/stable/40062334

Clement, P. W. (1994). Quantitative evaluation of 26 years of private practice. *Professional Psychology: Research and Practice, 25*, 173–176. doi:10.1037/0735-7028.25.2.173

Clement, P. W. (2008). Outcomes from 40 years of psychotherapy in a private practice. *American Journal of Psychotherapy, 62*, 215–239. doi:10.1037/0735-7028.25.2.173

Clement, P. W. (2013). Practice-based evidence: 45 years of psychotherapy's effectiveness in private practice. *American Journal of Psychotherapy, 67*(1), 23–46.

Crane, D. R., & Christensen, J. D. (2008). The medical offset effect: Patterns in outpatient services reduction for high utilizers of health care. *Contemporary Family Medicine, 30*(2), 127–138. doi:10.1007/s10591-008-9058-2

Crits-Christoph, P., & Mintz, J. (1991). Implications of therapist effects for the design and analysis of comparative studies of psychotherapies. *Journal of Consulting and Clinical Psychology, 59*(1), 20–26.

Cummings, N. A. (2007). Treatment and assessment take place in an economic context, always. In S. O. Lilienfeld & W. T. O'Donohue (Eds.), *The great ideas of clinical science: 17 principles that every mental health professional should understand* (pp. 163–184). New York, NY: Routledge.

Cummings N. A., Cummings, J. L., & Johnson, J. N. (1997). *Behavioral health in primary care: A guide for clinical integration*. Madison, CT: Psychosocial Press.

Cummings, N. A., O'Donohue, W. T., & Ferguson, K. E. (2002). *The impact of medical cost offset on practice and research: Making it work for you. Cummings Foundation on Behavioral Health: Healthcare Utilization and Cost Series* (Vol. 5). Reno, NV: Context Press.

Dawes, R. M. (1989). Experience and validity of clinical judgment: The illusory correlation. *Behavioral Sciences and the Law, 7*(4), 457–467. doi:10.1002/bsl.2370070404

Duncan, B. L., Miller, S. D., Wampold, B. E., & Hubble, M.A. (Eds.). (2010). *The heart and soul of change: Delivering what works in therapy* (2nd ed.). Washington, DC: American Psychological Association.

Dunning, D., Heath, C., & Suls, J. (2004). Flawed self-assessment: Implications for health, education, and the workplace. *Psychological Science in the Public Interest, 5*, 69–106. doi:10.1111/j.1529-1006.2004.00018.x

Dweck, C. S. (2006). *Mindset: The new psychology of success*. New York, NY: Random House.

Elaad, E. (2003). Effects of feedback on the overestimated capacity to detect lies and the underestimated ability to tell lies. *Applied Cognitive Psychology, 17*, 349–363. doi:10.1002/acp.871

Ericsson, K. A. (2006). The influence of experience and deliberate practice on the development of superior expert performance. In K. A. Ericsson, N. Charness, P. J. Feltovich, & R. R. Hoffman (Eds.), *The Cambridge handbook of expertise and expert performance* (pp. 683–703). Cambridge, UK: Cambridge University Press.

Ericsson, K. A. (2009a). *The development of professional expertise: Toward measurement of expert performance and design of optimal learning environments*. New York, NY: Cambridge University Press.

Ericsson, K. A. (2009b). Enhancing the development of professional performance: Implications from the study of deliberate practice. In K. A. Ericsson (Ed.), *The development of professional expertise: Toward measurement of expert performance and design of optimal learning environments* (pp. 405–431). New York, NY: Cambridge University Press.

Ericsson, K. A., Charness, N., Feltovich, P. J., & Hoffman, R. R. (Eds.). (2006). *The Cambridge handbook of expertise and expert performance*. New York, NY: Cambridge University Press.

Eysenck, H. (1952). The effects of psychotherapy: An evaluation. *Journal of Consulting Psychology, 16*(5), 329–324. PMID:13000035

Eysenck, H. (1955). The effects of psychotherapy: A reply. *Journal of Abnormal Psychology, 50*(1), 147–148.

Forand, N. R., DeRubeis, R. J., & Amsterdam, J. D. (2013). Combining medication and psychotherapy in the treatment of major mental disorders. In M. J. Lambert (Ed.), *Bergin and Garfield's handbook of psychotherapy and behavior change* (pp. 735–774). Hoboken, NJ: Wiley.

Garcia, J. A., & Weisz, J. R. (2002). When youth mental health care stops: Therapeutic relationship problems and other reasons for ending youth outpatient treatment. *Journal of Consulting and Clinical Psychology, 70*(2), 439–443. doi:10.1037/0022-006X.70.2.439

Gawande, A. (2004, December 6). The bell curve: What happens when patients find out how good their doctors really are? *New Yorker.* Retrieved from https://www.newyorker.com/magazine/2004/12/06/the-bell-curve

Gilbody, S., House, A., & Sheldon, T. (2002). Psychiatrists in the UK do not use outcome measures: National survey. *The British Journal of Psychiatry, 180*, 101–103. doi:10.1192/bjp.180.2.101

Goldberg, S. B., Rousmaniere, T., Miller, S. D., Whipple, J., Nielsen, S. R., Hoyt, W. T., & Wampold, B. E. (2016). Do psychotherapists improve with time and experience? A longitudinal analysis of outcomes in a clinical setting. *Journal of Counseling Psychology, 63*(1), 1–11. doi:10.1037/cou0000131

Gøtzsche, P. C., Young, A. H., & Crace, J. (2015). Does long term use of psychiatric drugs cause more harm than good? *BMJ, 350*, h2435. doi:10.1136/bmj.h2435

Grove, W. M., & Meehl, P. E. (1996). Comparative efficiency of informal (subjective, impressionistic) and formal (mechanical, algorithmic) prediction procedures: The clinical-statistical controversy. *Psychology, Public Policy, and Law, 2*(2), 293–323. doi:10.1037/1076-8971.2.2.293

Hannan, C., Lambert, M. J., Harmon, C., Nielsen, S. L., Smart, D. W., Shimokawa, K., & Sutton, S. W. (2005). A lab test and algorithms for identifying clients at risk for treatment failure. *Journal of Clinical Psychology: In Session, 61,* 155–163. doi:10.1002/jclp.20108

Hansen, N., Lambert, M. J., & Forman, E. M. (2002). The psychotherapy dose-response effect and its implication for treatment delivery services. *Clinical Psychology: Science and Practice, 9*(3), 329–343. doi:10.1093/clipsy.9.3.329

Hatfield, D. R., & Ogles, B. M. (2004). The use of outcome measures by psychologists in clinical practice. *Professional Psychology: Research and Practice, 35*(5), 485–491. doi: 10.1037/0735-7028.35.5.485

Howard, K. I., Kopta, S. M., Krause, M. S., & Orlinsky, D. E. (1986). The dose-effect relationship in psychotherapy. *American Psychologist, 41*(2), 159–164. doi:10.1002/jclp.10167

Hubble, M. A., Duncan, B. L., & Miller, S. D. (Eds.). (1999). *The heart and soul of change: What works in therapy.* Washington, DC: American Psychological Association.

Imel, Z. E., Wampold, B. E., Miller, S. D., & Fleming, R. R. (2008). Distinctions without a difference: Direct comparisons of psychotherapies for alcohol use disorders. *Journal of Addictive Behaviors, 22,* 533–543. doi:10.1037/a0013171

Kopta, S. M., Howard, K. I., Lowry, J. L., & Beutler, L. E. (1994). Patterns of symptomatic recovery in psychotherapy. *Journal of Consulting and Clinical Psychology, 62*(5), 1009–1016. doi:10.1037/0022-006X.62.5.1009

Kruger, J., & Dunning, D. (1999). Unskilled and unaware of it: How difficulties in recognizing one's own incompetence lead to inflated self-assessments. *Journal of Personality and Social Psychology, 77*(6), 1121–1134. doi:10.1037/0022-3514.77.6.1121

Lambert, M. J. (2004). Introduction and historical overview. In M. J. Lambert (Ed.), *Bergin and Garfield's handbook of psychotherapy and behavior change* (5th ed., pp. 3–15). Hoboken, NJ: Wiley.

Lambert, M. J. (2010). *Prevention of treatment failure: The use of measuring, monitoring, and feedback in clinical practice.* Washington, DC: American Psychological Association.

Lambert, M. J. (2013). The efficacy and effectiveness of psychotherapy. In M. J. Lambert (Ed.), *Bergin and Garfield's handbook of psychotherapy and behavior change* (pp. 169–218). Hoboken, NJ: Wiley.

Lambert, M. J., & Ogles, B. M. (2004). The efficacy and effectiveness of psychotherapy. In M. J. Lambert (Ed.), *Bergin and Garfield's handbook of psychotherapy and behavior change* (5th ed., pp. 139–193). Hoboken, NJ: Wiley.

Lambert, M. J., & Shimokawa, K. (2011). Collecting client feedback. *Psychotherapy, 48*(1), 72–79. doi:10.1037/a0022238

Laska, K. M., Guran, A. S., & Wampold, B. E. (2014). Expanding the lens of evidence-based practice in psychotherapy: A common factors perspective. *Psychotherapy, 51*(4), 467–481. doi:10.1037/a0034332

Law, D. D., Crane, D. R., & Berge, D. M. (2003). The influence of individual, marital, and family therapy on high utilizers of health care. *Journal of Marital and Family Therapy, 29*(3), 353–363.

Leo, J. (1985). A therapist in every corner: Harmony was the goal, but participants seemed out of tune. *Time, 126*(25), 59.

Lipsey, M. W., & Wilson, D. B. (1993). The efficacy of psychological, educational, and behavioral treatment: Confirmation from meta-analysis. *American Psychologist, 48,* 1181–1209.

Luborsky, L., Diguer, L., Seligman, D. A., Rosenthal, R., Krause, E. D., Johnson, S., . . . Schweizer, E. (1999). The researcher's own therapy allegiances: A "wild card" in comparisons of treatment efficacy. *Clinical Psychology: Science and Practice, 6,* 95–106. doi:10.1093/clipsy.6.1.95

Lutz, W., Leon, S. C., Martinovich, Z., Lyons, J. S., & Stiles, W. B. (2007). Therapist effects in outpatient psychotherapy: A three-level growth curve approach. *Journal of Counseling Psychology, 54,* 32–29. doi:10.1037/0022-0167.54.1.32

Madsen, W. C. (2007). *Collaborative therapy with multi-stressed families* (2nd ed.). New York: Guilford.

Meyer, H. (1980). Self-appraisal of job performance. *Personnel Psychology, 33,* 291–295. doi:10.1111/j.1744-6570.1980.tb02351.x

Miller, S. D. (2013). The evolution of psychotherapy: An oxymoron. Retrieved from http://www.slideshare.net/scottdmiller/evolution-of-psychotherapy-an-oxymoron

Miller, S. D., Duncan, B. L., & Hubble, M. A. (1997). *Escape from Babel: Toward a unifying language for psychotherapy practice.* New York, NY: W. W. Norton.

Miller, S. D., Wampold, B. E., & Varhely, K. (2008). Direct comparisons of treatment modalities for youth disorders: A meta-analysis. *Psychotherapy Research, 18*, 5–14. doi:10.1080/10503300701472131

Mukuria, C., Brazier, J., Barkham, M., Connell, J., Hardy, G., Hutten, R., ... Parry, G. (2013). Cost-effectiveness of an improving access to psychological therapies service. *The British Journal of Psychiatry, 202*(3), 220–227. doi:10.1192/bjp.bp.111.107888

Okiishi, J., Lambert, M. J., Nielsen, S. L., & Ogles, B. M. (2003). Waiting for supershrink: An empirical analysis of therapist effects. *Clinical Psychology and Psychotherapy, 10*(6), 361–373. doi:10.1002/cpp.383

O'Leary, K. D., & Borkovec, T. D. (1978). Conceptual, methodological, and ethical problems of placebo groups in psychotherapy research. *American Psychologist, 33*(9), 821–830. doi:10.1037/0003-066X.33.9.821

Ricks, D. (1974). Supershrink: Methods of a therapist judged successful on the basis of adult outcomes of adolescent patients. In D. Ricks, A. Thomas, & M. Roff (Eds.), *Life history research in psychopathology* (Vol. 3. pp. 275–297). Minneapolis: University of Minnesota.

Rosenzweig, S. (1936). Some implicit common factors in diverse methods of psychotherapy. *American Journal of Orthopsychiatry, 6*, 412–415. doi:10.1111/j.1939-0025.1936.tb05248.x

Rosenzweig, S. A. (1954). A transvaluation of psychotherapy: A reply to Hans Eysenck. *Journal of Abnormal Psychology, 49*, 298–304. doi:10.1037/h0061172

Rousmaniere, T., Goodyear, R., Miller, S. D., & Wampold, B. E. (2017). *Cycle of excellence: Using deliberate practice to improve supervision and training*. Washington, DC: American Psychological Association.

Rousmaniere, T. G., Swift, J. K., Babins-Wagner, R., Whipple, J. L., & Berzins, S. (2014). Supervisor effects on client outcome in routine practice. *Psychotherapy Research*, 1–10. doi:10.1080/10503307.2014.963730

Saptya, J., Riemer, M., & Bickman, L. (2005). Feedback to clinicians: Theory, research, and practice. *Journal of Clinical Psychology: In Session, 61*(2), 145–153.

Schuckard, E., Miller, S. D., & Hubble, M. A. (2017). Feedback-informed treatment: Historical and empirical foundations. In D. S. Prescott, C. L. Maeschalck, & S. D. Miller (Eds.), *Feedback-informed treatment in clinical practice: Reaching for excellence* (pp. 13–35). Washington, DC: American Psychological Association.

Segal, J. (Ed.). (1975). *Research in the service of mental health, report of the research task force of the National Institute of Mental Health* (DHEW Publication No. ADM 75-236). Washington, DC: U.S. Government Printing Office.

Seligman, M. E. P. (1995). The effectiveness of psychotherapy: The *Consumer Reports* study. *American Psychologist, 50*(12), 965–974. doi:10.1037/0003-066X.50.12.965

Shapiro, J. L. (1987). Message from the master on breaking old ground. The evolution of psychotherapy conference. *Psychotherapy in Private Practice, 5*(3), 65–72. doi:10.1300/J294v05n03_07

Skovholt, T. M., & Jennings, L. (2005). Mastery and expertise in counseling. *Journal of Mental Health Counseling, 27*(1), 13–18. doi:10.17744/mehc.27.1.gnblmy6g3dbqduq4

Skovholt, T. M., & Rønnestad, M. H. (1995). *The evolving professional self: Themes in counselor and therapist development*. New York, NY: Wiley.

Smith, M. L., & Glass, G. V. (1977). Meta-analyses of psychotherapy outcome studies. *American Psychologist, 32*(9), 752–760. doi:10.1037//0003-066X.32.9.752

Stefini, A., Salzer, S., Reich, G., Horn, H., Winkelmann, K., Behts, H., ... Kronmüeller, K. T. (2017). Cognitive-behavioral and psychodynamic therapy in female adolescents with bulimia nervosa: A randomized control trial. *Journal of the American Academy of Child and Adolescent Psychiatry, 56*(4), 329–335. doi:10.1016/j.jaac.2017.01.019

Strupp, H. (1963). The outcome problem in psychotherapy revisited. *Psychotherapy, 1*(1), 1–13. doi:10.1037/h0094491

Swift, J. K., Greenberg, R. P., Whipple, J. L., & Kominiak, N. (2012). Practice recommendations for reducing premature termination in therapy. *Professional Psychology: Research and Practice, 43*(4), 379–387. doi:10.1037/a0028291

Task Force on Promotion and Dissemination of Psychological Procedures (TFPP). (1995). Training in and dissemination of empirically-validated psychological treatment: Report and recommendations. *The Clinical Psychologist, 48*, 2–23.

Tetlock, P. E., & Gardner, D. (2015). *Superforcasting: The art and science of prediction*. New York, NY: Crown Publishing.

Walfish, S., McAlister, B., O'Donnell, P., & Lambert, M. J. (2012). An assessment of self-assessment bias in mental health providers. *Psychological Reports, 110*(2), 639–644.

Wampold, B. E. (2001). *The great psychotherapy debate: Models, methods, and findings*. Mahwah, NJ: Lawrence Erlbaum.

Wampold, B. E. (2007). Psychotherapy: The humanistic (and effective) treatment. *American Psychologist, 62*, 857–873. doi:10.1037/0003-066X.62.8.857

Wampold, B. E. (2010). *The basics of psychotherapy: An introduction to theory and practice.* Washington, DC: American Psychological Association.

Wampold, B. E. (2013). The good, the bad, and the ugly: A 50-year perspective on the outcome problem. *Psychotherapy, 50*(1), 16–24.

Wampold, B. E. (2015). How important are the common factors to psychotherapy: An update. *World Psychiatry, 14*, 270–277.

Wampold, B. E., & Brown, G. S. (2005). Estimating variability in outcomes attributable to therapists: A naturalistic study of outcomes in managed care. *Journal of Consulting and Clinical Psychology, 73*(5), 914–923. doi:10.1037/0022-006X.73.5.914

Wampold, B. E., & Imel, Z. E. (2015). *The great psychotherapy debate: The evidence for what makes therapy work* (2nd ed.). New York, NY: Routledge.

Wampold, B. E., Minami, T., Baskin, T. W., & Tierney, S. C. (2002). A meta-re(analysis) of the effects of cognitive therapy versus "other therapies" for depression. *Journal of Affective Disorders, 68*, 159–165. doi:10.1016/S0165-0327(00)00287-1

Wampold, B. E., Minami, T., Tierney, S. C., Baskin, T. W., & Bhati, K. S. (2005). The placebo is powerful: Estimating placebo effects in medicine and psychotherapy in randomized clinical trials. *Journal of Clinical Psychology, 61*(7), 835–854. doi:10.1002/jclp.20129

Wampold, B. E., Mondin, G. W., Moody, M., Stich, F., Benson, K., & Ahn, H. (1997). A meta-analysis of outcome studies comparing bona fide psychotherapies: Empirically, "All must have prizes." *Psychological Bulletin, 122*, 203–215. doi:10.1037/0735-7028.24.2.190

Warren, J. S., Nelson, P. L., Mondragon, S. A., Baldwin, S. A., & Burlingame, G. A. (2010). Youth psychotherapy change trajectories and outcomes in usual care: Community mental health versus managed care settings. *Journal of Consulting and Clinical Psychology, 78*(2), 144–155. doi:10.1037/a0018544

Webb, C. A., DeRubeis, R. J., & Barber, J. P. (2010). Therapist adherence/competence and treatment outcome: A meta-analytic review. *Journal of Consulting and Clinical Psychology, 78*, 200–211. doi:10.1037/a0018912

Wierzbicki, M., & Pekarik, G. (1993). A meta-analysis of psychotherapy dropout. *Professional Psychology: Research and Practice, 24*(2), 190–195. doi:10.1037/0735-7028.24.2.190

Zeig, J. K. (1987). Introduction. In J. K. Zeig (Ed.), *The evolution of psychotherapy* (pp. xv–xxviii). New York, NY: Brunner/Mazel.

Zimmerman, M., & McGlinchey, J. B. (2008). Why don't psychiatrists use scales to measure outcome when treating depressed patients? *The Journal of Clinical Psychiatry, 69*, 1916–1919. doi:10.4088/JCP.v69n1209

CHAPTER 2

Principles and Core Strategies of Effective Therapy

Research shows unequivocally that psychotherapy works. It is effective with individuals, couples, families, and groups for a myriad of concerns and problems. It is also evident that *who* provides the therapy is more important to eventual outcome than *what* model he or she chose to employ. In this chapter we expand our discussion as we consider nearly half a century of research to address two specific questions: What factors most influence therapy outcomes? And, how do these factors known to influence outcomes translate to effective practice? To answer these questions, I outline a perspective inclusive of a set of principles, core competencies, and processes that are not the province of any one therapeutic approach but instead are part of effective therapy, irrespective of the clientele or presenting concern. I refer to this as a *strengths-based* approach.

EVIDENCE-BASED PRACTICE AND EMPIRICALLY SUPPORTED TREATMENTS: ONE AND THE SAME?

Any effort to describe how to work effectively and improve as a psychotherapist is contingent on a rational, viable framework that is informed by research and includes guidance for practice. Two vastly different perspectives meet this criterion: empirically supported treatments (ESTs) (introduced in Chapter 1) and evidence-based practice (EBP). Although ESTs and EBP are substantially different, Laska, Gurman, and Wampold (2014) contend that professionals often cannot distinguish between the two, "There is much confusion for students, psychologists, and consumers of psychotherapy alike" (p. 467). In a survey of clinical psychology graduate students, the majority identified EBP as synonymous with ESTs (Luebbe, Radcliffe, Callands, Green, & Thorn, 2007). This confusion is easily corroborated through an Internet search of the terms "empirical-supported treatments" and "evidence-based practice." Many sites either inaccurately define the terms, describe them as the same, or use the terms interchangeably. Whether a student or experienced practitioner, it is important to be clear regarding the differences between ESTs and EBP.

Chambless and Hollon (1998) define ESTs as "clearly specified psychological treatments shown to be efficacious in controlled research with a delineated population" (p. 7). ESTs are based on the randomized controlled trial (RCT), in which two independent studies are required to demonstrate that a particular approach is efficacious for a specific disorder or condition, most commonly from the *Diagnostic and Statistical Manual of Mental Disorders (DSM)* currently in its fifth edition (*DSM-5*; American Psychiatric Association, 2013). The EST perspective is consistent with a prescriptive medical model in which an approach is chosen based on a client's diagnosis, then is methodically delivered in accordance with a treatment manual to ensure adherence and fidelity. Bohart (2000, p. 131) outlined the following model:

Treatment → operates on patient → to produce effects

In contrast to the EST movement, which is based exclusively on the study of treatment models and the RCT design, EBP is inclusive of meta-analyses, as well as naturalistic, process-outcome, and correlational studies, and delves into a broad array of factors such as the therapeutic relationship, client and therapist effects, and other elements thought to influence therapeutic outcomes. Proponents of ESTs criticized EBP, referring to its broader scope and acceptance of varied forms of research as "unscientific." Critics have argued,

> The treatment method is the only aspect in which psychotherapists can be trained, it is the only aspect that can be manipulated in a clinical experiment to test its worth, and, if proven valuable, it is the only aspect that can be disseminated to other psychotherapists. (Chambless & Crits-Christoph, 2006, p. 199)

Proponents of EBP disagree, citing evidence that models contribute little to the overall variance in outcome (Wampold, 2001; Wampold & Imel, 2015). An additional argument is that the EST perspective is fundamentally restrictive in its reliance on one form of research and disregard for factors influential to therapeutic change. Critics further contend that the unreliability of psychiatric diagnosis, a one-size-fits-all ideology, an absence of focus on the therapeutic relationship, issues with allegiance effects (as discussed in Chapter 1), and the lack of differential efficacy in comparative analyses between bona fide treatment approaches raise major issues regarding the EST movement (Wampold & Imel, 2015). The concern over lack of focus on the therapeutic relationship emerged largely as the result of efforts from the American Psychological Association's (APA) Division 29 (The Society for the Advancement of Psychotherapy). Division 29's Steering Committee (2001) concluded:

> The therapy relationship makes substantial and consistent contributions to psychotherapy outcome independent of the specific type of treatment.... Efforts to promulgate practice guidelines or evidence-based lists of effective psychotherapy

without including the therapy relationship are seriously incomplete and potentially misleading on both clinical and empirical grounds. (p. 495)

Laska et al. (2014) expressed particular concern over the EST ideology:

> We believe the prioritization of randomized controlled trials (RCTs) and ESTs over the last few decades has unintentionally limited the scope of EBP and may have ironically worked against the central purpose of psychotherapy research, that is, the improvement of practice, by limiting the variety of evidence deemed relevant to such an aim. (p. 467)

The researchers further observed that such a position is in accordance with philosophers of science such as Thomas Kuhn (1962). They concluded:

> Restricting the lens through which a phenomenon is examined (in this case, psychotherapy) restricts what can be observed and the manner in which "evidence" is interpreted. In other words, a restricted scientific aperture means less of the evidentiary picture is in focus. (p. 468)

There continues to be much debate about the practicality of ESTs from both a research standpoint and in terms of how psychotherapists practice in everyday, effectiveness-based (real-world) settings. However, beyond the points already raised, further discussion is outside the scope of this volume. Both new and experienced clinicians are encouraged to explore and discuss the full range of issues to draw their own conclusions (Wampold & Imel, 2015). The focus of this book is on the use of EBP, which will be discussed in detail next.

DEFINING EVIDENCE-BASED PRACTICE

The APA defines EBP as, "The integration of the best available research with clinical expertise in the context of patient characteristics, culture, and preferences" (APA Presidential Task Force on Evidence-Based Practice, 2006, p. 273). Two other major U.S. entities have similarly defined EBP. First, the Substance Abuse Mental Health Services Administration (SAMHSA, 2016) states, "EBPs integrate clinical expertise; expert opinion; external scientific evidence; and client, patient, and caregiver perspectives so that providers can offer high-quality services that reflect the interests, values, needs, and choices of the individuals served." A second entity, the Institute of Medicine (IOM), follows suit:

> Evidence based medicine is the conscientious, explicit, and judicious use of current best evidence in making decisions about the care of individual patients. The practice of evidence based medicine means integrating individual clinical expertise with the best available external clinical evidence from systematic research. (Sackett, Rosenberg, Muir Gray, Haynes, & Richardson, 1996, p. 71)

Each of the previous definitions shares consensus in three major areas: (a) best evidence or research; (b) clinical expertise; and (c) individual patient characteristics (values, needs, choices, etc.). These three areas offer guidance to behavioral healthcare professionals in terms of practice. It can be further argued that therapists have a responsibility to ensure that each area informs their clinical practice. It should be noted that for the purposes of this book, we will refer to the APA's definition of EBP to develop our understanding of how each of the aforementioned key areas translates to practice and informs a strengths-based approach.

Best Available Research

In Chapter 1, we learned about the two primary study designs used in psychotherapy research: RCT and meta-analysis. In practice, the challenge for psychotherapists is twofold. It is to determine what forms of external evidence, whether from RCTs or meta-analyses, are pertinent to: (a) becoming an effective psychotherapist overall; and (b) each, unique, individual client. A commitment to the best available research includes remaining up-to-date on empirical literature and synthesizing relevant findings in ways that improve practice, supervision, training, and policy.

Clinical Expertise

Another key idea from Chapter 1 is the role of the therapist in treatment outcomes. To recap, between 5% and 9% of the variance in outcome can be attributed to the person of the therapist (Crits-Christoph & Mintz, 1991; Wampold & Brown, 2005; Wampold & Imel, 2015). Clinical expertise draws attention to the proficiency and judgment acquired through clinical experience and practice, which includes the responsiveness of the therapist in each therapeutic encounter. According to the APA (2006), "Clinical expertise . . . entails the monitoring of patient progress (and of changes in the patient's circumstances—e.g., job loss, major illness) that may suggest the need to adjust treatment. . . . If progress is not proceeding adequately, the psychologist alters or addresses problematic aspects of the treatment (e.g., problems in the therapeutic relationship or in the implementation of the goals of the treatment) as appropriate" (pp. 276–277, 280).

The most effective therapists are attuned to the vicissitudes of the client–therapist relationship, remaining thoughtful and compassionate in their understanding of and response to individual clients' predicaments, rights, and preferences in making clinical decisions about their care (Bertolino, 2015). As such, there is a commitment to self-awareness, professional development, and the distilment of strategies that show benefit without holding allegiances to particular methods, approaches, or models. Central to clinical expertise is the use of routine outcome monitoring (ROM) to adjust services as needed. For therapists who are committed to improving their therapeutic effectiveness through ROM, feedback-informed treatment (FIT) provides excellent guidance with four core areas of competence as a starting point (Bertolino & Miller, 2013; Prescott, 2017). The four areas are:

1. *Research foundations:* This area of competence includes knowledge of the research on the therapeutic alliance, behavioral healthcare outcomes, and available research on expert performance and its application to clinical practice. Also included in this area is familiarity with valid, reliable, and feasible alliance and outcome measures.

2. *Implementation:* This includes the integration of consumer-reported outcome and alliance data into clinical work as well as the transparency with consumers about collecting feedback regarding the alliance and outcome. This area of competence ensures that the course and outcome of behavioral healthcare services are informed by consumer preferences and values.

3. *Meaning and reporting:* This area of competence involves documenting the therapeutic alliance and the outcomes of clinical services on an ongoing basis. In addition, emphasis is on providing details in reporting outcomes to assess the accuracy and generalizability of the results.

4. *Continuous professional improvement*: This includes clinicians' commitment to ongoing development by determining a baseline level of performance, comparing their level of performance to the best available norms, standards, or benchmarks. Clinicians then develop and execute plans for improvement of their performance, including the use of deliberate practice for achieving superior performance. (Bertolino & Miller, 2013; Prescott, 2017)

Patient Characteristics, Culture, and Preferences

The third key element of being evidence-based involves close attention, with attunement to a myriad of influences that represent the essence of each individual client. Patient (client) characteristics include, but are not limited to, age, gender, gender identity, ethnicity, race, social class, disability status, sexual orientation, development, and life stage. They also refer to client strengths, resources, beliefs, and factors that can influence change. Therapists who are mindful of client characteristics strive to understand the local knowledge and culture of each individual, including the individual's expectations, values, and preferences related to treatment. Through ongoing feedback, therapists adjust the therapy to provide a better fit and improve the possibilities for positive outcomes.

There is a further similarity between the most commonly accepted definitions of EBP. None of the definitions refer to specific approaches, models, methods, or techniques. Instead, the definitions collectively highlight the importance of being client centered, an acknowledgment that the relative benefits of therapist-derived interventions void of the three areas described will likely be diminished. As we now move into a strengths-based framework, we remain mindful that effective therapy is not comprised of a random set of ideas and methods; rather, it is founded on research and delivered by a skilled practitioner who is invested in both the *fit* and *effect* of the therapeutic practices. By *fit* we mean the chosen intervention is appropriate for the client. Does it fit the client's worldview, culture, and ideas about change? *Effect* refers to outcome. Did the intervention, at minimum, provide some benefit to the client (e.g., individually, relationally, and/or socially), and at best lead to a positive, measurable improvement in functioning?

COMMON FACTORS: A BRIEF HISTORY AND CONUNDRUM

As evidenced by the volume of books, chapters, and articles and conferences such as Evolution of Psychotherapy, divergent conversations regarding the proposed change mechanisms in psychotherapy continue. One perspective that has gained considerable and lasting attention is the idea of consistent or common elements among bona fide approaches that account for the majority of variance in treatment outcomes. This perspective stands in stark contrast to the EST movement and the idea that models have unique and specific elements responsible for change (see Chapter 1). In 1936, psychologist Saul Rosenzweig wrote a seminal paper entitled, "Some Implicit Common Factors in Diverse Models of Psychotherapy," in which he raised the idea that although diverse methods of psychotherapy could look different, they had the same effective factors. Rosenzweig stated:

> What ... accounts for the result that apparently diverse forms of psychotherapy prove successful in similar cases? Or if they are only apparently diverse, what do these therapies actually have in common that makes them equally successful? ... it is justifiable to wonder ... whether the factors that actually are in operation in several different therapies may not have much more in common than have the factors alleged to be operating. (pp. 412–413)

Shortly after, several prominent theorists assembled at the 1940 conference of the American Orthopsychiatric Society. One of the presentations, "Areas of Agreement in Psychotherapy," explored the concept of common factors, which was later published in the *American Journal of Orthopsychiatry* (Watson, 1940). The panelists agreed on four areas of commonality in therapy: (a) having similar objectives, (b) making sure that the relationship is central, (c) keeping the responsibility for choice on the client, and (d) enlarging the client's understanding of self. Watson elaborated:

> If we were to apply to our colleagues the distinction, so important with patients, between what they tell us and what they do, we might find that agreement is greater in practice than in theory. ... We have agreed further ... that our

techniques cannot be uniform and rigid, but vary with the age, problems and potentialities of the individual client and with the unique personality of the therapist ... A therapist has nothing to offer but himself. (p. 29)

Subsequent to Rosenzweig's paper and the 1940 conference, little followed to advance the idea of common factors. Heine (1953) published a study comparing the popular methods of the time, supporting Rosenzweig's analysis by concluding that a common factor(s) was operating in the different forms of psychotherapies investigated (Sparks, Duncan, & Miller, 2008). Equally intriguing, Heine indicated that theory and technique are less important than the characteristics of the individual applying them. Sparks et al. (2008) noted that this conclusion "reiterates the 1940 panel's assertions and has since gained much empirical support" (p. 455). Heine endorsed the idea that the field commit itself to developing a psychotherapy rather than a series of psychotherapies. Support for Rosenzweig and Heine's ideas came in 1955 when Hoch opined:

If we have the opportunity to watch many patients treated by many different therapists using different techniques, we are struck by the divergencies in theory and in practical application and similarity in therapeutic results.... There are only two logical conclusions ... first that the different methods regardless of their theoretical background are equally effective, and that theoretical formulations are not as important as some unclear common factors present in all such therapies. (p. 323)

In 1961, Jerome Frank took a formal step of describing components shared across models. Frank identified four features shared by all effective therapies: (a) an emotionally charged, confiding relationship with a helping person; (b) a healing setting; (c) a rationale, conceptual scheme, or myth that plausibly explains the patient's symptoms and prescribes a ritual or procedure for resolving them; and (d) a ritual or procedure that requires the active participation of both patient and therapist and that is believed by both to be the means of restoring the patient's health.

In the 1982 edited book *Converging Themes in Psychotherapy*, Goldfried and Padawer (1982) suggested that once the theoretical jargon of different therapeutic schools of thought was removed, one could discern principles at a level of abstraction somewhere between the observable methods of clinical intervention and the higher order, theoretical speculation about why these methods might be effective elsewhere. These common principles of change include (a) the presence of clients' expectations that change is possible, (b) the existence of an optimal therapeutic relationship, (c) providing feedback to help clients become more aware of aspects of themselves and others, (d) the encouragement of corrective experiences, and (e) facilitation of ongoing reality testing.

Around the same time, a parallel line of thinking could be found in the work of Prochaska and colleagues (Prochaska & DiClemente, 1985; Prochaska,

DiClemente, & Norcross, 1992), who were developing the transtheoretical model of change. In their work, primarily with persons experiencing addictive behaviors (i.e., cigarette smoking, alcohol abuse, and obesity), Prochaska et al. (1992) identified 10 processes of change "receiving the most theoretical and empirical support," stating, "There are striking similarities in the frequency with which the change processes were used across these problems" (p. 1107). The researchers concluded, "We have discovered robust commonalities in how people modify their behavior. From our perspective the underlying structure of change is neither technique-oriented nor problem specific" (p. 1110).

Other perspectives that either hinted at or directly addressed the idea of commonalities across models of psychotherapy followed. In 1986, Orlinsky and Howard proposed that five process variables are active in any psychotherapy: the therapeutic contract, therapeutic interventions, the therapeutic bond between therapist and patient, the patient's and therapist's states of self-relatedness, and therapeutic realization. Then, Grencavage and Norcross (1990) reviewed 50 separate publications between 1936 and 1989, which identified between one and 20 common factors each, for a collective total of 89. From the studies, the researchers grouped the factors into five areas: client characteristics, therapist qualities, change processes, treatment structure, and therapeutic relationship. Also in 1990, Beutler and Clarkin published their systematic treatment selection (STS) model, which attempted to integrate common and specific factors into a single model that therapists could use to guide treatment, considering variables of patient dimensions, environments, settings, therapist dimensions, and treatment types (Beutler & Clarkin, 1990).

Since Rosenzweig's paper in 1936, much had happened to draw attention to the potential of common factors. But it wasn't until researcher Michael Lambert (1992) used the meta-analytic design to identify four specific factors affecting outcome that the idea of common factors took shape. Lambert (2005) stated:

> Common factors are those dimensions of the treatment setting (therapist, therapy, client) that are not specific to any particular technique. Research on the broader concept of common factors investigates causal mechanisms such as expectation for improvement, therapist confidence, and a therapeutic relationship that is characterized by trust, warmth, understanding, acceptance, kindness, and human wisdom. . . . Common factors, no matter how unimportant they may be from the point of view of a particular theory (theoretically inert or trivial) are central to nearly all psychological interventions in practice, if not, theory. (p. 856)

S. D. Miller, Duncan, and Hubble (1997) later added:

> The evidence makes it clear that similarities rather than differences between therapy models account for most of the change that clients experience in treatment. What emerges from examining these similarities is a group of common

factors that can be brought together to form a more unifying language for psychotherapy practice: a language that contrasts sharply with the current emphasis on difference characterizing most professional discussion and activity. (p. 15)

Lambert (1992) estimated that the major contributors to outcome, in order of their significance, were *extratherapeutic change*, *the therapeutic relationship*, *expectancy and placebo*, and *model and technique*. *Extratherapeutic change (client) factors* are estimated to be responsible for approximately 40% of the variance in outcome (S. D. Miller et al., 1997). This category of factors refers to components in the life and environment of the client that affect the occurrence of change, such as the client's inner strengths, support system, environment, and spontaneous chance events outside of therapy. Specific examples of these factors include faith, resilience and protective factors, persistence, supportive family members, community involvement, employment, and having a change focus (Hubble, Duncan, & Miller, 1999).

The second factor is *the therapeutic relationship*, which accounts for 30% of the variance in outcome. This set of factors represents the strength of the therapeutic alliance between the therapist and client(s) (Lambert, 1992). This alliance is the joint product of the therapist and client together focusing on the work of therapy (Sprenkle & Blow, 2004). Perhaps the two most significant aspects of this factor are the quality of clients' participation and the degree to which they are motivated, engaged, and join in the therapeutic work (Orlinsky, Grawe, & Parks, 1994; Prochaska et al., 1992). Clients who are engaged and connected with therapists may benefit most from therapy. Relationship factors also include behaviors provided by the therapist, such as warmth, empathy, encouragement, and acceptance.

The third factor, *expectancy and placebo*, refers to the portion of improvement derived from clients' knowledge of being helped, the instillation of hope, and pretreatment expectancy (Lambert, 1992). It also includes the belief of both the client and therapist in the restorative power of the treatment, recognition of therapist confidence, enthusiasm, and use of credible methods and techniques. Simply expecting therapy to help can serve as a placebo and counteract demoralization, activate hope, and advance improvement (Frank & Frank, 1991). Lambert (1992) initially estimated that expectancy and placebo in therapy contributed approximately 15% of the variance in therapeutic outcome.

The fourth and final factor, *model and technique*, consists of the therapist's theoretical orientation, therapeutic methods, strategies, or tactics implemented to move clients to take some action to improve themselves or their situation (Hubble et al., 1999; Lambert, 1992). Lambert originally suggested that model and technique contribute the same percentage to outcome variance as do expectancy and placebo factors—about 15%. He acknowledged that "no statistical procedures were used to derive the percentages" and his findings were based on an interpretation of, not a statistical analysis of, 40 years of data (p. 98). Figure 2.1 illustrates Lambert's assignment of percentages to the common factors.

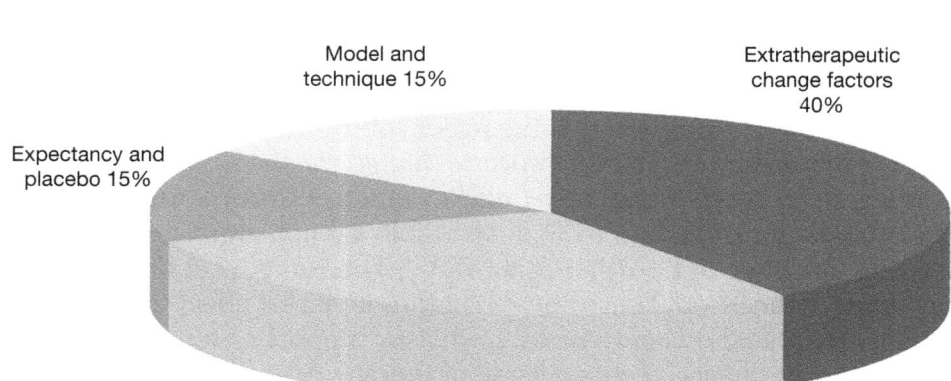

FIGURE 2.1 Common Factor.

The common factors perspective spawned numerous articles, chapters, and books including two comprehensive volumes, *The Heart and Soul of Change: What Works in Therapy?* (Hubble et al., 1999) and *The Heart and Soul of Change: Delivering What Works in Therapy* (Duncan, Miller, Wampold, & Hubble, 2010). The common factors certainly account for why psychotherapy works and in doing so answers the first question posed in this chapter, "What factors most influence therapy outcomes?" (Wampold & Imel, 2015). When it comes to the second question, however, "How do these factors known to influence outcomes translate to effective practice?" the common factors present a conundrum. Schuckard, Miller, and Hubble (2017) observed, "Clinicians want and need to know what to say and do to assist their clients" (p. 17). The common factors framework, as detailed in the literature, offers neither, and logically cannot. As soon as the shared elements of models are translated into method, techniques, and strategies, they cease to be common (Seidel, Miller, & Chow, 2014). In effect, the common factors become "specific ingredients," which as we have learned contribute very little to the variance in outcomes.

EVOLVING FROM THE COMMON FACTORS

To address the common factors conundrum, we refer to the research of psychologist Bruce Wampold (2001), who nearly a decade after Lambert (1992) completed a scientific evaluation and statistical analysis of the data. Wampold found that Lambert had correctly interpreted that the significant portion of the variance in psychotherapeutic outcomes is due to client/extratherapeutic factors or nonspecific effects. Wampold suggested that 87% of the outcome variance is related to those elements of the intervention not specified or directed by the theory, such as patient expectations for improvement, the credibility of the person providing the treatment, and credibility of the treatment being delivered; these factors often influence study outcomes, even though they are not usually specified as active ingredients in the intervention.

Wampold further found that ingredients such as model effects accounted no more than 8% of the variance (as compared to Lambert's estimation of 15%) and that only 1% of the overall variance could be assigned to a specific technique. This leaves approximately 22% in variance unexplained. According to Wampold (2001), this variability is due in part to client differences:

> Whatever the source of the unexplained variance, it is clearly not related to specific ingredients.... Lest there be any ambiguity about the profound contrast between general and specific effects, it must be noted that the 1% of the variability in outcomes due to specific ingredients is likely a gross upper bound. Clearly, the preponderance of the benefits of psychotherapy are due to factors incidental to the particular theoretical approach administered and dwarf the effects due to theoretically derived techniques. (pp. 207–209)

Wampold (2001, 2015; Wampold & Imel, 2015) offers initial guidance for navigating the common factors landscape. Based on his meta-analysis, he concluded that common factors are relevant and essential to therapeutic outcomes and "the choice of model does not affect conclusions about the impact of these factors" (p. 270). However, specific ingredients do play a role in psychotherapy outcome. As stated in the opening chapter, "Models are essential to effective psychotherapy, just not in ways originally conceived." According to Wampold (2015),

> Specific ingredients not only create expectations . . . but universally produce some salubrious actions. That is, the therapist induces the patient to enact some healthy actions, whether that may be thinking about the world in less maladaptive ways, and relying less on dysfunctional schemas (cognitive-behavioral treatments), improving interpersonal relations (interpersonal psychotherapy and some dynamic therapies), being more accepting of one's self (self-compassion therapies, acceptance and commitment therapy), expressing difficult emotions (emotion-focused and dynamic therapies), taking the perspective of others (mentalization therapies), and so on. (p. 272)

The task of the therapist is to effectively engage clients through such factors as the working alliance, empathy, expectancy, psychoeducation about the disorder, and the like, which are robustly related to outcome. Those therapists who can form an alliance with a range of patients, have a sophisticated set of facilitative interpersonal skills, worry about their effectiveness, and make deliberate efforts to improve are the therapists who achieve better outcomes. As discussed, the concepts "fit" and "effect" are of critical importance as we determine whether and to what degree our attempts at intervention fit with a particular client and the effect of those interventions as measured by client benefit.

Our next step is to consider Wampold's preliminary guidance to further address the question: How do these factors translate to effective practice? Building on what we have learned to this point, we now explore a strengths-based framework, which incorporates best available research, clinical expertise, and client characteristics, culture, and preferences, the three cornerstones of EBP.

THE THIRD WAVE: A STRENGTHS-BASED PERSPECTIVE

Psychotherapy could be considered as evolving in three waves (Bertolino & O'Hanlon, 2002). The first wave began with Sigmund Freud in the early 1900s and rested on the notion that mental illness was the result of intrapsychic pathology. The therapist was considered the expert, responsible for identifying and remediating pathology by delving into the patient's past to releasing repressed material held captive by the unconscious. Psychoanalysis was the primary methodology of the time. Through principles of classical and operant conditioning, behaviorism was thought to provide an alternative to psychoanalysis; however, it too was reliant on the therapist as expert. Whereas psychoanalysis was largely based on interpretation and considered profoundly subjective, behaviorism was roundly criticized for being dehumanizing and overly mechanistic.

The second wave, which began in the 1950s, initially brought about a shift in focus from pathology to problems. Cognitively oriented therapies and systems theory began to gain popularity, which represented a paradigm shift by suggesting that problems existed not with people but between people. An emphasis on client interaction also brought about a new nomenclature. Terms such as *neurosis*, *narcissistic*, and *complex* were replaced with *enmeshment*, *hierarchy*, and *homeostasis* (Bertolino & O'Hanlon, 2002). As the second wave matured, a notable shift in psychotherapy resulted with the rise of humanistic psychology. Theorists including Abraham Maslow, Carl Rogers, and Rollo May rose to prominence with a focus on growth and self-actualization, which stood in stark contrast to the deficit and pathology-focused perspective developed by Freud (1909/1953), who once remarked, "I have found little that is good about human beings. In my experience, most of them are trash" (p. 56).

A further example of evolvement during the second wave could be found in the work of psychiatrist Milton Erickson, considered by some to be the first competence-based practitioner. Erickson developed an approach based on utilization, which involved actively using what the patient brought to the therapeutic encounter as part of the change process. According to Erickson (1954), "The purpose of psychotherapy should be the helping of the patient in that fashion most adequate, available, and acceptable. In rendering the patient aid, there should be full respect for and utilization of whatever the patient presents" (p. 127). Even with the efforts of Erickson and the humanists, many of the approaches developed during the second wave were largely problem-focused and reliant on the therapist as the expert (Bertolino, 2010).

It wasn't until the late 1970s that therapists began to take notice of their biases and blinders. Sexism and other forms of prejudice existed in some of the more prominent theories of the time and had gone largely unchallenged (Bertolino & O'Hanlon, 2002). The feminist critique in particular drew attention to the importance of gender inequities and sociocultural issues, which had existed in psychotherapy since its inception, and their impact on clients (Goldner, 1985). Bertolino and O'Hanlon (2002) wrote, "Many commonly-used practices of the first- and second-wave theories and practices marginalized women and minorities while all but avoiding the larger social context within which 'problems' occurred" (p. 3).

The changes that began to take root during this time represented a third wave, a dramatic shift in ideology from pathology and problems to competency. Prior to this shift, it was commonly accepted that the therapist's role was to identify client deficits and implement strategies to ameliorate those deficits which were typically expressed in symptoms and behaviors. The third wave not only redirected attention toward strengths, it redefined the posture of the therapist to that of a collaborator. Therapists became cocreators in the therapeutic process in which both the client and the therapist had expertise: The client was considered an expert on his or her life, what hasn't worked, what might work in the future, and what "fit" best intervention-wise. The therapist was considered an expert in terms of education, experience, and creativity in developing possibilities to positive change.

The collaborative nature of therapy was underscored by constructivism, the idea that there are multiple ways of viewing and experiencing the world, and social constructionism, which emphasizes the role of language and interaction, within which both problems and solutions are constructed. Not only are there countless ways for clients to view their lives and situations, there are also multiple pathways to change (Berger & Luckmann, 1966; Maturana, 1978). In accordance, a host of new "constructive" models accompanied the third wave, in particular, solution-focused and solution-oriented therapies and narrative therapy (Hoyt, 1994, 1996, 1998).

Research Comes of Age

It would take time for research to catch up with and substantiate what theorists had long believed. While there exists no evidence that a focus on pathology is necessary for or facilitates positive change, numerous studies show the benefits of identifying and building on client competencies (Duncan et al., 2010). In 2000, then president of the APA Martin Seligman and his coauthor Mihaly Csikszentmihalyi (2000) wrote:

> What we have learned over 50 years is that the disease model does not move us closer to the prevention of these serious problems. Indeed the major strides in prevention have largely come from a perspective focused on systematically building competency, not correcting weakness. . . . Much of the task of

prevention in this new century will be to create a science of human strength whose mission will be to understand and learn how to foster these virtues in young people. Working exclusively on personal weakness and on the damaged brains, however, has rendered science poorly equipped to do effective prevention. We need now to call for massive research on human strength and virtue. We need to ask practitioners to recognize that much of the best work they already do in the consulting room is to amplify strengths rather than repair the weaknesses of their clients. (pp. 6–7)

Strengths represent a key part of the 87% of the variance in outcome related to the client and the client's life (Wampold, 2001). Simply, clients are the engineers of change. When factored in with available research and knowledge regarding the role of the therapist, the therapeutic alliance, expectancy, and other factors known to be associated with positive outcomes, a more complete picture of how to work effectively takes shape.

The Strengths-Based Approach Defined

As in Chapter 1 with personal philosophies, let's now translate what we have learned from the best available research into working philosophy. What follows is a definition of a strengths-based approach to counseling and psychotherapy:

> A strengths-based perspective emphasizes the abilities and resources people have within themselves and their support systems to more effectively cope with life challenges. When combined with new experiences, understandings, and skills, these abilities and resources contribute to improved well-being and outcome, which is comprised of three areas of functioning: individual, interpersonal relationships, and social role. Strengths-based practitioners value relationships and convey this through respectful, culturally-sensitive, collaborative practices that support, encourage, and empower. Routine outcome monitoring (ROM) is used to create and maintain a culture of feedback—a responsive, consumer-driven climate to ensure the greatest benefit of services.

There are several interrelated components to this definition. First is the cornerstone of a strengths-based perspective—a focus on abilities (i.e., strengths, competencies). A strengths-based perspective is two-pronged, involving both the activation and utilization of latent or underemployed abilities *and* the teaching of new ones. How to actively evoke and utilize client strengths will be discussed shortly.

A second component of a strengths-based perspective is *well-being*. Well-being is a construct comprised of several elements. For example, weather is made up of temperature, barometric pressure, humidity, and the like. Each is important but does not in and of itself define weather. Similarly, well-being is inclusive of three elements or areas: *individual, interpersonal*, and *social role functioning*.

Individual functioning includes positive emotion, engagement, meaning, and accomplishment (Seligman, 2011). In brief, positive emotion includes, but is not limited to, happiness and life satisfaction. Engagement relates to subjective absorption through experiences in the present. For example, a client could become immersed in an activity such as reading, in which he or she experiences pleasure, loses track of time, and feels experientially absorbed. Meaning equates to belonging to and serving something that is believed to be bigger than one's self. Accomplishment or achievement is the pursuit of something for its own sake and is commonly seen in the pursuit of success, competence, or mastery.

An additional facet of well-being is *interpersonal functioning*, which refers to close, often intimate, positive interactions with others. Most frequently this category includes caregivers, family, and those who play significant roles in clients' lives. The final area is *social role functioning*, a category that captures the impact of employment, school, community support, and other more general yet important forms of support. As with the elements of weather, each of the three areas of functioning is important but does not by itself define well-being; it is their collective value that forms well-being. To conclude, in psychotherapy, improved well-being equates to improved outcome.

A third component of a strengths-based perspective is a focus on the therapeutic relationship. Therapists value each interaction as an opportunity to work together toward a hoped-for future. To this end, strategies used to strengthen the alliance and promote change are provided with respect to the culture of the client. The therapeutic alliance, which will be discussed in detail later in this chapter, is arguably the most vigorously studied variable in psychotherapy literature (Norcross, 2011).

As discussed in the opening chapter, the final component of a strengths-based perspective is ROM to create a culture of feedback to evaluate the impact and benefit of services. ROM is composed of two forms of measurement: *outcome* and *alliance*. *Outcome* refers to the impact of services, from the client's perspective, on major areas of functioning: individual, interpersonal, and social role. *Alliance* or process measurement involves elicitation of the client's perceptions of the therapeutic relationship. Routine (i.e., each session or meeting) and ongoing (i.e., from the start of services to discontinuation) monitoring improves the effectiveness of services by allowing the client and his or her experiences to serve as a guide. Studies involving the use of real-time feedback demonstrate that it as much as doubles the effect size of services, decreases deterioration and dropout rates, and reduces psychiatric hospitalizations and costs of care (Bertolino, Bargmann, & Miller, 2013).

What Strengths-Based Is *Not*

Any discussion of a perspective, framework, or model is at risk of being misunderstood. To this end, strengths based is not about positive thinking or seeing the proverbial glass as being half full, both of which represent oversimplifications.

Instead, being strengths based involves looking beyond what is immediately observed or believed to be true and making the investment in clients to know more about them. Madsen (2007) has referred to this through the notion of being "appreciative allies," a concept that translates to first acknowledging the negative emotional reactions we may have to clients whose actions we find intolerable or offensive. In doing so, we open ourselves up to finding something, however small, that we can appreciate and respect about clients. These granules contribute to the foundation for subsequent work and reflect our faith that positive change and successful outcome are possible even in the most challenging situations. Such a perspective can circumvent services by freeing therapists from predetermined theoretical restraints that suggest impossibility.

Next, some so-called competency-based and collaborative frameworks focus almost exclusively on strengths. The idea is that clients have all the strengths they need to resolve the problems they encounter. This idea is not only a misrepresentation of what it means to be strengths based, it can also be invalidating to those who desperately need therapists to thoroughly understand the different hardships and risks they are facing. Being strengths based does not mean being "problem phobic" nor does it suggest forcing an agenda that focuses only on solutions or what works. Clients are not bottomless reservoirs of ability who have every answer to every life problem. Overlooking serious threats to the well-being of clients is unrealistic and potentially hazardous. A strengths-based perspective does not involve downplaying or altogether ignoring real-life difficulties, pain, and suffering of clients. Rather, it translates to acknowledging and attending to the hardships that clients face and identifying threats while focusing on both the evocation of strengths and education in the service of change. The latter relates to creating situations in which clients can acquire new information and develop new skills, which reflects an emphasis on lifelong learning.

STRENGTHS-BASED PRINCIPLES: FROM EVIDENCE TO PRACTICE

Founded on the research covered so far in this volume and other findings yet to be discussed, a strengths-based perspective is not considered a theoretical model, but instead an overarching framework that informs effective practice, regardless of the choice of model. Therefore, the forthcoming principles are not the province of any particular approach. They collectively reflect and shape therapy through known mechanisms of change.

There are a few additional thoughts before we explore the strengths-based principles. The principles that follow are in accordance with Castonguay and Beutler (2006) who stated, "We think that psychotherapy research has produced enough knowledge to begin to define the basic principles that govern therapeutic change in a way that is not tied to any specific theory, treatment model, or narrowly defined set of concepts" (p. 5). Next, the principles are in accord with the APA definition of EBP. Each principle stands on its own in terms of its contribution to successful services; however, each principle is but one pillar. It is the collective tapestry of the principles that creates the foundation of a strengths-based perspective.

The principles will be described using a three-level structure. The first level is the principle itself. The second is the "key competency" associated with the principle. The key competency represents the overall skill for therapists to develop and continue to improve on. The third level includes key tasks associated with the primary competency.

Principle 1: Expectancy and Hope Are Catalysts of Change

Key Competency: Demonstrate faith in the restorative effects of services

At first glance, it would seem that factors such as expectancy and hope would rank lower on a list of principles of effective therapy. But both the presence or absence and diminishment of this class of factors is far-reaching. Surgeon Atul Gawande (2007), the author of *Better: A Surgeon's Notes on Performance*, has said that the worst thing a physician can do is give up hope on a patient. Consider the words of Emil "Jay" Freireich, who started college at the age of 16 with $25 given by a friend of his mother and began medical school at 18. Dr. Freireich helped discover the cure for childhood leukemia before he was 40 and became the champion of clinical research to alleviate the suffering of thousands of cancer victims. Dr. Freireich is very candid about the impact of hope:

> There's no possibility of being pessimistic when people are dependent on you for their only optimism. On Tuesday morning, I make teaching rounds, and sometimes medical fellows say, "This patient is eighty years old. It's hopeless." Absolutely not! It's challenging. It's not hopeless. You have to come up with something. You have to figure out a way to help them, because people must have hope to live. (quoted in Gladwell, 2013, p. 139)

Take a moment to refer back to your responses to the questions posed about personal philosophy in Chapter 1. Now, consider how your underlying beliefs about people and change might affect what you do as a therapist. As we have learned, our personal philosophies are precursors to theory. We are constantly influencing our clients and, reciprocally, being influenced by clients. There is a responsibility to stay attuned to the influence we have on our expectations of clients, therapy, our methods, and the prospects of change. In turn, we must remain aware of clients' views of these influences. Although therapists have long been cognizant of the role of hope and expectancy, research was slow to describe and validate their collective influence. Even today, it remains one of the more elusive factors in outcome.

In the 1960s several researchers began formal exploration of both clients' and therapists' expectations on treatment outcomes (Frank, 1961, 1968; Goldstein, 1962). In his book *Persuasion and Healing: A Comparative Study of Psychotherapy*, Jerome Frank (1961) explored the concept of common factors, one of which was client expectations. Frank was particularly interested in expectation, initially referred to as placebo effects, with the use of psychopharmacology and, later, psychotherapy. Rosenthal and Frank (1956) observed, "The giving of any medication may have certain meanings for a patient in terms of his relationship to his physician which may benefit his condition irrespective of the pharmacological action of the drug" (p. 296).

Frank's work eventually led to a more refined and expansive discussion of expectancy to reflect the portion of improvement derived from clients' knowledge of being helped, the instillation of hope, recognition of therapist confidence, enthusiasm, and use of credible methods and techniques. Expectancy also includes the belief of both the client and the therapist in the restorative power of the treatment, including its procedures. Simply expecting therapy to help can serve as a placebo and counteract demoralization, activate hope, and advance improvement.

Expectations about therapy are crucial, especially at the beginning. People would not bother with therapy if they did not believe it could be beneficial in some way. This factor is commonly referred to as pretreatment or preservices expectancy (Mueller & Pekarik, 2000; Safren, Heimberg, & Juster, 1997; Schneider & Klauer, 2001). Pretreatment expectancy is important for therapists as well as clients.

Although specific methods and techniques contribute little to the variance in outcomes, all therapeutic processes involve techniques or rituals (Frank & Frank, 1991). As discussed, the important aspects in bringing about change are (a) the processes and practices therapists use that contribute to the expectancy for change and increase in hope, (b) clients' and practitioners' belief in the treatments and the rationales behind them, and (c) the fit between methods and clients' perspectives about their problems and possibilities for solution.

Consider that in the largest study ever completed on the treatment of persons with depression, the Treatment of Depression Collaborative Research Program (TDCRP), the most effective psychiatrists achieved better outcomes administering a placebo than the least effective psychiatrists administering antidepressant medication (McKay, Imel, & Wampold, 2006). An attitude of pessimism or an emphasis on psychopathology or the long-term process of change can negatively affect hope. In contrast, therapists' attitudes that positive change can and does occur even in difficult situations coupled with an emphasis on possibilities and improvement can instill and promote hope. Processes and practices that are respectful, collaborative, honor clients' ideas about change, and, ultimately, build on, create, and/or rehabilitate hope increase the prospects of change. Therapists using such processes and practices expect and anticipate positive change and continuously monitor for it.

Expectancy and hope offer a remedy to impossibility. When things are going poorly, most people would like their lives, at some level, to improve, at least minimally. Hope for this improvement is not about people looking at the world through rose-colored glasses but recognizing that if people have choices, most prefer things to be better. An underlying pessimism or negativity—unless to empathize with the client—can represent the difference between clients having a positive experience and continuing services.

Client expectations that services are, at minimal, safe and, at best, able to change their lives for the better help to act as a placebo to counteract demoralization, activate hope, and advance improvement (Frank & Frank, 1991; S. D. Miller et al., 1997). Similarly, therapists who have the attitude that positive change can occur even in difficult situations coupled with an emphasis on possibilities tend to instill and promote hope in every interaction, however small. Processes and practices that are respectful, collaborative, honor clients' ideas about change increase the prospects of change.

Lambert (1992; Asay & Lambert, 1999) initially estimated that expectancy and placebo in therapy contributed approximately 15% of the variance in therapeutic outcome. Recent estimates suggest that expectancy and hope contribute about 4% to the overall variance in outcome. Dew and Bickman (2005) suggest that expectancy is related to both client improvement and the therapeutic alliance (Principle 3), which are inextricably intertwined. What follows is a series of strategies therapists can use to maximize the contributions of clients in therapy.

- Maintain the belief that clients are motivated and capable of proactive change.
- Demonstrate faith in clients and their caregivers to achieve positive change.
- Demonstrate faith in the restorative effects of services.
- Build on preservice expectancy (i.e., the expectations clients and others may have at the *start of services*).
- Create expectancy for change by focusing on what is possible and changeable.
- Create expectancy for change by using language that is respectful and emanates hope.
- Accommodate clients' expectations of therapy.
- Believe and demonstrate faith in the procedures and practices utilized.
- Show interest in the results of the therapeutic procedure, orientation, or method.
- Ensure that the procedure or orientation is credible from the client's or caregiver's frame of reference.
- Ensure that the procedure or orientation is connected with or elicits the client's previously successful experiences.

- Work in ways that enhance or highlight the client's feelings of personal control.
- View clients as people, not as their problems or difficulties or in ways that depersonalize them.

Principle 2: Clients Are the Most Significant Contributors to Outcome

Key Competency: Evoke and utilize client contributions to change

Based on his meta-analysis, Wampold (2001) suggested that client/extratherapeutic factors as well as unexplained and error variance account for approximately 87% of the variability in outcome. It is reasonable to suppose that a substantial portion of the unexplained variance is due to the client (Bohart & Tallman, 2010).

This set of factors involves the client's *internal strengths* and *external resources*. *Internal strengths* include optimism, persistence, resilience, protective factors, coping skills, creativity, and the ability to self-express or disclose. Resilience and protective factors are qualities and actions that allow clients to meet the difficulties and challenges of life (Bohart & Tallman, 2010). Growth and maturation relate to the ability of clients to move through or mature out of individual and life cycle developmental phases, manage the trials and tribulations of life, overcome problems, and cope with trauma (Bertolino, 2014).

External resources refer to relationships, social networks, and systems that provide support and opportunities. Examples are family, friendship, employment, educational, community, and religious supports. Other external resources can include affiliation or membership in groups or associations that provide connection and stability. Client support systems are central in maintaining long-term change; focusing on processes that tap into, develop, and encourage such capacities is central to a strengths-based perspective (Bertolino, 2014, 2015).

Client contributions also include opportunities for new learning and skill development. Psychoeducational and experiential activities are used to help clients to develop a more encompassing repertoire of skills. A combination of already existing strengths and the addition of new skills is a formidable duo that provides clients with a broader range of options and responses for coping with life challenges.

Extratherapeutic factors further involve characteristics or qualities of clients that influence change, such as level of motivation, commitment to change, spontaneous recovery, and influential happenings outside of therapy that play a major role in change. Whether clients choose to discuss these events in therapy or not, they inevitably influence the process (Bohart & Tallman, 2010; Duncan & Miller, 2000). We want to know: How have clients experienced past change, with or without the support of psychotherapy? For example, a growing number of studies on client change demonstrate that many alcoholics recover without treatment (W. R. Miller & Rollnick, 2013). Researchers have also found that 40% to 60% of people who experience traumas either recover on their own or even grow from the trauma (Calhoun & Tedeschi, 2013; Tedeschi, Park, & Calhoun, 1998). This "recovery" has become known as *posttraumatic growth*.

The idea of self-change is further supported through two additional examples. First is a study by Prochaska, Norcross, and DiClemente (1994) who found that many individuals are able to overcome problems such as smoking on their own. Second, a Gallup poll found that 90% of a random sample of 1,000 individuals reported that they had overcome a significant health, emotional, addiction, or lifestyle problem in the last year (Gurin, 1990). And as it turns out, individuals who are not in therapy often use the same healing processes employed by psychotherapists.

According to Bohart (2000), much of the mystery around client factors disappears if one considers therapy from a different vantage point. The researcher contends:

> In contrast to the idea that healing power primarily comes from therapists and their interventions, it is clients who are the healers. Clients are intelligent, thinking beings who are not merely operated on by supposedly "potent" interventions and treatments which change them. Rather, clients are active agents who operate on therapist input and modify it and use it to achieve their own ends. (p. 132)

What follows is a list of processes and strategies therapists can use to make the most of client contributions to change. Because this list is not exhaustive, as a reader you are encouraged to keep track of the processes and strategies that you find beneficial. Upcoming chapters will offer additional ways of developing this class of factors.

- Communicate the belief that clients are competent and capable.
- Enlist, promote, and utilize client abilities and skills related to resilience, coping, and protective factors.
- Identify abilities and past solutions typically utilized in contexts other than the problem area(s) and link them to present situations.
- Identify and assist clients in developing systems of support, community resources, and social networks (e.g., family, friends, educators, employers, religious/spiritual advisors, groups, and other outside helpers and community members).
- Learn what clients do to get their everyday needs met (i.e., whom they seek out for support, where they go for support).
- Identify what resources clients *already* have in their lives that may be used actively in the present.
- Identify moments (exceptions) in the past or present—even if fleeting—when the client's problems were less present or absent altogether.
- Explore moments in the past or present when clients have made beneficial decisions.

- Even when external influences factor into change (psychotherapy, medication, etc.) or clients assign change to influences outside of their control (e.g., luck, chance), attribute the majority of change to their own qualities and actions.
- Create opportunities for clients to acquire and develop new skills.
- When others closely aligned with clients have made positive contributions to their lives, share the credit for change with such persons.
- Assist clients with evaluating the benefits of positive change.
- Identify ways that clients can utilize abilities to face future challenges.
- Explore ways that clients can extend change into other areas of life.
- Encourage personal agency and accountability.

Principle 3: The Therapeutic Alliance Makes Substantial and Consistent Contributions to Outcome

Key Competency: Engage clients through the working alliance

No aspect of psychotherapy has been studied in more or in greater detail than the therapeutic relationship. To date, over 1,100 studies have been completed on the therapeutic relationship as a whole or one or more components of it (Norcross, 2011). These studies have helped to identify and describe in detail the alliance, which is considered an expansion of the therapeutic relationship. Bordin (1979) originally delineated three components regarding the affective quality of the client–therapist relationship: (a) trust, warmth, and caring; (b) the tasks; and (c) the goals of therapy. The therapeutic alliance has been expanded to comprise four empirically established components: (a) the client's view of the relationship; (b) agreement on the goals, meaning, or purpose of the treatment; (c) agreement on the means and methods used in treatment; and (d) accommodation of the client's preferences (see Figure 2.2). Each of these will be discussed next.

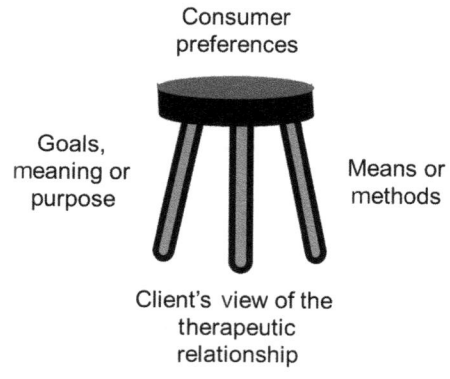

FIGURE 2.2 Components of the Therapeutic Alliance.

1) *The client's view of the relationship (including perceptions of the provider as warm, empathic, and genuine).* Simply, client ratings of the therapeutic relationship are significantly related to outcome and are widely considered the best and most consistent process predictor of improvement (Bachelor & Horvath, 1999; Baldwin, Wampold, & Imel, 2007; Horvath & Bedi, 2002; Orlinsky et al., 1994; Orlinsky, Rønnestad, & Willutzki, 2004). In fact, client ratings of providers as empathic, trustworthy, and nonjudgmental are better predictors of positive outcome than are provider ratings, diagnosis, approach, or any other variable (Horvath & Symonds, 1991; Lambert & Bergin, 1994). Clients who are engaged and connected with therapists and those affiliated with services are likely to benefit most.

It is important to note that several key relational variables including empathy, positive regard, and congruence can be traced back to Carl Rogers' (1957) seminal article, "The Necessary and Sufficient Conditions of Therapeutic Personality Change." Truax and Carkhuff (1967) built on Rogers' idea, defining empathy as the therapist's ability to be "accurately empathic, be with the client, be understanding, or grasp the client's meaning" (p. 25). Positive regard, which Rogers referred to as unconditional positive regard, is "the extent that the therapist finds himself experiencing a warm acceptance of each aspect of the client's experience as being a part of that client" (p. 98). Congruence or genuineness speak to the therapist's ability to relate transparently and honestly with the client, casting aside the façade of the professional role.

Because client ratings of the therapeutic alliance are the best and most consistent process predictor of outcome, Rogers' "core conditions" are contingent on a fit with the client. For example, Bachelor's (1988) study of client perceptions of empathy found that this factor had different meanings for different clients. Therefore, relational factors should not be viewed or practiced as universal constructs, but instead as experiences to be understood through the experience of individual clients.

2) *Agreement on the goals, meaning, or purpose of the treatment.* Orlinsky et al. (2004) observe, "The quality of the patient's participation . . . [emerges] as the most important [process] determinant in outcome" (p. 324). It is of little debate that clients who are engaged and involved in services and treatment processes are likely to receive greater benefit. This finding is consistent with the *Consumer Reports* study that found clients who reported being more actively involved in therapy benefited the most (Seligman, 1995). Involving clients in the purpose of services and goals can affect the degree of engagement and, therefore, eventual outcome. Negative outcome is often traced to the exclusion of the client from service decisions. Duncan, Hubble, and Miller (1997) stated, "Impossibility . . . is at least partly a function of leaving clients out of the process, of not listening or of dismissing the importance of their perspective" (p. 30).

3) *Agreement on the means and methods used in treatment.* In addition to involving clients in determining the purpose of services and goals, it is also important that clients be in agreement on *how* to improve functioning and

well-being (outcome). In any given problem situation there are multiple options available in terms of how to approach it. Essential to the success of techniques, methods, and interventions is the degree to which they *fit* with clients. Effective therapists stay clear of prescriptive, one-size-fits-all methods, instead involving clients in therapy-related processes.

4) *Accommodation of the client's preferences.* A growing number of studies have identified the role of client expectations and personal preferences on the alliance (Norcross, 2011). Although moderate and strong preferences differ in terms of their influence on the client–provider connection, what is important is that therapists attend to the values, beliefs, worldviews, and service expectations of clients. Key areas for clients include, but are not limited to, who should be involved with services, when and where to meet, the length of sessions, and so on.

Each component in the therapeutic alliance serves a role in strengthening relationships not only with clients but with those who may be involved in the lives of clients. Because the strength of the alliance is an excellent predictor of eventual outcome, it is imperative that therapists attune themselves to practices that enhance engagement. Although the strength of the therapeutic bond is not highly correlated with the length of treatment (Horvath & Luborsky, 1993), there are threats (e.g., distrust of professionals, previous experiences in therapy, expectations) to the bond between therapists and clients.

The most effective practitioners continuously work on their relationships with clients, understanding the importance of forming stable connections and gaining feedback about both the alliance and the outcome (i.e., fit and effect), which we explore in detail in Chapter 3. In fact, the most significant difference between average and above average therapists is in their ability to form, nurture, and sustain alliances with a diverse range of clients (Baldwin et al., 2007). The following is an array of strategies for strengthening the therapeutic relationships with clients.

- Use active listening and attending skills to connect with clients while recognizing that caution toward professionals may be an appropriate response based on their past experiences.
- Create space for the client to tell his or her story through a discovery-oriented approach.
- Collaborate with caregivers, family members, outside helpers, and community resources to create strong social networks and systems of support for the client.
- Collaborate with clients in setting goals.
- Incorporate the views of involved helpers (i.e., extended family, social service workers, medical personnel, educators, law enforcement, educators) in setting goals and determining directions.
- Collaborate with clients on tasks to accomplish goals.

- Attend to the contributions of the therapist to the alliance including possible negative effects.
- Incorporate an outcome orientation as a means to monitor the benefit of services from the perspective of clients and other stakeholders.
- Use respectful, nondepersonalizing, and nonpathologizing language when describing clients and the concerns of clients.
- Learn about the preferences and expectations of clients and as best as possible accommodate services to those preferences and expectations.
- Offer options and choices in services and processes.
- Discuss with clients possible benefits and side effects of services.
- Discuss with clients parameters of confidentiality and informed consent.
- Provide rationale for services.
- Incorporate real-time feedback processes to learn and respond to clients' views of relationships.
- Learn and adapt to the ways in which clients use language.
- Demonstrate concern for the well-being, feelings, and interests of clients.
- Compliment clients for positive intentions and actions.
- Consider clients as experts on their lives, learning about and respecting their ideas.
- Develop and increase awareness regarding personal biases and viewpoints and how they can affect relationships and services.

Principle 4: Culture Influences and Shapes All Aspects of Human Life

Key Competency: Communicate respect for clients and their cultures

Recall that the third component of an evidence-based approach is "client, characteristics, culture, and preferences." Culture specifically refers to a system of shared beliefs, values, customs, behaviors, and artifacts among various groups within a community, institution, organization, or nation. From generation to generation, members of society use their cultural references to cope with their world and with one another. Hays (2007) suggested the acronym ADDRESSING as a way to identify different aspects of culture: age, developmental and acquired disability, religion, ethnicity, social class, sexual orientation, indigenous heritage, national origin, and gender/sex. Brown (2008) expanded on Hays' perspective to include other social locations such as vocational and recreational choices, partnership status, parenthood (or not), attractiveness, body size and shape, and state of physical health. Culture is a powerful filter through which behavior can be understood; however, no one aspect provides a comprehensive explanation of it (Sue, Arredondo, & McDavis, 1992). Culture is inclusive of client characteristics (Principle 1) and one's community.

Cultural competence is a cornerstone of a strengths-based perspective. As therapists, we work with clients, family members, coworkers, and others who are culturally different from ourselves. Such persons come from an array of backgrounds, and their customs, thoughts, ways of communicating, values, traditions, and institutions vary accordingly. In our work with clients we emphasize awareness and learning, forming new patterns of response and ways to effectively apply those responses to appropriate settings. Further, therapists with diverse backgrounds can draw on their experiences and their general cultural knowledge to match clients' ideas about problems, possibilities, and potential solutions. Thus, knowledge of different cultures and perspectives is beneficial by allowing therapists to view situations differently without having to align with any one viewpoint. This knowledge also brings with it an expanded repertoire of methods to use that may be helpful in delivering services.

There is considerable overlap between culture and other aspects associated with this particular principle. It is simply not possible to be culturally attuned in therapy without attention to expectancy and hope, client contributions, the therapeutic alliance, and growth, development, and well-being, which will be discussed next. The following are points of awareness and processes for therapists to reflect on and incorporate in practice.

- Maintain self-awareness and sensitivity to one's own cultural heritage, background, and experiences and their influence on personal attitudes, values, and biases.
- Recognize limits of multicultural competency and expertise.
- Recognize sources of personal discomfort with differences that may exist between ourselves as therapists and clients in terms of race, ethnicity, culture, gender, and other influences.
- Acknowledge that specific racial and cultural factors influence service-oriented processes—understand and respect the client's cultural heritage and practices.
- Develop a multilevel understanding of clients, family, community, helping systems, and other associated relational or systemic influences.
- Consult others who share cultural similarities and expertise with clients being served.
- Create safe and nurturing cultural, physical, psychological, and social environments and settings.
- Use assessment processes that identify concerns, risks, and threats to cultural safety and well-being.
- Acknowledge and address risks and issues related to cultural safety.

- Acknowledge caregivers as capable of keeping their children safe.
- Create culturally meaningful experiences in services-based activities.
- Use person-first language.
- Individualize services and avoid "one-size-fits-all" approaches.
- Acknowledge clients as teachers and experts on their own lives and experiences.
- Emphasize capacities of clients to adapt, change, and grow.
- Empower clients and others by using practices that identify and employ their unique capabilities.
- Identify, assess, address, and monitor barriers to services, particularly those cultural barriers associated with accessibility.
- Create plans of action that are culturally sensitive.
- Exercise care in matching methods (i.e., techniques, interventions) with clients.
- Utilize strategies that are respectful and reflective of differences.
- Explore exceptions to risks and incorporate them into action plans.
- Employ proactive (as opposed to reactive) systems of response.
- Use culturally sensitive methods of research and evaluation.
- Manage the dynamics of difference.
- Acquire and institutionalize cultural knowledge.
- Adapt to the diversity and cultural contexts of the individuals, families, and communities served.

Principle 5: Effective Services Promote Growth, Development, Well-Being, and Functioning

Key Competency: Utilize strategies that support and empower clients to achieve meaningful improvement

Despite the growing number of psychotherapies, each with an explanation about the nature of problems and how to remedy those problems, psychotherapy outcomes have remained flat for the past 40 years (Wampold & Imel, 2015). In a documentary about his life, *Wizard of the Desert*, Milton Erickson was asked why he did not talk in any classic analytical terms. The psychiatrist replied:

> Every year it seems the president of the American Psychological Association comes out with a brand new comprehensive theory of psychology. There'll be another one next year. Psychiatrists comes out with a brand new comprehensive

(theory) . . . and everybody wants to make a name for himself by attaching his name to a hypothetical, theoretical system. And I think you should bear in mind that a human being is a human being and that's been the case for millions of years. Any patient who comes to you is strictly an individual whom you don't know and he doesn't know you and the interaction between you and him is something to be discovered, and not approved by the Adlerian, Freudian, Stekelian, Rogerian, or Myerian, existentialist, and so on. (Vesely, 2014)

There exists no evidence that the provision of explanations about the nature of problems or pathology in general improves therapy outcomes. In contrast, as we will learn, explanations that are individualized, adaptive, fit with, and are acceptable to clients provide rationale and *are* part of effective therapy. Further, evidence suggests that a focus on growth, development, and well-being is beneficial to clients (Duncan et al., 2010).

Clients are better served when therapists concentrate their efforts on the identifying and mobilizing factors responsible for change and, in doing so, view change as a process as opposed to providing explanations or theories of causality. S. D. Miller et al. (1997) described the role of mental health professionals as one of enhancing "the factors responsible for change-in-general rather than on identifying and then changing the factors a theory suggests are responsible or causing problems-in-particular" (p. 127).

As described earlier, an orientation toward growth, development, and well-being correlates with improvement in individual, interpersonal, and social role functioning, which is indicative of improved outcome. To assist with improvement of functioning, we consider *how* clients can flourish in society by concentrating on exceptions to problems—times when things have gone better in relation to challenges—and building on those often subtle differences in the present and future. Focusing on exceptions and the prospects of future change does not mean dismissing past events. Just as some will prefer to search for explanations to problems, some may prefer to study the past and past events. From a strengths-based perspective, therapists acknowledge the role of the past and other potential influences as much or as little as clients and those associated with clients want while placing attention on the prospects of an improved future.

A focus on improvement necessitates keeping an eye out for positive change from the start of therapy. Factors such as the severity of symptoms, personality characteristics, and the strength of support systems will influence rates of improvement in services; however, research makes it clear that the process of change begins early in services (S. D. Miller et al., 1997). Some clients may respond and make appreciable gains more slowly than others; as a result, the most significant portion of change will be demonstrated over the long term, but this appears to be more the exception than the norm. Research suggests that as treatment progresses, a reliable course of diminishing returns occurs with more and more effort required to obtain barely noticeable differences in improvement (Howard, Kopta, Krause, & Orlinksy, 1986).

Even though the amount of change decreases over time, as long as progress is being made, services can remain beneficial. Furthermore, if clients experience meaningful change early on, the probability of positive outcome significantly increases (Haas, Hill, Lambert, & Morrell, 2002; Percevic, Lambert, & Kordy, 2006; Whipple et al., 2003). In contrast, when clients show little or no improvement or experience a worsening of symptoms early on in treatment, they are at significant risk for negative outcome and dropout (Bertolino et al., 2013; Duncan et al., 2010; Howard et al., 1986; Howard, Moras, Brill, Martinovich, & Lutz, 1996). As an aside, lack of benefit early in services is likely to contribute to greater frustration and loss of faith in services, for both clients *and* therapists.

The previous findings underscore the importance of ROM, which will be discussed in greater detail in the next chapter. Through ROM, therapists can become more attuned to client experiences by learning what minimally needs to happen in each session or interaction, throughout the course of services, to bring about meaningful and noticeable improvement. Here are some areas to emphasize in therapy to promote growth, development, and well-being.

- Focus on meeting clients' basic needs (i.e., food, water, sleep, safety).
- Listen for and honor clients' ideas about directions for therapy/services.
- View meaningful change as attainable and problems as barriers to progress, not fixed pathology.
- View growth, development, and maturation as part of the change processes.
- Consider individual, interpersonal, and social role functioning as robust indicators of benefit of services.
- Focus on maximizing the impact of each interaction and/or session.
- Monitor change from the outset of services, recalling that change tends to occur early in services.
- In lieu of positive change, engage clients in conversations earlier rather than later to make adjustments in services.
- Emphasize possibilities for change through a future focus.
- Explore exceptions to problems and how change is already happening with clients.
- Focus on creating small changes, which can lead to bigger ones.
- Scan the lives of clients for spontaneous change and build on those changes.
- Approach assessment processes as opportunities to initiate positive change.
- Allow reentry or easy access to future services as needed.
- Use methods that positively reinforce healthy behaviors and functioning.
- Use methods that contribute to the clients' sense of self-esteem, self-efficacy, and self-mastery.

The principles described in this chapter are present across all effective therapies. Each principle is also consistent with EBP, grounded in empirical research, and aimed at enhancing human relationships, development, and well-being. But it is the collective influence of the principles that truly influences outcomes.

As we have learned, the therapeutic endeavor is reliant on therapists who maintain a philosophy characterized by an unwavering belief in client capacities, close attunement to the nuances of the therapeutic alliance, cultural awareness, an expectation of and belief in change, hope, a commitment to ROM to ensure the benefit of services, and ongoing efforts to improve individual effectiveness. To this end, the most effective therapists share a series of qualities and actions, which are evidence based and reflective of the strengths-based principles outlined in this chapter. These qualities and actions will be described next.

PUTTING THE PIECES TOGETHER: QUALITIES AND ACTIONS OF EFFECTIVE THERAPISTS

Not unlike those who pursue excellence in other disciplines and fields, the most effective psychotherapists have a passion for developing a knowledge of current research, using strategies aligned with empirical evidence, and a commitment to improving their performance. But they also share several qualities and actions specific to psychotherapy that are detailed throughout this chapter. Based on best available evidence as well as theory and policy, psychologist Bruce Wampold (2014) has compiled a list that serves as a guide for therapists committed to excellence (see Anderson, Ogles, Patterson, Lambert, & Vermeersch, 2009; APA Presidential Task Force on Evidence-Based Practice, 2006; Baldwin et al., 2007; Duncan et al., 2010; Lambert, Harmon, Slade, Whipple, & Hawkins, 2005; Norcross, 2011; Wampold, 2007). According to Wampold (2014), effective therapists:

1. Have a sophisticated set of interpersonal skills that includes verbal fluency, perceptiveness, expressiveness, warmth and acceptance, and empathy. Therapists are able to focus attention on clients and listen for nuanced communication.

2. Have clients who feel understood, trust their therapist, and believe their therapists can help them. Therapists create these conditions in the first moments of the interaction through verbal and (importantly) nonverbal behavior. During initial contacts, clients are very sensitive to cues of acceptance, understanding, and expertise. Although these conditions are necessary throughout therapy, they are particularly critical in the initial interaction to ensure engagement in the therapeutic process.

3. Are able to form a working alliance with a broad range of clients. The working alliance involves the therapeutic bond, but also importantly agreement about the task of goals of therapy. The effective therapist

builds on the client's initial trust and belief to form this alliance and the alliance becomes solidly established early in therapy.

4. Provide acceptable and adaptive explanations for each client's particular distress. There are several considerations involved in providing explanations. First, an explanation must be consistent with the healing practice—in psychotherapy, the explanation is psychological. Second, an explanation must be acceptable and accepted by the client, a process that involves compatibility with clients' attitudes, values, culture, and worldview. Third, an explanation must be adaptive—that is, an explanation provides the means by which clients can overcome their difficulties. This induces positive expectations that clients can master what is needed to resolve difficulties. Fourth, the scientific truth of explanations is unimportant relative to client acceptance. Therapists are aware of client contexts in the development and presentation of explanations. Acceptance of the explanation leads to purposeful collaborative work.

5. Provide a treatment plan that is consistent with the explanation provided to their clients. Once a client accepts the explanation, the treatment plan will make sense and client compliance will be increased. The treatment plan must involve healthy actions—effective therapists facilitate clients to do something that is in their best interest. Different treatment approaches involve different actions, but the commonality is that all such actions are psychologically healthy.

6. Are influential, persuasive, and convincing. Effective therapists present explanations and treatment plans in ways that convince clients that such explanations are correct and that compliance with the treatment will benefit clients. This process leads to client hopefulness, increased expectancy for mastery, and enactment of healthy actions. These characteristics are essential for forming a strong working alliance.

7. Continuously monitor client progress in an authentic way. This monitoring may involve the use of instruments or scales or checking in with the patient regularly. Authenticity refers to communication to clients that therapists truly want to know how clients are doing. Administration of scales—for instance, without a discussion with clients—is insufficient; effective therapists will integrate progress evidence into treatment. Therapists are particularly attentive to evidence that their clients are deteriorating.

8. Are flexible and will adjust therapy if resistance to the treatment is apparent or clients are not making adequate progress. Although effective therapists are persuasive, clients may not accept the explanations and/or treatments or may not be making adequate progress given the nature of the problem. Therapists are aware of verbal and nonverbal cues that clients may be resistant to explanation or treatments, and use the evidence gleaned from assessing therapeutic progress with outcome instruments. Effective therapists take in new information, test hypotheses about their

clients, and are willing to be wrong. Adjustments might involve subtle differences in the manner in which a treatment is presented, use of a different theoretical approach, referral to another therapist, or use of adjunctive services.

9. Do not avoid difficult material in therapy and use such difficulties therapeutically. It is not unusual that clients will avoid material that is difficult. Effective therapists can infer when such avoidance is taking place and does not collude to avoid the material; rather, therapists will facilitate a discussion of the difficult material and in therapy will address core client problems. Such discussions are typically emotional and thus effective therapists are comfortable with interactions with strong affect. When the difficult material involves the relationship between therapists and clients, effective therapists address the interpersonal process in a therapeutic way.

10. Communicate hope and optimism. This communication is relatively easy for motivated clients who are making adequate therapeutic progress. However, those with severe and/or chronic problems typically experience relapses, lack of consistent progress, or other difficulties. Effective therapists acknowledge these issues but continue to communicate hope that the client will achieve realistic goals in the long run. This communication is not Pollyannaish optimism, but rather a firm belief that together therapists and clients will work successfully. This hopefulness is about both clients' and therapists' capabilities. In addition, effective therapists mobilize client strengths and resources to facilitate their abilities to solve their problems. Moreover, effective therapists emphasize client attributions—that it is clients, through their work, who are responsible for therapeutic progress, creating a sense of mastery.

11. Are aware of clients' characteristics and context. Client characteristics refer to the culture, race, ethnicity, spirituality, sexual orientation, age, physical health, motivation for change, and so forth. Context involves available resources, family and support networks, vocational status, cultural milieu, and concurrent services. Therapists work to coordinate care of clients with other psychological, psychiatric, physical, or social services. Furthermore, effective therapists are aware of how their own backgrounds, personalities, and statuses interact with those of clients, in terms of clients' reactions to therapists, therapists' reactions to clients, and to their interaction.

12. Are aware of their own psychological process and do not inject their own material into the therapy process unless such actions are deliberate and therapeutic. Effective therapists reflect on their own reactions to clients (i.e., countertransference) to determine if these reactions are reasonable given client presentations or are based on therapist issues.

13. Are aware of the best research evidence related to each particular client, in terms of treatment, problems, social context, and so forth. Particularly

important is understanding the biological, social, and psychological bases of the disorder or problem experienced by the client.

14. Seek to continually improve. Development of skill in an area involves intensive practice with model-based feedback. Feedback on the progress of clients is critical to improvement but the feedback is most useful if imbedded in a coherent model of therapy so that therapists can make specific changes and determine the outcomes produced by such changes. Evidence that clients are not making satisfactory progress is useful but knowledge that clients are not making satisfactory progress and that there is insufficient agreement about the goals of therapy provides information that therapists can use in a particular case. Moreover, therapists can use such information across clients to detect general patterns. The essential point here is that effective therapists, by definition, are therapists who achieve expected or more than expected progress with their clients, generally, and who are continually improving.

In the next chapter we take a substantial step by detailing ways that therapists can begin to put the principles described in this chapter to work through processes that facilitate client engagement.

REFERENCES

American Psychiatric Association. (2013). *Diagnostic and statistical manual for mental disorders* (5th ed.). Arlington, VA: American Psychiatric Publishing.

American Psychological Association, Presidential Task Force on Evidence-Based Practice. (2006). Evidence-based practice in psychology. *American Psychologist, 61*(4), 271–285. doi:10.1037/0003-066X.61.4.271

Anderson, T., Ogles, B. M., Patterson, C. L., Lambert, M. J., & Vermeersch, D. A. (2009). Therapist effects: Facilitative interpersonal skills as a predictor of therapist effects. *Journal of Clinical Psychology, 65*(7), 755–768. doi:10.1002/jclp.20583

Asay, T. P., & Lambert, M. J. (1999). The empirical case for the common factors in therapy: Quantitative findings. In M. A. Hubble, B. L. Duncan, & S. D. Miller (Eds.), *The heart and soul of change: What works in therapy* (pp. 33–56). Washington, DC: American Psychological Association.

Bachelor, A. (1988). How clients perceive therapist empathy: A content-analysis of received empathy. *Psychotherapy, 25*, 227–240. doi:10.1037/h0085337

Bachelor, A., & Horvath, A. (1999). The therapeutic relationship. In M. A. Hubble, B. L. Duncan, & S. D. Miller (Eds.), *The heart and soul of change: What works in therapy* (pp. 133–178). Washington, DC: American Psychological Association. doi:10.1037/11132-004

Baldwin, S. A., Wampold, B. E., & Imel, Z. E. (2007). Untangling the alliance-outcome correlation: Exploring the relative importance of therapist and patient variability in the alliance. *Journal of Consulting and Clinical Psychology, 75*(6), 842–852. doi:10.1037/0022-006X.75.6.842

Berger, P. L., & Luckmann, T. (1966). *The social construction of reality: A treatise in the sociology of knowledge*. New York, NY: Anchor Books.

Bertolino, B. (2010). *Strengths-based engagement and practice: Creating effective helping relationships*. Boston: Allyn & Bacon.

Bertolino, B. (2014). *Thriving on the front lines: Strengths-based youth care work*. New York, NY: Routledge.

Bertolino, B. (2015). *Working with children and adolescents in residential care: A strengths-based approach*. New York, NY: Routledge.

Bertolino, B., Bargmann, S., & Miller, S. D. (2013). Manual 1: What works in therapy: A primer. In B. Bertolino & S. D. Miller (Eds.), *The ICCE manuals of feedback informed treatment*. Chicago, IL: International Center for Clinical Excellence. Retrieved from https://scott-d-miller-ph-d.myshopify.com/collections/fit-manuals/products/manual-1-what-works-in-therapy-a-primer

Bertolino, B., & Miller, S. D. (Eds.). (2013). *The ICCE manuals of feedback informed treatment* (Vols. 1–6). Chicago, IL: International Center for Clinical Excellence. Retrieved from https://scott-d-miller-ph-d.myshopify.com/collections/fit-manuals

Bertolino, B., & O'Hanlon, B. (2002). *Collaborative, competency-based counseling and therapy*. Boston, MA: Allyn & Bacon.

Beutler, L. E., & Clarkin, J. (1990). *Systematic treatment selection: Toward targeted therapeutic interventions*. New York, NY: Brunner/Mazel.

Bohart, A. C. (2000). The client as active self-healer: Implications for integration. *Journal of Psychotherapy Integration, 10*(2), 127–149. doi:10.1037/11436-018

Bohart, A. C., & Tallman, K. T. (2010). Clients: The neglected common factor in psychotherapy. In B. L. Duncan, S. D. Miller, B. E. Wampold, & M. A. Hubble (Eds.), *The heart and soul of change: Delivering what works in therapy* (2nd ed., pp. 83–111). Washington, DC: American Psychological Association.

Bordin, E. S. (1979). The generalizability of the psychoanalytic concept of the working alliance. *Psychotherapy: Theory, Research, and Practice, 16*, 252–260. doi:10.1037/h0085885

Brown, L. S. (2008). *Cultural competence in trauma therapy: Beyond the flashback*. Washington, DC: American Psychological Association.

Calhoun, L. G., & Tedeschi, R. G. (2013). *Posttraumatic growth in clinical practice*. New York, NY: Routledge.

Castonguay, L. G., & Beutler, L. E. (2006). Common and unique principles of therapeutic change: What do we know and what do we need to know? In L. G. Castonguay & L. E. Beutler (Eds.), *Principles of therapeutic change that work* (pp. 353–369). New York, NY: Oxford University Press. doi:10.1093/med:psych/9780195156843.003.0018

Chambless, D. L., & Crits-Christoph, P. (2006). The treatment method. In J. C. Norcross, L. E. Beutler, & R. F. Levant (Eds.), *Evidence-based practices in mental health* (pp. 191–200). Washington, DC: American Psychological Association.

Chambless, D. L., & Hollon, S. D. (1998). Defining empirically supported therapies. *Journal of Consulting and Clinical Psychology, 66*, 7–18. doi:10.1037/0022-006X.66.1.7

Crits-Christoph, P., & Mintz, J. (1991). Implications of therapist effects for the design and analysis of comparative studies of psychotherapies. *Journal of Consulting and Clinical Psychology, 59*(1), 20–26.

Dew, S. E., & Bickman, L. (2005). Client expectancies about therapy. *Mental Health Services Research, 7*(1), 22–33. doi:10.1007/s11020-005-1963-5

Duncan, B. L., Hubble, M. A., & Miller, S. D. (1997). Stepping off the throne. *Family Therapy Networker, 21*(4), 22–31, 33.

Duncan, B. L., Miller, S. D., Wampold, B. E., & Hubble, M.A. (Eds.). (2010). *The heart and soul of change: Delivering what works in therapy* (2nd ed.). Washington, DC: American Psychological Association.

Erickson, M. H. (1954). Special techniques of brief hypnotherapy. *Journal of Clinical and Experiential Hypnosis, 2*, 109–129. doi:10.1080/00207145408409943

Frank, J. D. (1961). *Persuasion and healing: A comparative study of psychotherapy*. Baltimore, MD: Johns Hopkins Press.

Frank, J. D. (1968). The influence of patients' and therapists' expectations on the outcome of psychotherapy. *British Journal of Medical Psychology, 41*(4), 349–356. doi:10.1111/j.2044-8341.1968.tb02043.x

Frank, J. D., & Frank, J. B. (1991). *Persuasion and healing: A comparative study of psychotherapy* (3rd ed.). Baltimore, MD: Johns Hopkins Press.

Freud, S. (1953). *Some general remarks on the nature of hysterical attacks: Vol. 7. Collected papers* (pp. 257–268). London, UK: Hogarth Press. (Original work published 1909)

Gawande, A. (2007). *Better: A surgeon's notes on performance*. New York, NY: Henry Holt and Company. ISBN: 9780312427658

Gladwell, M. (2013). *David and Goliath: Underdogs, misfits, and the art of battling giants*. New York, NY: Little, Brown and Company.

Goldfried, M. R., & Padawer, W. (1982). Current status and future directions in psychotherapy. In M. R. Goldfried (Ed.), *Converging themes in psychotherapy: Trends in psychodynamic, humanistic, and behavioral practice* (pp. 3–49). New York, NY: Springer Publishing.

Goldner, V. (1985). Feminism and family therapy. *Family Process, 24*(1), 31–47. doi:10.1111/j.1545-5300.1985.00031.x

Goldstein, A. P. (1962). Participant expectancies in psychotherapy. *Psychiatry, 25*(1), 72–79.

Grencavage, L. M., & Norcross, J. C. (1990). Where are the commonalities among the therapeutic common factors? *Professional Psychology: Research and Practice, 21*(5), 372–378. doi:10.1037/0735-7028.21.5.372

Gurin, J. (1990, March). Remaking lives. *American Health*, 50–52.

Haas, E., Hill, R. D., Lambert, M. J., & Morrell, B. (2002). Do early responders to psychotherapy maintain treatment gains? *Journal of Clinical Psychology, 58*(9), 1157–1172. doi:10.1002/jclp.10044

Hays, P. A. (2007). *Addressing cultural complexities in practice: Assessment diagnosis and therapy* (2nd ed.). Washington, DC: American Psychological Association.

Heine, R. W. (1953). A comparison of patients' reports on psychotherapeutic experience with psychoanalytic, nondirective and Adlerian therapists. *American Journal of Psychotherapy, 7*, 16–23.

Hoch, P. (1955). Aims and limitations of psychotherapy. *American Journal of Psychiatry, 112*, 321–327. doi:10.1176/ajp.112.5.321

Horvath, A. O., & Bedi, R. P. (2002). The alliance. In J. C. Norcross (Ed.), *Psychotherapy relationships that work: Therapist contributions and responsiveness to patient needs* (pp. 37–69). New York, NY: Oxford University Press.

Horvath, A. O., & Luborsky, L. (1993). The role of the therapeutic alliance in psychotherapy. *Journal of Consulting and Clinical Psychology, 61*(4), 561–573. doi:10.1037/0022-006X.61.4.561

Horvath, A. O., & Symonds, B. D. (1991). Relation between working alliance and outcome in psychotherapy: A meta-analysis. *Journal of Consulting and Clinical Psychology, 38*(2), 139–149. doi:10.1037/0022-0167.38.2.139

Howard, K. I., Kopta, S. M., Krause, M. S., & Orlinsky, D. E. (1986). The dose-effect relationship in psychotherapy. *American Psychologist, 41*(2), 159–164. doi:10.1037/0003-066X.41.2.159

Howard, K. I., Moras, K., Brill, P. L., Martinovich, Z., & Lutz, W. (1996). Evaluation of psychotherapy: Efficacy, effectiveness, and patient progress. *American Psychologist, 51*(10), 1059–1064. doi:10.1037/0003-066X.51.10.1059

Hoyt, M. F. (Ed.). (1994). *Constructive therapies.* New York, NY: Guilford Press.

Hoyt, M. F. (Ed.). (1996). *Constructive therapies 2.* New York, NY: Guilford Press.

Hoyt, M. F. (Ed.). (1998). *The handbook of constructive therapies: Innovative approaches from leading practitioners.* San Francisco, CA: Jossey-Bass.

Hubble, M. A., Duncan, B. L., & Miller, S. D. (1999). *The heart and soul of change: What works in therapy?* Washington, DC: American Psychological Association.

Kuhn, T. S. (1962). *The structure of scientific revolutions.* Chicago, IL: University of Chicago Press.

Lambert, M. J. (1992). Implications of outcome research for psychotherapy integration. In J. C. Norcross & M. R. Goldfried (Eds.), *Handbook of psychotherapy integration* (pp. 94–129). New York, NY: Basic Books.

Lambert, M. J. (2005). Early response in psychotherapy: Further evidence for the importance of common factors rather than "placebo effects." *Journal of Clinical Psychology, 61*(7), 855–869. doi:10.1002/jclp.20130

Lambert, M. J., & Bergin, A. E. (1994). The effectiveness of psychotherapy. In A. E. Bergin & S. L. Garfield (Eds.), *Handbook of psychotherapy and behavior change* (4th ed., pp. 143–189). New York, NY: Wiley.

Lambert, M. J., Harmon, C., Slade, K., Whipple, J. L., & Hawkins, E. J. (2005). Providing feedback to psychotherapists on their patients' progress: Clinical results and practice suggestions. *Journal of Clinical Psychology: In Session, 61*(2), 165–174. doi:10.1002/jclp.20113

Laska, K. M., Gurman, A. S., & Wampold, B. E. (2014). Expanding the lens of evidence-based practice in psychotherapy: A common factors perspective. *Psychotherapy, 51*(4), 467–481. doi:10.1037/a0034332

Luebbe, A. M., Radcliffe, A. M., Callands, T. A., Green, D., & Thorn, B. E. (2007). Evidence-based practice in psychology: Perceptions of graduate students in scientist practitioner programs. *Journal of Clinical Psychology, 63*, 643–655. doi:10.1002/jclp.20379

Madsen, W. C. (2007). *Collaborative therapy with multi-stressed families* (2nd ed.). New York, NY: Guilford Press.

Maturana, H. R. (1978). Biology of language: Epistemology of reality. In G. Miller & E. Leneberg (Eds.), *Psychology and biology of language and thought* (pp. 27–63). New York, NY: Academic Press.

McKay, K. M., Imel, Z. E., & Wampold, B. E. (2006). Psychiatrist effects in the psychopharmacological treatment of depression. *Journal of Affective Disorders, 16*, 236–242. doi:10.1016/j.jad.2006.01.020

Miller, S. D., Duncan, B. L., & Hubble, M. A. (1997). *Escape from Babel: Toward a unifying language for psychotherapy practice.* New York, NY: W. W. Norton.

Miller, W. R., & Rollnick, S. (2013). *Motivational interviewing: Helping people to change* (3rd ed.). New York, NY: Guilford Press.

Mueller, M., & Pekarik, G. (2000). Treatment duration prediction: Client accuracy and its relationship to dropout, outcome, and satisfaction. *Psychotherapy: Theory, Research, Practice, Training, 37*(2), 117–123. doi:10.1037/h0087701

Norcross, J. C. (Ed.). (2011). *Psychotherapy relationships that work: Evidence-based responsiveness* (2nd ed.). New York, NY: Oxford University Press.

Orlinsky, D. E., Grawe, K., & Parks, B. K. (1994). Process and outcome in psychotherapy—Noch einmal. In A. E. Bergin & S. L. Garfield (Eds.), *Handbook of psychotherapy and behavior change* (4th ed., pp. 270–378). New York, NY: Wiley.

Orlinsky, D. E., & Howard, K. I. (1986). Process and outcome in psychotherapy. In S. L. Garfield & A. E. Bergin (Eds.), *Handbook of psychotherapy and behavior change* (3rd ed., pp. 311–381). New York, NY: Wiley.

Orlinsky, D. E., Rønnestad, M. H., & Willutzki, U. (2004). Fifty years of process-outcome research: Continuity and change. In M. J. Lambert (Ed.), *Bergin and Garfield's handbook of psychotherapy and behavior change* (5th ed., pp. 307–390). Hoboken, NJ: Wiley.

Percevic, R., Lambert, M. J., & Kordy, H. (2006). What is the predictive value of responses to psychotherapy for its future course? Empirical explorations and consequences for outcome monitoring. *Psychotherapy Research, 16*(3), 364–373. doi:10.1080/10503300500485524

Prescott, D. S. (2017). Feedback-informed treatment: An overview of the basics and core competencies. In D. S. Prescott, C. L. Maeschalck, & S. D. Miller (Eds.), *Feedback-informed treatment in clinical practice: Reaching for excellence* (pp. 37–52). Washington, DC: American Psychological Association.

Prochaska, J. O., & DiClemente, C. C. (1985). Common processes of change in smoking, weight control, and psychological distress. In S. Shiftman & T. Wills (Eds.), *Coping and substance abuse* (pp. 345–363). San Diego, CA: Academic Press.

Prochaska, J. O., DiClemente, C. C., & Norcross, J. C. (1992). In search of how people change: Applications to addictive behaviors. *American Psychologist, 47*(9), 1102–1114. doi:10.1037/0003-066X.47.9.1102

Prochaska, J. O., Norcross, J. C., & DiClemente, C. C. (1994). *Changing for good: The revolutionary program that explains the six stages of change and teaches you how to free yourself from bad habits*. New York, NY: Morrow.

Rapp, C. A., & Goscha, R. J. (2012). *The strengths-model: A recovery-oriented approach to mental health* (3rd ed.). New York, NY: Oxford University Press.

Rogers, C. R. (1957). The necessary and sufficient conditions of therapeutic personality change. *Journal of Consulting Psychology, 21*(2), 95–103. doi:10.1037/h0045357

Rosenthal, D., & Frank, J. D. (1956). Psychotherapy and the placebo effect. *Psychological Bulletin, 53*(4), 294–302. doi:10.1037/h0044068

Rosenzweig, S. A. (1936). Some implicit common factors in diverse methods of psychotherapy. *American Journal of Orthopsychiatry, 6*, 412–415. doi:10.1111/j.1939-0025.1936.tb05248.x

Sackett, D. L., Rosenberg, W. M. C., Muir Gray, J. A., Haynes, R. B., & Richardson, W. S. (1996). Evidence based medicine: What it is and what it isn't: It's about integrating individual clinical expertise and the best external evidence. *BMJ, 312*(7023), 71–72. doi:10.1136/bmj.312.7023.71

Safren, S., Heimberg, R., & Juster, H. (1997). Clients' expectancies and their relationship to pretreatment symptomatology and outcome of cognitive-behavioral group treatment for social phobia. *Journal of Consulting and Clinical Psychology, 65*, 694–698. doi:10.1037/0022-006X.65.4.694

Schneider, W., & Klauer, T. (2001). Symptom level, treatment motivation, and the effects of inpatient psychotherapy. *Psychotherapy Research, 11*(2), 153–167. doi:10.1080/713663888

Schuckard, E., Miller, S. D., & Hubble, M. A. (2017). Feedback-informed treatment: Historical and empirical foundations. In D. S. Prescott, C. L. Maeschalck, & S. D. Miller (Eds.), *Feedback-informed treatment in clinical practice: Reaching for excellence* (pp. 13–35). Washington, DC: American Psychological Association.

Seidel, J. A., Miller, S. D., & Chow, D. L. (2014). Effect size calculations for the clinician: Methods and comparability. *Psychotherapy Research, 24*, 470–484. doi:10.1080/10503307.2013.840812

Seligman, M. E. P. (1995). The effectiveness of psychotherapy: The *Consumer Reports* study. *American Psychologist, 50*(12), 965–974. doi:10.1037//0003-066X.50.12.965

Seligman, M. E. P. (2011). *Flourish: A visionary new understanding of happiness and well-being*. New York, NY: The Free Press.

Seligman, M. E. P., & Csikszentmihalyi, M. (2000). Positive psychology: An introduction. *American Psychologist, 55*(1), 5–14. doi:10.1037/0003-066X.55.1.5

Sparks, J., Duncan, B., & Miller, S. D. (2008). Common factors in psychotherapy. In J. Lebow (Ed.), *Twenty-first century psychotherapies: Contemporary approaches to theory and practice* (pp. 453–497). Hoboken, NJ: Wiley.

Sprenkle, D., & Blow, A. (2004). Common factors and our sacred models. *Journal of Marital and Family Therapy, 30*, 113–129.

Steering Committee. (2001). Empirically supported therapy relationships: Conclusions and recommendations of the Division 29 Task Force. *Psychotherapy, 38*(4), 495–497. doi:10.1037/0033-3204.38.4.495

Substance Abuse and Mental Health Services Administration. (2016, January 6). Evidence-based practices web guide. Retrieved from https://www.samhsa.gov/ebp-web-guide

Sue, D. W., Arredondo, P., & McDavis, R. J. (1992). Multicultural counseling competencies and standards: A call to the profession. *Journal of Counseling and Development, 70*(4), 477–486. doi:10.1002/j.1556-6676.1992.tb01642.x

Tedeschi, R. G., Park, C. L., & Calhoun, L. G. (1998). *Posttraumatic growth: Positive transformations in the aftermath of crisis.* Mahwah, NJ: Lawrence Erlbaum.

Truax, C. B., & Carkhuff, R. R. (1967). *Toward effective counseling and psychotherapy.* Chicago, IL: Aldine.

Vesely, A. (Director). (2014). *Wizard of the desert: An Alex Vesely film* [Motion picture]. United States: Noetic Films.

Wampold, B. E. (2001). *The great psychotherapy debate: Models, methods, and findings.* Mahwah, NJ: Lawrence Erlbaum.

Wampold, B. E. (2007). Psychotherapy: The humanistic (and effective) treatment. *American Psychologist, 62*(8), 857–873. doi:10.1037/0003-066X.62.8.857

Wampold, B. E. (2014). Qualities and actions of effective therapists. Continuing Education in Psychology. American Psychological Association. Retrieved from https://www.apa.org/education/ce/effective-therapists.pdf

Wampold, B. E. (2015). How important are the common factors in psychotherapy? An update. *World Psychiatry, 14,* 270–277. doi:10.1002/wps.20238

Wampold, B. E., & Brown, G. S. (2005). Estimating variability in outcomes attributable to therapists: A naturalistic study of outcomes in managed care. *Journal of Consulting and Clinical Psychology, 73*(5), 914–923. doi:10.1037/0022-006X.73.5.914

Wampold, B. E., & Imel, Z. E. (2015). *The great psychotherapy debate: The evidence for what makes therapy work* (2nd ed.). New York, NY: Routledge.

Watson, G. (1940). Areas of agreement in psychotherapy: Section meeting, 1940. *American Journal of Orthopsychiatry, 10,* 698–709. doi:10.1111/j.1939-0025.1940.tb05736

Whipple, J. L., Lambert, M. J., Vermeersch, D. A., Smart, D. W., Nielsen, S. L., & Hawkins, E. J. (2003). Improving the effects of psychotherapy: The use of early identification of treatment and problem-solving strategies in routine practice. *Journal of Counseling Psychology, 50*(1), 59–68. doi:10.1037/0022-0167.50.1.59

CHAPTER 3

Early Client Engagement

Chapters 1 and 2 provided a foundation for effective practice through exploration of current findings related to the effectiveness of psychotherapy, evidence-based practice, foundational principles and strategies that underscore effective practice, what it means to be strengths based, and qualities and actions of effective therapists. In this chapter, we begin to more actively translate research into practice. To do so, we will learn about ways to effectively engage clients, starting with initial contacts that extend throughout the course of therapy.

THE ALLIANCE–OUTCOME CORRELATION

The best *process* predictor of outcome is the quality of the client's participation in therapy (Orlinsky, Rønnestad, & Willutzki, 2004). By process, we mean that the alliance is not static; it is highly malleable and subject to sudden change. A responsibility of the therapist is to continuously monitor the client–therapist alliance, checking in regularly, and being responsive to client feedback. To this end, better alliances yield better outcomes. In fact, in an extraordinary study by Baldwin, Wampold, and Imel (2007), the researchers determined that 97% of the variance in outcome was due to therapists' ability to form a good alliance with clients. In another study, researchers found that therapists' ability to handle difficult interpersonal encounters predicted therapists' success in terms of outcomes (Anderson, Ogles, Patterson, Lambert, & Vermeersch, 2009). Research makes it clear that therapist development is contingent on finding ways to assist therapists to better connect with their clients, particularly those clients that therapists find most challenging. Failure to develop strong alliances leads to higher dropout and negative outcomes in therapy.

A FEW WORDS ABOUT WORDS: STRENGTHS-BASED LANGUAGE AND CONVERSATIONS

The role of language will be continuous throughout this book. This is because the primary way that therapists can effect change is through language and interaction. Although there is no evidence that a pathology focus facilitates positive change or improves outcomes, a nomenclature that emphasizes client deficiency, lack of motivation, and the absence of ability remains. As described in Chapter 1, therapists who adopt a language that is situated on deficit and pathology typically have personal philosophies rooted in corresponding beliefs that clients are both damaged and incapable. Such a focus can have far-reaching implications. In addition to the potential of disrespect toward clients, emphasis on pathology can leave a wake of negative aftereffects that can follow clients for years to come. For example, clients can be stigmatized and viewed as "incompetent," "unmotivated," and "impossible." But studies suggest that language has an even far greater impact on well-being and physical health than expected. Although there is a long-established correlation between optimism and health (Boehm & Kubzansky, 2012), recent studies by the University of Pennsylvania have demonstrated a link between language used on social media (Facebook, Twitter, etc.) and heart disease (Eichstaedt, Schwartz, Kern, Labarthe, et al., 2015; Eichstaedt, Schwartz, Kern, Park, et al., 2015). Eichstaedt and colleagues (Eichstaedt, Schwartz, Kern, Labarthe, et al., 2015; Eichstaedt, Schwartz, Kern, Park, et al., 2015) found that expressions of negative emotions such as anger, stress, and fatigue in tweets were associated with higher risk of heart disease.

In contrast, Eichstaedt et al. (Eichstaedt, Schwartz, Kern, Labarthe, et al., 2015; Eichstaedt, Schwartz, Kern, Park, et al., 2015) also found that positive emotions like excitement and optimism were associated with lower risk of heart disease. Ireland, Schwartz, Chen, Ungar, and Albarracin (2015) studied the prevalence of HIV and learned that sexually transmitted infection rates and references to risky behavior on Twitter were associated with a higher prevalence of HIV in all counties except those with high rates of future orientation. Data-driven analyses likewise showed that words and phrases referencing the future (e.g., tomorrow, would be) correlated with a lower prevalence of HIV. Said differently, future-oriented messages also appeared to buffer health risk.

Similarly, the language of optimism and competence positively affects client experiences in therapy, strengthens the alliance, and increases the likelihood of success. These benefits are elevated through language that not only builds on client capacities, but also invites collaboration with clients and instills hope. In this section, we explore ways that language can advance conversations, assist with communicating respect, identify what is working, and create opportunities for future change. How therapists use language will not only influence their effectiveness but strengthen their alliances with clients. A starting point then is for therapists to trade in vocabularies that are jargon filled, potentially disrespectful, and can inhibit change for a strengths-based vocabulary that emphasizes human

TABLE 3.1

PATHOLOGY- AND STRENGTHS-BASED VOCABULARIES

Pathology-Based		Strengths-Based
Fix	→	Empower
Weakness	→	Strength
Limitation	→	Possibility
Pathology	→	Health
Problem	→	Solution
Insist	→	Invite
Closed	→	Open
Shrink	→	Expand
Defense	→	Access
Expert	→	Partner
Control	→	Nurture
Backward	→	Forward
Manipulate	→	Collaborate
Fear	→	Hope
Cure	→	Growth
Stuck	→	Change
Missing	→	Latent
Resist	→	Utilize
Past	→	Future
Hierarchical	→	Horizontal
Diagnose	→	Appreciate
Treat	→	Facilitate
End	→	Beginning
Judge	→	Respect
Never	→	Not yet
Limit	→	Expand
Defect	→	Asset
Rule	→	Exception

potential and possibility (Bertolino, 2014). Table 3.1 provides illustrations of both pathology and strengths-based vocabularies.

Mindfulness of the influence of language on therapy is a first step. A next step is to begin to use language in ways that facilitate change. Strengths-based words provide a way to do this by highlighting competencies, descriptions of behavior, and ways to construct collaborative conversations. Table 3.2 further illustrates the differences between traditional, pathology-based conversations and collaborative, strengths-based conversations.

When we introduce new and respectful ways of talking with and about clients, we enhance those factors that account most for positive outcomes.

TABLE 3.2

CONTRASTS IN PATHOLOGY- AND STRENGTHS-BASED CONVERSATIONS

Pathology-Based Conversations	Strengths-Based Conversations
Conversations for explanations	Conversations for change/difference
■ Searching for evidence of functions for problems	■ Highlighting changes that have occurred in clients' problem situations
■ Searching for or encouraging searches for causes and giving or supporting messages about determinism (biological/developmental/psychological)	■ Presuming change will and is happening
	■ Searching for descriptions of differences in the problem situation
■ Focusing or allowing a focus on history as the most relevant part of the client's life	■ Introducing new distinctions or highlighting distinctions with clients
	Conversations for competence/abilities
■ Engaging in conversations for determining diagnosis, categorization, and characterization	■ Presuming clients' competence/ability
	■ Searching for contexts of competence away from the problem situation
■ Supporting or encouraging conversations for identifying pathology	■ Eliciting descriptions of exceptions to the problem or times when clients dealt with the problem situation in a way they liked
Conversations for inability	
■ Searching predominantly or exclusively for what clients cannot do and lack in terms of skill or ability	Conversations for possibilities
Conversations for insight/understanding	■ Focusing the conversation on the possibilities of the future/goals/visions
■ Focusing primarily or exclusively on insight	■ Introducing new possibilities for doing/viewing into the problem situation
Conversations for expressions of emotion	Conversations for goals/results
■ Focusing primarily or exclusively on elicitation of clients' expressions of feelings and on feelings	■ Focusing on how clients or supportive others will know that they've achieved their therapeutic goals
Conversations for blame and recrimination	Conversations for accountability/personal agency
■ Making attributions of bad/evil personality or bad/evil intentions	■ Holding clients or supportive others accountable for their actions
Adversarial conversations	■ Presuming actions derive from clients' intentions/selves
■ Believing that clients and/or supportive others have hidden agendas that keep them from cooperating with treatment goals/methods	Conversations for actions/description
	■ Channeling the conversation about the problem situation into action descriptions
■ Using trickery/deceit to get clients to change	■ Changing characterizational/theoretical talk into descriptive words
■ Believing that other professional staff are experts and clients and caregivers or supportive others are nonexperts	■ Focusing on actions clients or supportive others can take that make a difference in the problem situation

Collaborative, strengths-based language also increases therapist creativity. This is because, as discussed in the opening chapter, clients and therapists alike are operating from a growth mindset (Dweck, 2006). To test this, write down as many options as you can think of for working with a client who has been labeled as "oppositional," "argumentative," and "manipulative." Next, write down as many options as you can for working with a client who is described as "energetic," "openly expresses self," and "independent." What becomes clear is the way we use language dramatically influences options for helping clients. Therapists can use language that either closes down or opens up possibilities. Table 3.3 provides examples of ways that we can use solution-talk to reframe common concerns that are typically described through problem-talk and in pathological terms.

As we progress in this volume, we will consider various ways in which language can be used as a vehicle for change. It should be stated that the use of strengths-based language does not in any way remove or preclude clients from being responsible for their actions. In fact, it can be argued that language, when used effectively, can be used to invite accountability. This is because clients tend to experience therapists as allies in the change process. In the next section, we will explore four specific ways of using language to invite clients into collaborative relationships and ultimately strengthen the alliance.

TABLE 3.3

PROBLEM-TALK VERSUS SOLUTION-TALK

Problem-Talk	Solution-Talk
Hyperactive	Very energetic at times
Attention deficit disorder	Short attention span sometimes
Bipolar	Has significant ups and downs
Anger problem	Gets upset sometimes
Depressed	Sad
Oppositional	Argues a point often
Rebellious	Developing his/her own way
Codependent	People are important to him/her
Disruptive	Often forgets the rules in class
Family problems	Worries about his or her own life
Dissociative	Protects self emotionally when feeling unsafe
Shy	Takes a little time to know people
Negative peer pressure	People try to influence him/her
Isolating	Likes being by himself/herself

STRENGTHENING THE ALLIANCE THROUGH COLLABORATION KEYS

There are numerous ways to establish and strengthen the alliance between the therapist and the client. However, some efforts are more critical than others, particularly in early encounters. Given the high rates of client dropout, we want to do our best to effectively engage clients from the outset. Shortly we will learn that there is some evidence that relationships that have some "fits and starts" (i.e., small issues between clients and therapists) but improve over time have better outcomes. However, we do not want to leave the solidarity of our relationships with clients up to chance. Instead, we want to actively engage clients from the outset and over the course of therapy. To do this, we can employ five "collaboration keys" (Bertolino, 2010, 2014; Bertolino & O'Hanlon, 2002).

In addition to early engagement of clients, a further purpose of the collaboration keys is to increase transparency. The more clients understand therapy processes, the more comfortable they are likely to be with the therapist and how he or she works. Because better alliances yield better outcomes, we want to consider any factors that may interfere with clients' experiences in therapy, particularly early on, and take corrective actions as needed. Doing so requires putting thought into details of how we practice. As with the principles of a strengths-based perspective, the collaboration keys are interrelated. While they will be discussed as independent entities, therapists aim to maximize their collective influence. Lastly, the order of the collaboration keys in practice is something for each therapist to determine through thought, action, and reflection (TAR; Bertolino & Miller, 2013).

Collaboration Key 1: Orient Clients to Information-Gathering Processes

In healthcare and behavioral healthcare, information is being gathered at a historic rate. For some clinicians, as much as 60% of their time is spent gathering information and filling out forms. It is understood that given the safety and well-being of clients, information is critical in behavioral health services. And yet it is also clear that much of the information collected has little or no bearing on services. Therapists therefore face the challenge of determining what kind of information to gather and how that information will impact the direction of services.

Information gathering is a multifaceted process of collecting data either by phone, via web services, or through in-person contacts and can involve standardized instruments (e.g., assessments, inventories, surveys), service plans, authorization forms, and other forms of data collection. Information gathering may occur on a one-time basis, periodically, or as in the case of routine outcome monitoring (ROM; see Collaboration Key 2), in each therapeutic encounter.

To be purposeful and deliberate, we want to ensure the majority of the information gathered is useful, with an understanding that some information will be non–service-related but necessary to meet funding, accreditation, or licensing requirements. We also want to know: Is the documentation feasible from the client's point of view? That is, is it overly-lengthy? Easily understandable? Redundant? One way to remain client-focused is through a periodic review of procedures—in this case, those pertaining to forms. Doing so not only helps to streamline (i.e., remove, update, shorten) paperwork but also helps to avoid redundancy with information collected, which can reduce the amount of time spent filling out forms and/or have clients repeat themselves.

Streamlining documentation is particularly important given that many clients begin therapy in a state of distress. Extensive paperwork can prolong client suffering and dampen expectations of therapy. Formal review of information-gathering processes can also help with identification of inefficiencies that can lead to more and perhaps unnecessary work and user error. Periodic quality reviews provide a way to monitor what documentation is used, how it is presented to clients, and how data are stored.

Some documentation forms will need to be completed before services can begin. Others can be completed as services progress. Therapists can begin to build good alliances by being mindful of clients' experiences with forms and information gathering. This can be done by preparing clients ahead of time by having forms available for completion online, by sending a packet with forms to be completed prior to the start of services, and/or by asking clients to come to their first appointments a few minutes early to complete necessary documentation. Doing so can reduce the amount of time spent in sessions on forms.

Another process that can help to prepare clients for information gathering is acknowledging that filling out forms is necessary but that efforts have been made to make the process as simple as possible. This can be done by saying to the client:

> (If completing forms in a waiting room prior to or during the opening moments of a session) As you have probably experienced in other settings, we have some forms to complete before we talk about what brought you in today. I/We have made the process as straightforward as possible, understanding that you have things on your mind that you'd like to get to. I'm going to go over each of the forms, but if I move too quickly please let me know. I'll be happy to explain things better. If you need to pause or take a break, please do so. Is that okay?

Another consideration when introducing forms such as assessments, questionnaires, and surveys is to normalize the process so clients understand that the information they are giving is going to be used as part of the therapy. Here's one way to do this:

> The questions on the forms are ones that I/we ask of everyone. The information you provide will help me/us to understand more about you. Some questions are to the point and for more informational purposes. But we also want to know about things that you have gone through or experienced, how things are going with you including what you're concerned about and how that's affected you, what you'd like to see change, what has and hasn't worked for you in trying to manage your

concerns, and how we can be of help to you. And as you complete the forms, if you need a break please take one. If you feel like we've missed something, please be sure to let me/us know. And if you'd prefer to tell me/us about something rather than write about it, that's okay. We want to make sure that we fully understand what you need and how we can best help you. How does that sound?

In some settings, the paperwork is minimal and it may not be necessary to say as much to clients. However, it is always good practice to acknowledge the purpose of information gathering. Always listen first, which is how good alliances are formed. If more information is needed, try to wait until the end of the visit, then review the paperwork, fill in missing data, and complete any remaining forms.

Similarly, it is also good practice to advise clients that further information, either in written or verbal form, may be requested as therapy progresses. This may seem obvious given that therapy involves conversation; however, therapy can look dramatically different depending on the therapist's approach, the office staff's demeanor, and/or the client's disposition. Clients will be far more patient and flexible when therapists exercise transparency.

Collaboration Key 2: Introduce Routine Outcome Monitoring

A cornerstone of evidence-based practice and a strengths-based perspective is the use of ROM. The benefits of ROM are extensive, with studies indicating that its use increases the effect size of services, decreases deterioration and dropout rates, and reduces psychiatric hospitalizations and costs of care (Bertolino, Bargmann, & Miller, 2013). More importantly, ROM creates a culture of feedback that helps therapists to learn about clients' perceptions and the impact of services to make adjustments in real time.

Recall the story of Cincinnati Children's Hospital (CCH) in Chapter 1. CCH monitored its outcomes in patients with cystic fibrosis (CF) and compared those outcomes with other treatment programs. As a result, CCH learned that its outcomes were average in terms of life expectancy and in the lower quartile when it came to lung functioning, the most critical variable in life expectancy in patients with CF (Gawande, 2004). With specific, as opposed to general, outcome data on its patients, CCH narrowed its focus to these factors, including lung functioning, that were most highly correlated with treatment outcomes. This narrowing of focus is in accordance with the 80/20 rule of the Pareto principle, named after Italian economist Vilfredo Pareto (see Juan & De Feo, 2010). The 80/20 rule suggests that 80% of the results or value comes from 20% of the source or focus. In behavioral health, best available research indicates that ROM is part of the 20% of information needed by clinicians to improve their outcomes. The 80/20 rule will be discussed in greater detail in Chapter 4.

A central part of the definition of strengths-based provided in Chapter 2 is, "ROM is used to create and maintain a culture of feedback—a responsive, consumer-driven climate to ensure the greatest benefit of services." This statement represents one of the most important developments in the fields of health and behavioral healthcare in the last 20 years. For decades, therapists have asked the public and third-party payers to continue to reimburse for services without really having data to back up the effectiveness of psychotherapy. But just as CCH has had to provide data related to its outcomes, how do we really know, beyond anecdotally, if a therapist, a program, or a service is truly effective? It is critically important that therapists make concerted efforts to more clearly delineate their outcomes and *how* those outcomes are measured.

Behavioral health studies over the past 50 years have found that a combination of a client's rating of the therapeutic alliance with the experience of meaningful change in the initial stages of services is a highly reliable predictor of eventual treatment outcome (Duncan, Miller, & Sparks, 2004). Further, best available research reveals that ROM provides a meaningful method for documenting the benefit of services. The American Pychological Association Presidential Task Force on Evidence-Based Practice (2006) concluded, "Providing clinicians with real-time patient feedback to benchmark progress in treatment" is one of the "most pressing research needs" (p. 278).

As discussed, ROM is composed of two forms of measurement: *outcome* and *alliance*. Let's take a moment to expand on the descriptions of each offered in Chapter 2. *Outcome* is comprised of three aspects of functioning: individual, interpersonal, and social role. Outcome measurement involves capturing clients' reports of the subjective benefit of services at the *beginning* of meetings (or sessions or interactions). This includes the idiosyncratic meaning attached by the client. Through ongoing monitoring of outcomes, clinicians are able to learn from clients whether and to what degree services provided are beneficial. Further, discussions about progress, lack thereof, or deterioration will be more data driven as the outcomes are graphed and monitored. It should be noted that more so than diagnosis, the severity of the client's distress at intake predicts eventual outcome. Clients with higher levels of distress are more likely to show measured benefit from treatment than those with lower levels or those who present as non-distressed (Duncan, Miller, Wampold & Hubble, 2010). Knowledge about client distress can inform decisions regarding the dose and intensity of services.

Alliance measurement involves monitoring the four components of the alliance described in Chapter 2: the client's view of the relationship (including perceptions of the provider as warm, empathic, and genuine); agreement on the goals, meaning, or purpose of the treatment; agreement on the means and methods used; and the client's preferences. Formal alliance measurement takes place at the *end* of each meeting (or session or interaction) to learn how the client experienced the conversation. However, alliance monitoring also involves periodically checking in. We want to know: Are clients feeling heard and understood? Are they satisfied with the direction of services? Do they feel the means used to achieve goals are a good fit? As meetings/sessions progress and end, therapists check with clients to learn their perceptions of interactions, again learning what worked well, what did not, and to make any necessary adjustments to accommodate their preferences.

There are numerous options in terms of choices of outcome and alliance measures, each with benefits and drawbacks. Selection and implementation of measures should be made with great care and will be discussed in the next chapter, along with details about how to effectively use ROM. At this juncture, we want to begin by making a commitment to measuring the benefit of services in a reliable and valid way. With such a commitment we introduce and explain the role of ROM to clients. Here is an example of how to do this:

Introduction

I/We are committed to helping you to have the best experience possible and achieve the results you want from our work together. To ensure these things I/we have a way of working that may be a little different than other practices/agencies. For example, I/we will check in with you periodically to get a sense of your experience. I/we will ask about what has been helpful, what has not, what is working, and what is not. This feedback will help me/us to make adjustments in our work together.

Along with checking in with you, there are two (brief) measures that can help me/us to learn from you whether our work together is benefitting you and if the way we are working together is a good fit for you. The first, _____, is completed at the start of our sessions. Research shows that if we are going to be successful in our work together, we should see signs of improvement earlier rather than later. If what we're doing works, then we'll continue. If not, then I'll/we'll try to change or modify the therapy. If things still don't improve, then I'll/we'll work with you to find an option for you to get the help you want. Does it make sense to you?

The second measure, _____, is completed near the end of our sessions and will let me/us know more about how the meeting (or session or interaction) went for you and what I/we can do differently in future sessions should you decide to continue services here. Research indicates that your experience of our work together is a good predictor of whether we'll be successful. I'm not aiming for a perfect score with this measure. Life isn't perfect, and neither am I. What I'm hoping for is feedback about even the smallest things—things that may seem unimportant—so that we can adjust our work and make sure we don't get off course. Whatever your feedback might be, I promise I won't take it personally. I'm always learning and am curious about what I can learn from getting this feedback from you that will in time help me improve my skills. How does that sound to you?

Once consent has been acquired, the therapist says:

Thank you for your openness in helping me/us learn how I/we can best help you with your concerns. I/we would like to ask that you be as open and forthcoming as you are comfortable when I/we check in and when you complete the questionnaires. I/we also welcome any feedback you might have at any point during our work together. It is important that you achieve the results you hope for and if not, we will discuss options to provide further opportunities for you to experience the outcome you desire.

"We" can be substituted in practices where there are multiple providers, when service teams are involved, and/or when clients are in concurrent services or programs.

ROM, a central component of which is real-time feedback, ultimately serves two purposes: to determine the benefit and fit of services. Based on real-time feedback, decisions about type of service or approach, dosage form (i.e., frequency and length of meetings), and/or referral can be made. Real-time feedback also provides rationale for service decisions. For example, the level of distress reported by clients can play a vital role in determining what type of service represents the best fit at that moment in time. Measuring distress increases accountability and stewardship because it informs therapists of how the client is functioning. As discussed, the use of real-time feedback can help in selecting the best available type of service and dosage form, which if provided in a timely, efficient, and cost-effective manner can help to get clients back on track with their lives (Bertolino, 2017; Chiles, Lambert, & Hatch, 1999; Kraft, Puschner, Lambert, & Kordy, 2006).

It is understood that some therapists and administrators may be skeptical about the promise of ROM. There is a long-standing belief among behavioral healthcare professionals that they "know real change" when they see it. As we learned in the first two chapters, the findings are quite the opposite. At the same time, the news is rather promising when therapists accept the challenge of demonstrating, through reliable and valid means, that therapy makes significant and lasting contributions to individuals, relationships, and society. In upcoming chapters we will continue to explore how to implement ROM in clinical practice, respond to feedback, improve our individual effectiveness as clinicians, and subsequently, achieve better outcomes.

Collaboration Key 3: Create Space

At its core, therapy is a conversation between two or more people. As Rogers (1957) stated, one person, the client, is in a state of incongruence or distress. Central to therapy, then, is creating space for the client who is in distress to detail what he or she most wants the therapist to know. The therapist's job is to establish a safe, respectful, and open context through which that can occur.

Engagement involves careful listening and attention to clients. Of the keys to collaboration, none is more essential than creating space—room for clients to share stories through their experiences, points of view, concerns, and hopes for change. For some, sharing their stories will be the most important part of services. This is because many clients have heard the voices of blame, marginalization, and negativity in previous therapy experiences.

To create space, therapists ask general questions. Examples include:

- Where would you like to start?
- What would you like to talk about?
- What is most important for me to know about you and/or your situation/concern?
- Are there certain things that you want to be sure we talk about?
- What is your understanding of therapy (or our services) and how I (or we) work with others?
- What ideas do you have about how coming to see me might be helpful?
- In what ways do you see me as helping you with your situation?
- What are your best hopes for our work together?
- What do you feel/think you need from me right now?

Therapy isn't always initiated by clients, as is the case with children and youth, or those mandated to therapy. In these instances, it remains important to ask questions such as those in the previous list. We want to invite clients to tell us about themselves and their situations—including any dissatisfaction they may have about the choice of involvement with services. The more clients are left out of conversations, the more service-oriented relationships are likely to suffer. At the same time, therapists will seek moments to explain, as needed, the purpose of services, their role, and so on.

Therapists pay especially close attention to clients' statements and responses, taking care not to dismiss their internal experience(s) by pushing for change, trying to get them to move on, being too positive, or using other methods that clients may experience as being insensitive or disrespectful. Therapists remain attuned to the inherent cultural biases that may exist toward redemptive stories. We try not to change, reframe, or invalidate clients' non-redemptive, unhappy-ending stories too quickly and without properly attending to their emotional experience. Doing so means avoiding the use of glib explanations (e.g., "I wonder what you are meant to learn from this?" or "What part of you needs or benefits from this pain?") and platitudes (e.g., "Everything will work out"; "God doesn't give you more than you can handle"; and "You are going to be all right."). The use of explanations, interpretations, and metaphors based on clinicians' personal assumptions and biases can alienate clients and close avenues to change.

Recall that one of the three key elements of evidence-based practice is client "characteristics, culture, and preferences" (American Pychological Association Presidential Task Force on Evidence-Based Practice, 2006, p. 273). Any efforts to engage clients in thoughtful understanding of their lives and situations must be done with consideration of our personal biases as helping professionals. We adopt a position of cultural curiosity by asking clients about their cultures, contributing to a cross-cultural interaction in a mutually influencing relationship (Madsen, 2007). Cultural curiosity involves elicitation, instead of assignment of meaning. Therapists evoke from clients and others the meanings they have attached to events, situations, and relationships as opposed to ascribing some professional explanation or meaning.

To prepare for engaging clients in conversations, psychologist Julie Tilsen (2013) has proposed a set of questions to consider as clinicians. These questions can help us to clarify where we stand, what we believe and think, and how we feel before stepping into relational territory. They are meant to shine light on how we position ourselves in our relationships with clients. Although Tilsen's questions were originally geared toward those who work with youth, they are relevant to all therapists and have been modified as such.

- *How do you think of yourself in relationship to clients, and clients in relationship to you?*
  This central question focuses on how we position ourselves with clients regarding cultural and ethical matters. We explore: How do we view the role of authority, professional power, and influence? What is your perspective on self-disclosure? We also reflect further on philosophical issues as to how we expect change to occur, whether we, as a therapist, think that we also learn and change as we work with others,

- *How do you think about the purpose of your relationship?*
  We clarify: What is our role in therapy? What is the role of our clients? How do we define what we are doing in our work with clients? What are the results, outcomes, and by-products of this relationship? And what are the implications—meaning and effects—of thinking this way?

- *How do you think about your relationship with external institutions of authority (e.g., licensing boards, professional guilds, third-party payers, corrections/law enforcement, social service systems, medical authorities, education systems, etc.)?*
  This question spawns others that reveal our position on external entities that may be involved with the care, oversight, and treatment of clients. Whom do you work for and account to? What authorities or institutions do you turn to for information and direction? How do you use that information? How do you feel about and use diagnosis and/or labels? How do you communicate with and share information with collateral service providers? How do you talk with clients about this process? How do we manage multiple perspectives?

- *How do you think of yourself in relationship to prevailing cultural discourses?*
  In what ways do you consider the impact of your social location on your identity as a therapist, and in relationship to the social location of clients? How do you think services are influenced by social discourses and local

politics? In what ways do you explore prevailing discourses and their effects in you, clients, and your work?

- *How do you decide to communicate (or not communicate) with clients the ways in which you view all of these relationships?*
  What are your thoughts on transparency? How is transparency different than self-disclosure? What are ethical implications of your stance on transparency? (pp. 3–4)

Learning involves ongoing reflection, which the previous questions are intended to encourage. Lack of thought about issues pertinent to relationships can contribute to relationship problems, which in turn can affect eventual outcome. In addition, because such questions draw attention to ethics and accountability, there is an increased risk of misunderstanding when these things have not been thought out. One way to reflect on these questions is by talking about them in small groups. Doing so will provide an opportunity to flesh out thoughts and feelings and to hear multiple, and often very different, points of view.

Collaboration Key 4: Address Expectations

Clients both seek and begin services with ideas shaped by multiple influences. Media (television, film, radio, magazines), social relationships, previous service experiences, and interactions with professionals all represent possible sources of information which can at best educate and at worst produce paralyzing fears. Some will express apprehension or fear, others will not. Regardless of whether services are by choice or not, it is critical that therapists invite clients to ask questions and share their thoughts in terms of expectations. This can include what might help clients to feel more comfortable, what could contribute to a positive experience, what they hope to accomplish, and any ideas as to what might help to get the services or program off to a good start. Client expectations of services can affect how services progress and the degree to which they can be beneficial (Frank & Frank, 1991). Beyond asking straightforward questions about the expectations of clients, we can strengthen the alliance through active listening, exploring beliefs, and being transparent in answering questions.

A major step is just asking for help, which can bring a host of feelings and worries to the forefront. These feelings may be intensified and contribute to a sense of being "one-down" in relation to the provider, potentially contributing to distrust and suspicion. One way to neutralize any ill feelings as well as myths about how things will unfold is to ensure that those involved are able to ask questions *prior to the start of services*—during phone calls, for example. These "pre-interviews" provide an early opportunity to answer general questions and alleviate anxiety (Bertolino, 2003).

It is worth mentioning that the word *interviewing* may seem antithetical to a collaborative stance, suggesting an asymmetrical relationship. Interviewing in this sense refers to therapists being open, flexible, and genuine. The following examples offer ideas about how to approach initial contacts:

Dialogue Example 3.1: Attending to Expectations

Caller: I'm calling about the possibility of seeing a therapist. But I really don't know if you can help me. I haven't had much success with therapy.

Therapist: I'm glad you called. I'm sorry you haven't had much success with therapy. How did you hope I might help with your situation?

Caller: I'm just not sure what you do. Do you see people like me, who are struggling?

Therapist: Yes, I do see people who are struggling. And I understand that each situation is different.

Caller: It is and I'm trying to figure out what to do. I'm not sure whether it's worth trying therapy again.

Therapist: It sounds like you're at a real point of decision. How can I help you with that decision?

Caller: I'm not sure if I have any specific questions. I'm just on the fence about it.

Therapist: It's an important decision for you. It's okay to want to just get a feel for things and sometimes it's helpful to do just what you're doing, call someone up and check them out.

Caller: That's really it. That makes me feel better.

Therapist: I'm glad to hear that.

Caller: I'd like to go ahead and make an appointment.

Therapist: I would be happy to help you with that.

[Sets appointment with client and gathers basic information]

Therapist: If between now and the time you come in you have any questions feel free to call back.

Caller: I will. Thank you.

Dialogue Example 3.2: Attending to Expectations

Therapist: We can talk in depth when you come in for your appointment, but is there anything that you'd like to know about how I work with people before then?

Caller: Now that you mention it, I've never been to therapy before and I'm a little worried that you are going to analyze me and well, tell me what's wrong with me. I mean, if that's what you do . . . but I don't think that's what I need.

Therapist: I'd like to try and understand what your hopes are for therapy and how I can best help you. We'll work together in deciding what is right for you. How does that sound?

Caller: That sounds good. It's a relief. I'm looking forward to our appointment.

Therapist: Great. See you then.

Dialogue Example 3.3: Attending to Expectations (Youth)

Caller (Youth): Yeah, my mom told me to call you. I have to see a therapist.

Therapist: Thanks for calling. So, your mom told you to call?

Youth: Yeah. I don't have a choice.

Therapist: You mean you don't have a choice about seeing a therapist?

Youth: Yeah.

Therapist: It must have taken a lot on your part to call. I admire that. How can I help you with this?

Youth: I guess . . . well, what do you do when you meet with people?

Therapist: Well, the main thing is I want each person to know that I respect him or her. I also want to take the time to make sure that I understand where each person is coming from. After that, I find out what people who choose to continue working want and how we can get that to happen.

Youth: Would you take their side?

Therapist: You mean your parents?

Youth: Yeah.

Therapist: I respect each person's opinion. Because your parents are your parents and they care about you and are responsible for you, they're going to have opinions about what is best for you. I'll support them. I'll also support you because you're entitled to your opinion. You don't have to agree with what your parents want for you, you just have to accept that that's how they see it. Do you know what I mean?

Youth: Yeah. That's cool. Well, what if I don't like therapy? Will you tell them I don't have to come any more?

Therapist: If you were to choose to see me and you found that you didn't like it, I'd certainly want to know. Knowing what's going on helps me to learn what's working and what's not and make adjustments so you feel better about coming to therapy. So, if you felt it wasn't working out, I'd want to talk about it. As far as not having to come back, I wouldn't claim to know what's best for you and your family. I can only say that I would want things to work out for all of you. If you didn't like therapy, I'd support you the same way that I would support your parents. I would help you and your family to arrive at a decision that makes sense for all of you.

Youth: Okay . . . do I have to tell you everything?

Therapist: You have to tell me only what you feel comfortable with. So that's for you to decide.

Youth: Okay, I'll give it a try.

Initial contacts are vitally important as they present an opportunity to flesh out expectations. There are situations in which initial contacts may be limited or, perhaps, not possible, but in most cases there will be room for clients to ask clarifying questions. What is clear is that the more comfortable our clients are, the more likely they are to follow through with and benefit from services.

A final area of therapy expectations is the preexisting beliefs clients have about therapy or like services. Clients' past experiences can influence the effectiveness of services rendered. Said differently, reputation matters. One way to address this issue is to directly ask clients what they know about the organization or agency, program, setting, and so on. Another is to ask about any previous experiences with services. Answers to these questions offer therapists the opportunity to dispel any myths and clarify what actually happens during service delivery. The following case example illustrates this point.

Case Example 3.1: Attending to Past Therapy Experiences

Anne, an 18-year-old female, came to see me due to problems with substance abuse. During our initial appointment she stated that she had recently seen a social worker at a local community mental health center. When I asked what her experience had been like Anne stated, "The social worker I saw was very nice. She listened really well." When I asked Anne how she knew the social worker had been listening to her she responded, "She would say 'uh huh' and nod her head." I followed, "Is that what you feel you need?" To this Anne replied, "That's not all I need. I didn't go back after a few sessions because I didn't think we were getting anywhere. I need someone to help me come up with some answers." I said, "Let me see if I follow you. Are you saying that what you need is someone who listens really well and also works with you to come up with answers?" "That's right. I need both," Anne replied. Although I had a good idea what would indicate to her that I was listening well, following her response, I spent time learning more from the young woman about how she thought I might help her in coming up with answers. Through the remainder of our time together I continued to check in with Anne to ensure that she was getting what she needed, to determine if any changes or modifications were necessary, and if the ways in which we were approaching her situation were right for her.

It is important to bear in mind that the preexisting beliefs of clients can affect the entire course of services. Clients whose experiences with a particular organization, program, or provider have been positive are more likely to be involved with and benefit from services. Conversely, negative experiences (e.g., feeling devalued, invalidated, being left out of discussions about services) can affect the degree to which clients benefit from current and future services (both within a practice/organization and with current or future outside helpers). The questions that follow can help learn about the expectations of those seeking services:

- Do you have any questions about what therapy is or is not?
- Do you have any questions about how I work with persons such as yourself?
- Do you have any questions about what I do here?
- What do you know about our program?
- Do you have any concerns about our program?
- Is there anything you would like to know about therapy or what I do here and the possible benefits or drawbacks?
- Is there anything I can do to help you feel more comfortable in starting therapy?
- (If the client has received services previously) What has been your experience with therapy in the past?
- (If the client experienced previous services as negative) What can we do differently here to ensure that things go better for you this time? (Bertolino, 2010)

Introducing other factors that may influence how clients expect services to proceed can also prove helpful. These can include, but are not limited to, intake processes, paperwork and documentation, payment processes, phone calls after hours, crises and emergencies, and referrals. Clients may have more or fewer questions about specific procedures and processes, but providing information in written form that can be followed up on during sessions is generally good practice. Informational materials should reflect the philosophy and language of the practice and include how clients will be referred to ("Clients," "Patients,"

Consumers," etc.), how therapists will be referred to (by surname, "Dr., Mr., Ms.," first name, etc.), and the general language that will be used with clients, in conversations with other professionals outside the setting, in reports and publications, and in community relations (e.g., fund-raisers and interviews).

Collaboration Key 5: Attend to Preferences

As discussed in Chapter 2, one of the four empirically supported components of the therapeutic alliance is *accommodating the client's preferences* (see Principle 3). Clients who seek services will often have preferences, making it important that therapists attend to such nuances and remain flexible in their practices. Positive change can be inhibited when a therapist's practice preferences run counter to or do not match those of clients. There are several ways of tuning into preferences. Examples include asking questions related to physical space and the setting of meetings/sessions, who should be involved with therapy, and the format of meetings/sessions (individual or joint meetings, length of meetings, etc.). The following case examples illustrate how to attend to client preferences.

Case Example 3.2: Attending to Physical Space Preferences

Mariah sought therapy after experiencing several panic attacks while out socially. Near the end of the initial phone call, she nervously inquired,

"Would it be possible to meet in a room where it isn't too loud? I don't mean just loud with sound. I mean a room where there aren't many things on the walls . . . it's not cluttered. It's quiet. Is that possible?"

"Sure," I replied.

"We have an office that has a couch and two chairs, a bookcase, and a desk, but there are very few other things in it—just one picture. I can show it to you when you come for your appointment. And if you don't find it comfortable, I have another in mind as well."

Case Example 3.3: Attending to Setting Preferences

Brian, a 15-year-old, was placed in an emergency shelter where I was a therapist. Prior to meeting with him, his mother informed me, "Therapy won't work with Brian. We've already tried it." When asked to elaborate, the mother would only say, "He hates to sit and talk. And even if he does sit down with you, he won't say anything more than 'yes' or 'no' to your questions."

Before my first meeting with Brian for therapy, I asked him if he preferred to talk inside the house or in an office, outside in the yard, or on a walk around the neighborhood. With a surprised look, Brian responded, "Can we really go outside and talk?" "Sure," I responded.

Brian and I ended up talking outside on the stairs of the emergency shelter. During that time, he expressed himself perhaps for the first time and talked about what he had been experiencing. In future meetings we shot baskets, walked down to the local waterfront, and even talked inside in an office.

Involvement in meetings can be especially sensitive for some clients. This is because in situations such as couples or family therapy one or more members may identify another as "the problem" and as a result expect such persons to be "fixed" and/or for them to be seen separately. It is imperative that therapists proceed carefully, acknowledging different perspectives while maintaining an open mind. However, therapists who attain multiple viewpoints are likely to have a more encompassing view of the concern(s) at hand. Therefore, therapists should not hesitate to firmly encourage participation, doing so in a respectful manner. The following is an example of a dialogue between a therapist and caller demonstrating how to attend to such a situation.

Dialogue Example 3.4: Attending to Preferences Around Session Attendance

Caller: My daughter is causing problems. Should I bring just her? Or should I bring the whole family? I've never done this before.

Therapist: We can approach this in different ways. Because I can never know you or your family the way you do, I'd first like to know whether you or anyone else in your family has a preference about who should come to the first session.

Caller: I know my daughter needs to come; she's the one who started all of this. But I know she'll go only if I make her because she already told me, "I don't need a shrink!"

Therapist: Okay. One possibility is to invite those you think can help with the concerns that you or your family are having. Another is to ask each person involved if he or she would like to come. You could also just make a decision yourself as to who should come in. We can always make adjustments later by including more or fewer people.

Caller: I really don't know. What do you recommend?

Therapist: From what you've described, it sounds like what's been happening with your daughter has had an effect on everyone in your family to some degree, so my inclination would be to see your whole family. This way I'll be able to hear different points of view and then we can go from there. How does that sound?

Caller: That sounds good. I'd like for both of my kids and my husband to come. But I do have another question. Can this still work even if everyone doesn't come? I mean, I don't know if my husband will come. He thinks there's a problem but he just thinks our daughter needs to change her attitude. So he may or may not be willing to come.

Therapist: There are going to be times when people might not be able to make it. Some might not be able to because of a scheduling conflict or, like your husband, may just not want to be involved. It's your call as to whether or not you push the issue or if you want me to talk with someone. Even if we start with certain people, we can always make changes in future sessions. Therapy can work without every family member being present. I'm confident that we can move toward the change you want with those who do come in.

Caller: That sounds good. I think we should start with all of us, and if my husband refuses to come, so be it. That makes the most sense to me. Let's set an appointment.

At times it can be helpful to suggest expanding sessions to include other persons (e.g., family members, friends, outside helpers). Adding people might generate more ideas that can help overcome client hurdles or impasses in services. It is important to let clients determine whether such suggestions are acceptable. In approaching these situations, therapists offer ideas about expanding the system rather than imposing them. Bertolino and O'Hanlon (2002) stated:

> The difference here is that a collaborative therapist would not hold or present the idea that this must occur or that this is the only way that positive change will take place. Instead, the therapist might suggest that bringing in another voice might offer a new perspective or lead to the generation of some new ideas. Ultimately, clients decide whether such ideas are acceptable to them and whether they are within their personal theories about how change will come about. (p. 32)

"Family" therapy can involve part of a family just as "couples" therapy can occur with just one member of a couple. Positive change is possible whether the therapist is working with an individual, one member of a couple, three members of a five-person family, or some other "nontraditional" configuration. Because client preferences, situations, and problems change, who attends therapy can change from session to session, calling for ongoing dialogue between the therapist and client to determine best procedures. By inviting clients into conversations that honor their preferences, therapists continue to strengthen the therapeutic relationship alliance. Here is a further example of how a therapist might attend to preferences around the format of a session.

Dialogue Example 3.5: Attending to Preferences About Session Format

Caller: I'm calling because I have an appointment to bring my son in tomorrow. My worry is that we tried this once before and he refused to talk.

Would it be possible for him to talk with you individually for just a few minutes? I don't think he'll talk if I'm in the room.

Therapist: Thank you for taking the time to call to let me know about your concern. Yes, I can meet with your son separately if you think that helps him to open up. I will want to check with him when you arrive tomorrow to make sure he's alright with that. I want him to know he has some choice in things too. Not necessarily about coming to therapy. That's your decision. But about our meeting arrangements. Are you okay if I ask him about it?

Caller: Sure. That's fine. I don't want him to think he's being forced into it. I just think it might help him to talk.

Therapist: That makes good sense to me. Is there anything else we ought to consider for your meeting?

Caller: No, that's it. It's a relief knowing that we can be flexible about this.

Therapist: Absolutely. If anything changes you can let us know by calling ahead of time or at the time of the meeting.

Therapists should exercise caution regarding preconceived meeting arrangements that may negatively affect the therapeutic alliance, hinder therapy, and lead to premature dropout and/or a negative outcome. Flexibility in making adjustments to meet client preferences can make large differences. Because preferences are subject to change, ongoing dialogue is necessary. The following example illustrates how a therapist can open up dialogue to determine if adjustments are in order for a first session.

Dialogue Example 3.6: Attending to First Session Preferences

Therapist: There aren't any right or wrong ways about how we work together. We could keep everyone together or I could spend some individual time with each of you, or we could do a combination of both. Whatever we decide, we can also change. Does anyone here have an opinion about how we should start?

Parent: Well, we tried meeting together in therapy and it didn't work. I think it's because we argued so much and talked over each other that we really couldn't get anywhere. So my vote is that we do something else.

Therapist: What might be a good way to start?

Parent: I think we should try meeting like this, but if we start arguing, maybe we should talk with you separately. That might be a good idea anyway—to talk to us separately once in a while.

Therapist: Okay. Who else agrees or has another idea?

(Two of the family members agree, and one does not give a verbal response.)

Therapist: Okay, so two of you agree. Luke, you didn't say anything, but I saw your shoulders drop. What do you think?

Youth: I don't care. This is stupid. I don't have anything to say anyway.

Therapist: That's fine. I just want to be sure that if you have an opinion you are able to share it. Will it be okay with you if you and I spend a few minutes together once in a while?

Youth: I guess.

In addition to the examples given, here are some questions to help in learning from clients their preferences about session attendance:

- Whom would you like to invite to the first session/meeting?
- (If a client is unsure about whom to invite or who ought to attend) I'd like to recommend that you invite the people to attend who you think will be most helpful in resolving the concern/problem.
- (If someone cannot/will not attend) For a variety of reasons, one or more persons may not be able or will not want to attend sessions/meetings. Change is constant and is possible even in very difficult situations. Having said that, I'll work with whoever is present to achieve positive change.
- I want to be sure that we explore avenues that might help to improve things with you/your situation. If it's okay with you, I'd like to offer an idea. What do you think about the idea of inviting [name(s) of person(s)] to attend a session sometime in the future?
- What conditions would make it comfortable with you to have [name(s) of person(s)] present at a meeting/session?
- (If client does not wish to include another person or expand the system) That's okay. I respect your decision not to include [name(s) of person(s)]. Will you please let me know if at any time you think bringing in another person might help move things along for you or your situation?
- (If clients have had previous experiences with social/psychological/health services) In the past, what groupings have worked best for you?
- (If a couple or family) What do you think about meeting together like this? Or: How would it be for each of you if we were to split up and I was to meet with each of you separately at times?
- Would it be okay with you if we occasionally vary who meets? For example, sometimes we might all meet together and at other times we might split up with two of you meeting with me at a time. How would that or some other variation be for you?
- Would you let me know if, at any point, you have any ideas—new or old ones—about how we should meet?

There are of course extenuating circumstances that require therapists to take more directive routes. For example, if a client uses verbally abusive statements about another and the therapist's immediate efforts do not end such behavior, it may be necessary to dismiss one or more persons from the situation. In such cases, clients may be brought back together when they agree to treat others more respectfully. Another situation would be prior knowledge of potential aggressive behavior or when meeting with certain combinations of people could increase risk of harm; in such situations, the therapist must respond accordingly. Safety and well-being are always a primary consideration.

Safety is also expressed in terms of physical space and settings within which therapy is provided. Physical space includes the design, setup, and accessibility of areas that clients and others may utilize (e.g., reception areas, hallways, stairs, ramps, elevators, waiting rooms, therapy offices, restrooms, parking). Setting also involves pictures and wall fixtures, reading materials (both leisure and educational), toys, and other physical elements that reflect respect for culture, ethnicity, and family background.

The fourth principle of a strengths-based perspective is, "Culture influences and shapes all aspects of clients' lives." The key competency within that principle is to *communicate respect for clients and their cultures*. Addressing client preferences such as the physical environment is one of the more visible ways of conveying cultural safety. It also conveys to our clients that we are listening and want them to feel safe. Although space restrictions, the timing of sessions, and so on, can provide barriers to some setting options, oftentimes acknowledging a preference and then making more subtle changes will help.

Studies suggest that setting variables, often referred to as an aspect of "site" effects, influence the variance in client outcomes (Greenberg, 1999). Said differently, attending to the preferences of clients lets them know we care. Although further research is needed to better understand how setting variables truly affect services, most of us can relate to the idea of feeling more or less comfortable in some settings versus others. Choices offer flexibility, which can strengthen the alliance, thereby increasing the likelihood of follow-through. At the same time, we want to hold those with whom we work accountable for their choices and actions (i.e., missing or being late for appointments, etc.). We maintain a flexible posture whenever possible and yet we fully expect clients to follow through with what has been agreed on.

Collectively, the five collaboration keys provide research-based means for building and strengthening the client–therapist alliance from the outset of services. They also help to build expectancy and hope, tap into client strengths, align with clients' cultures, and orient therapy toward future change. Therapists best serve their clients when they incorporate their voices and experiences throughout the course of therapy while keeping an eye on outcome.

In the next chapter, we explore processes related to gathering information and ways to use language to further encourage change. We'll also learn how to actively use ROM to measure the benefit of services.

REFERENCES

American Pychological Association Presidential Task Force on Evidence-Based Practice. (2006). Evidence-based practice in psychology. *American Psychologist, 61*(4), 271–285. doi:10.1037/0003-066X.61.4.271

Anderson, T., Ogles, B. M., Patterson, C. L., Lambert, M. J., & Vermeersch, D. A. (2009). Therapist effects: Facilitative interpersonal skills as a predictor of therapist effects. *Journal of Clinical Psychology, 65*(7), 755–768. doi:10.1002/jclp.20583

Baldwin, S. A., Wampold, B. E., & Imel, Z. E. (2007). Untangling the alliance-outcome correlation: Exploring the relative importance of therapist and patient variability in the alliance. *Journal of Consulting and Clinical Psychology, 75*(6), 842–852. doi:10.1037/0022-006X.75.6.842

Bertolino, B. (2003). *Change-oriented psychotherapy with adolescents and young adults: The next generation of respectful and effective therapeutic processes and practices.* New York, NY: W. W. Norton.

Bertolino, B. (2010). *Strengths-based engagement and practice: Creating effective helping relationships.* Boston, MA: Allyn & Bacon.

Bertolino, B. (2014). *Thriving on the front lines: Strengths-based youth care work.* New York, NY: Routledge.

Bertolino, B. (2017). Feedback-informed treatment in an agency serving children, youth, and families. In D. S. Prescott, C. L. Maeschalck, & S. D. Miller (Eds.), *Feedback-informed treatment in clinical practice: Reaching for excellence* (pp. 187–209). Washington, DC: American Psychological Association.

Bertolino, B., Bargmann, S., & Miller, S. D. (2013). Manual 1: What works in therapy: A primer. In B. Bertolino & S. D. Miller (Eds.), *The ICCE manuals of feedback informed treatment.* Chicago, IL: International Center for Clinical Excellence.

Bertolino, B., & Miller, S. D. (Eds.). (2013). *The ICCE manuals of feedback informed treatment* (Vols. 1–6). Chicago, IL: International Center for Clinical Excellence.

Bertolino, B., & O'Hanlon, B. (2002). *Collaborative, competency-based counseling and therapy.* Boston, MA: Allyn & Bacon.

Boehm, J. K., & Kubzansky, L. D. (2012). The heart's content: The association between positive psychological well-being and cardiovascular health. *Psychological Bulletin, 138*(4), 655–691. doi:10.1037/a0027448

Chiles, J., Lambert, M. J., & Hatch, A. L. (1999). The impact of psychological interventions on medical cost offset: A meta-analytic review. *Clinical Psychology, 6*(2), 204–220. doi:10.1093/clipsy.6.2.204

Duncan, B. L., Miller, S. D., & Sparks, J. A. (2004). *The heroic client: A revolutionary way to improve effectiveness through client directed, outcome-informed therapy* [Revised paperback edition]. San Francisco, CA: Jossey-Bass.

Duncan, B. L., Miller, S. D., Wampold, B. E., & Hubble, M.A. (Eds.). (2010). *The heart and soul of change: Delivering what works in therapy* (2nd ed.). Washington, DC: American Psychological Association.

Dweck, C. S. (2006). *Mindset: The new psychology of success.* New York, NY: Ballantine.

Eichstaedt, J. C., Schwartz, H. A., Kern, M. L., Labarthe, D. L., Merchant, R. M., Jha, S., . . . Seligman, M. E. P. (2015). Psychological language on Twitter predicts county-level heart disease mortality. *Psychological Science, 26*(2), 1–11. doi:10.1177/0956797614557867

Eichstaedt, J. C., Schwartz, H. A., Kern, M. L., Park, G., Labarthe, D. R., . . . Seligman, M. E. P. (2015). Psychological language on Twitter predicts county-level heart disease mortality. *Psychological Science, 26*(2), 159–169. doi:10.1177/0956797614557867

Frank, J. D., & Frank, J. B. (1991). *Persuasion and healing: A comparative study of psychotherapy* (3rd ed.). Baltimore, MD: Johns Hopkins Press.

Gawande, A. (2004, December 6). The bell curve: What happens when patients find out how good their doctors really are? *New Yorker.* Retrieved from https://www.newyorker.com/magazine/2004/12/06/the-bell-curve

Greenberg, R. P. (1999). Common factors in psychiatric drug therapy. In M. A. Hubble, B. L. Duncan, & S. D. Miller (Eds), *The heart and soul of change: What works in therapy* (pp. 297–328). Washington, DC: American Psychological Association.

Ireland, M. E., Schwartz, H. A., Chen, Q., Ungar, L. H., & Albarracin, D. (2015). Future-oriented tweets predict lower county-level HIV prevalence in the United States. *Health Psychology, 34*, 1252–1260. doi:10.1037/hea0000279

Juran, J. M., & De Feo, J. A. (2010). *Juran's quality control handbook: The complete guide to performance excellence* (6th ed.). New York, NY: McGraw-Hill.

Kraft, S., Puschner, B., Lambert, M. J., & Kordy, H. (2006). Medical utilization and treatment outcome in mid- and long-term outpatient psychotherapy. *Psychotherapy Research, 16*(2), 241–249. doi:10.1080/10503300500485458

Madsen, W. C. (2007). *Collaborative therapy with multi-stressed families* (2nd ed.). New York, NY: Guilford.

Orlinsky, D. E., Rønnestad, M. H., & Willutzki, U. (2004). Fifty years of process-outcome research: Continuity and change. In M. J. Lambert (Ed.), *Bergin and Garfield's handbook of psychotherapy and behavior change* (5th ed., pp. 307–390). Hoboken, NJ: Wiley.

Rogers, C. R. (1957). The necessary and sufficient conditions of therapeutic personality change. *Journal of Consulting Psychology, 21*(2), 95–103.

Tilsen, J. (2013). *Therapeutic conversations with queer youth: Transcending homonormativity and constructing preferred identities*. New York, NY: Aronson.

CHAPTER 4

Active Client Engagement (ACE)

Information-Gathering Processes

In this chapter, we take a significant step in understanding the role of the therapist as an active partner in the change process through exploration of strategies aimed at gaining a deeper understanding of clients' and their lives. To do this, we use active client engagement (ACE), an approach to gathering information, establishing a context of collaboration, and learning about client strengths, which will assist with establishing goals (Chapter 5) and in formulating strategies to help clients achieve their desired change. ACE is composed of three components:

1. *Acquisition of information*: This involves beginning therapy with a mindset of maintaining both structure and flexibility. By structure, we mean that the therapist is prepared for each session in terms of documentation requirements, ways to gather information relevant to the therapy, and a purpose of the therapeutic encounter. *Flexibility* refers to a willingness to depart from any plans, processes, or methods that are not working or do not fit with a particular client.
2. *Creating a context of collaboration*: Here, we refer to the partnership between the therapist and the client, in which each has expertise essential to a successful outcome. The therapist endeavors to create a context in which the client's voice is the key driver throughout therapy, beginning with initial information gathering.
3. *Evocation of strengths and resources*: This involves a commitment to learning about each client's internal abilities and competencies and external systems of support and using those resources in the service of change.

As with the strengths-based principles, each facet of ACE works in concert with and is dependent on the others. Together the three components assist with creating a focus in therapy and strengthening the therapeutic alliance. In addition, the three aspects of ACE are interventive. Our aim with all client interactions is to be as helpful as possible with an understanding that most change happens early in therapy (S. D. Miller, Duncan, & Hubble, 1997). If clients experience meaningful change early, the probability of positive outcome significantly increases (Haas, Hill, Lambert, & Morrell, 2002; Percevic, Lambert, & Kordy, 2006; Whipple et al., 2003). Therefore, information gathering is not simply about asking choreographed questions and filling out forms; rather, it is about using conversations to stimulate change and effort to maximize the benefit of each interaction, beginning with strengths-based information-gathering processes.

THE 80/20 RULE IN ACTION: PREPARING FOR CHANGE

In the Chapter 3, we explored a series of Collaboration Keys, the first of which is "Orient Clients to Information-Gathering Processes." As we know, many therapists spend an inordinate amount of time filling out forms, completing documentation, and so on. We learned that one approach to reducing paperwork is through periodic review of forms and documentation requirements. Here, we continue our conversation on information gathering by examining ways of being purposeful through our efforts to understand clients, their situations, and their lives.

Recall the 80/20 rule—the idea that 80% of the results or value comes from 20% of the source or focus. Here, we use the 80/20 rule as a way of determining what information brings the most value to clients and how it can be used to both monitor the effectiveness of services and improve outcomes. To orient toward this idea, consider Dr. Brendan Reilly, who in 1990 as chairman of Chicago's Cook County Hospital's Department of Medicine, saw a need for change within the Emergency Department, which was flooded with 250,000 patients annually. Many of those seeking treatment complained of chest pain, which the emergency room (ER) doctors took very seriously. The ER physicians were careful about diagnosis and care for these patients for fear of misdiagnosis and malpractice.

With the hospital ER inundated, Dr. Reilly faced the very difficult challenge of how to more efficiently and effectively make treatment decisions about patients. The physician turned to the work of Dr. Lee Goldman. In the 1970s, Dr. Goldman developed an algorithm reliant on three risk factors and an ECG. Three questions were asked to determine the risk: (a) Is the patient's pain stable or unstable? (b) Is there fluid in the patient's lungs? and (c) Is the patient's systolic blood pressure below 100 mm Hg? Coupled with the ECG, this information provided doctors with a more definitive answer in diagnosing chest pain. Dr. Reilly then used those risk factors to develop a decision tree.

For 2 years, Dr. Reilly collected data at Cook County Hospital that compared doctors' own judgment in evaluating heart attacks compared to Dr. Goldman's algorithm and decision tree. In the end, the results weren't even close. Left to their conventional methods—which doctors believed to be accurate despite substantial variability in their ratings of the seriousness of patients presenting with symptoms of heart attack—doctors *guessed* accurately with the most serious cardiac patients between 75% and 89% of the time. In contrast, the Goldman method produced accuracy rates of 95%. His staff was able to accurately recognize the patients who were not having a heart attack 70% better using the algorithm and decision tree than using their own judgment and previous standards by which to diagnose chest pain. Dr. Goldman's algorithm and decision tree demonstrated that asking more questions, running more tests, and gathering more information may not be an advantage. Results in hand, Dr. Reilly implemented the Goldman algorithm full time, making Cook County Hospital one of the first in the country to do so (Gladwell, 2005).

Dr. Goldman's algorithm helped to more effectively identify patients who were experiencing heart attacks, which saved lives. In addition, the efficiency with which cardiac patients were treated improved. There was clarity about what level of care should be provided to whom, under what circumstances. Further were the cost savings that would have been incurred had patients been unnecessarily admitted. Finally, the guesswork of doctors in the ER was reduced. Less guessing equaled more reliability.

As it turns out, when it comes to gathering *useful* information, there are similarities between ERs and psychotherapy. In both cases, having the most relevant information is vital to delivering the best possible care. Because both physicians and therapists have a responsibility to respond to those most at risk in a timely manner while managing scarce resources, time wasted on gathering information that is not pertinent to immediate care puts patients and clients in jeopardy and wastes valuable time. To be clear, in both healthcare and behavioral healthcare, certain information is required for reimbursement and safety purposes. The water becomes murky in behavioral health when clinicians' personal theoretical frameworks and curiosities contribute to extra forms, surveys, and questionnaires that they see as essential to practice.

We now come full circle to the 80/20 rule. A central focus of this chapter is on the 20% of information that therapists gather that informs and contributes to effective services. Just like the doctors at Cook County Hospital, much has been learned about the kind of information most important in psychotherapy. Although there are certainly instances in which more information is necessary to make informed choices, particularly when there is a threat of harm to the client or another, little evidence supports the idea that gathering more information as a standard of practice improves the quality and benefit of services to clients. Paperwork and standards should facilitate rather than impede clinical work.

We now explore methods for gathering information to increase our understanding of clients' distress, strengthening the alliance, and selecting and matching intervention strategies in ways that provide a good fit and positively effective outcomes. Central to our information gathering are the strengths-based principles outlined in Chapter 2 and the Collaboration Keys described in Chapter 3. Consistent with a collaborative stance, we primarily use the term *information gathering* to reflect a collaborative partnership between clients and therapists.

STRENGTHS-BASED INFORMATION GATHERING

The information-gathering process begins with serious thought being given to the relationship between documentation processes (written and electronic) and the purpose(s) of therapy. We want to know: Do the means used to collect information justify the ends—what we hope to achieve therapeutically with clients? We increase the likelihood of gathering useful information by reviewing our information-gathering methods to determine their purpose in treatment.

In this chapter, we examine two different processes for gathering information: (a) routine outcome monitoring (ROM) in practice (including feedback-informed treatment [FIT]) and (b) interviewing for strengths. Each process helps us to hone in on the 20% of information that, according to research, has the most return on investment in terms of psychotherapy outcomes. In accordance, the processes detailed in this chapter are meant to make early contacts and what follows treatment-wise seamless. Separating the two does not save time and increases costs. Our aim is to engage consumers by making processes around information gathering, particularly paperwork, as easy as possible. The first visit is critical and is a large determinant of whether clients continue or drop out.

Whether referring to information gathering or another aspect of the therapeutic encounter, the therapist's role is that of a co-expert and collaborator. As discussed in Chapter 2, both clients and therapists have expertise essential to the success of therapy. Clients are experts on their lives. They have had experiences inclusive of successes and failures and in many circumstances already know what does not work, what works to any degree, and what might work in the future. Equally important is that clients know what feels right, even if they have not been in therapy before. Clients' life experiences inform their responses and are to be appreciated, not passed over. Therapists' expertise exists in their education and training, work with clients, and commitment to bettering the lives of others. Effective therapists understand their influence in therapy and invite clients into active partnerships with an understanding both that client expectations and the role of the therapist can vary from culture to culture (Jennings & Skovholt, 2016).

Effective therapists are also clear that there is a purpose to therapy. They are structured in their approach, yet flexible. Although the structure of therapy depends largely on the therapist, client feedback assists with determining what is working and what is not and inform potential changes. The duality of structure and flexibility is ongoing. Research has shown that a lack of structure in therapy can lead to negative outcome (Mohr, 1995), whereas other findings indicate that therapists who remain flexible achieve the best outcomes (Wampold & Imel, 2015). Therapists who are client-driven, paying close attention to clients' expectations and preferences through ROM, are likely to achieve a balance in structure and flexibility.

PROCESS 1: ROM IN PRACTICE: PARTNERS FOR CHANGE OUTCOME MANAGEMENT SYSTEM

The final sentence of the definition of a strengths-based perspective reads, "Routine outcome monitoring (ROM) is used to create and maintain a culture of feedback—a responsive, consumer-driven climate to ensure the greatest benefit of services." The benefits of ROM are well established in both healthcare and behavioral healthcare. Studies demonstrate that the provision of ongoing feedback to therapists improves outcomes, increases retention, and reduces rates of deterioration (Lambert et al., 2001, 2002). A first step, then, is a commitment to using ROM. There is a critical second step without which ROM loses its efficacy. As discussed in Chapter 1, some therapists consistently outperform others (Okiishi, Lambert, Nielsen, & Ogles, 2003; Schuckard, Miller, & Hubble, 2017). This is because simply implementing a form of ROM does not in and of itself improve outcomes. Therapists must learn how to respond effectively to the feedback generated from ROM and continue to develop their knowledge and skills over time (Prescott, Maeschalck, & Miller, 2017). Given that therapist effects account for between 5% and 9% of the variance in outcome, it is imperative that clinicians fully embrace their role as change agents (Crits-Christoph & Mintz, 1991; Wampold & Brown, 2005; Wampold & Imel, 2015).

The second collaboration key detailed in Chapter 3 is to "Introduce Routine Outcome Monitoring." Doing so establishes with the client that monitoring both the outcome of services and the strength of the therapeutic alliance will be part of treatment. With this commitment, the therapist must choose and use measures that are reliable, valid, feasible, and cost-effective for the clientele and setting. In agency settings, the choice of measurement should involve direct service providers, supervisors, and administrators (Bertolino, 2017; Bertolino, Axsen, Maeschalck, Miller, & Babbins-Wagner, 2013; Moss & Mousavizadeh, 2017).

There are numerous measures and ROM packages available. Examples of outcome measures include the Outcome Questionnaire 45 (OQ-45; Burlingame, Lambert, Reisinger, Neff, & Mosier, 1995; Lambert & Burlingame, 1996; Lambert & Finch, 1999; Lambert et al., 1996), Youth Outcome Questionnaire (Y-OQ; Burlingame, Wells, & Lambert, 1996; Burlingame et al., 2001; Burlingame, Wells, Lambert, & Cox, 2004; Dunn, Burlingame, Walbridge, Smith, & Crum, 2005), Clinical Outcomes in Routine Management (CORE; Barkham, Mellor-Clark, Connell, & Cahill, 2006; Evans et al., 2002), and the Outcome Rating Scale (ORS; S. D. Miller & Duncan, 2000; S. D. Miller, Duncan, Brown, Sparks, & Claud, 2003). Examples of alliance measures are the Revised Helping Alliance Questionnaire (HAq-II; Luborsky et al., 1996), the Working Alliance Inventory (WAI; Horvath & Greenberg, 1989), and the Session Rating Scale (SRS; Duncan et al., 2003). Some measures are free or available at a cost per administration basis or a monthly or annual licensing fee. Drapeau (2012) provides a discussion of 10 measures/systems for tracking mental health changes in routine care for those interested.

For the purposes of discussion and for the remainder of this book, the ORS and SRS measures will be used as an example of ROM. The ORS and SRS measures, collectively known as the *Partners for Change Outcome Management System (PCOMS)*, have met the rigorous standards set by the U.S. Substance Abuse and Mental Health Services Administration (SAMHSA) and are listed on the National Registry of Evidence-Based Programs and Practices (NREPP) (www.nrepp.samhsa.gov). The basics of the measures are described here, but those interested are encouraged to explore the full psychometric properties and applications of the measures, which are available in detail elsewhere (Bertolino & Miller, 2013; Schuckard et al., 2017).

After a discussion of the measures, we explore how PCOMS is integrated into clinical practice through FIT, which involves the routine solicitation of feedback from clients regarding the therapeutic alliance and outcome of care and the use of this feedback by the therapist to inform the delivery of services to the client (Bertolino & Miller, 2013; Schuckard et al., 2017). FIT is of critical importance for reasons already discussed, particularly in light of the difficulties clinicians have exhibited in detecting when their cases are off-track and at risk of dropout or deterioration despite being exposed to feedback (Lambert, 2010; S. D. Miller, Duncan, & Hubble, 2004).

Overview of the ORS and the SRS

The ORS and SRS are brief, self-report measures for tracking client functioning/well-being (outcome) and the quality of the therapeutic alliance. Each measure takes less than a minute for clients to complete and for service providers to score and interpret. The ORS has been shown to be sensitive to change among those receiving services. Numerous studies have documented concurrent, discriminative, criterion-related, and predictive validity, test–retest reliability, and internal consistency reliability for the ORS and SRS (Schuckard & Miller, 2016). The impact of using these measures on the outcome of services has similarly been well documented (e.g., Anker, Dunkin, & Sparks, 2009; S. D. Miller, Duncan, Brown, Sorrell, & Chalk, 2006; Reese, Norsworthy, & Rowlands, 2009; Schuckard & Miller, 2016).

The ORS

The ORS is a brief, client-rated, four-item visual analogue scale that measures the client's experience of well-being in individual (personal), interpersonal, and social functioning. The individual domain measures symptomatic distress and personal well-being. The interpersonal domain measures how well the client is getting along in intimate or very close relationships. The third domain, social role, measures satisfaction with work and/or school and relationships outside of the home. The fourth and final domain captures the client's rating of overall life. The ORS takes less than 1 minute to administer, score, and interpret.

The ORS is designed and normed for adults and adolescents (ages 13+). The CORS is a children's version (CORS) that has been normed for ages 6 to 12.

The YCORS is a "clinical engagement" tool for children below 6 years, which although not scored, is used to provide very young children a way of expressing their well-being and satisfaction with a meeting or session along with the older children and/or adults with whom they may be in services. These tools are available in more than 19 languages, and a script is available for the oral administration of the ORS (www.scottdmiller.com). Samples of the ORS, CORS, and YCORS are provided in the Appendix, and individual licenses are available for free at www.scottdmiller.com.

Clinical Cutoff for the ORS

Determining the clinical cutoff for an outcome measure accomplishes two related objectives: (a) It defines the boundary between a normal and clinical range of distress, and (b) it provides a reference point for evaluating the severity of distress for a particular client or client sample. When the method described by Jacobson and Truax (1991) is used, the clinical cutoff for the ORS was determined to be 25 (S. D. Miller et al., 2003). The sample on which this score is based is quite large ($n = 34,790$) and comparison with other well-established measures shows it to be a reasonable differentiator between "normal" and "clinical" levels of distress. For example, the clinical cutoff score for the OQ-45 falls at the 83rd percentile of the nontreatment sample, and the clinical cutoff for the ORS falls at the 77th percentile of the nontreatment sample. Miller and colleagues have reported between 25% and 33% of people seeking treatment score above the clinical cutoff at intake (S. D. Miller & Duncan, 2000; S. D. Miller, Duncan, Sorrell, & Brown, 2005). Although the clinical cutoff for adults is 25, younger clients tend to score themselves higher. Therefore, the clinical cutoff for youth (ages 13–18) is 28, and for children (ages 6–12), the cutoff is 32. The clinical cutoff is an important statistical numeration because it helps therapists to determine a client's level of distress at the start of services, which is considered the most consistent predictor of eventual outcome (Duncan, Miller, Wampold, & Hubble, 2010).

Introducing the ORS

Following a general discussion of ROM and the measures with the client (described in Chapter 3, Collaboration Key 2) is the specific introduction of the ORS and, near the end of the session, the SRS. The ORS is completed at the beginning of sessions because we want to capture the current degree of distress experienced by clients. Below is an example of how to introduce the ORS:

> My/Our first priority is to make sure that you get the results you want. For this reason, it is very important that you are involved in monitoring our progress throughout therapy. I/We like to do this formally by using a measure called the Outcome Rating Scale or ORS. Basically, you fill it out at the beginning of each session, and then we talk about the results. A fair amount of research shows that if we are going to be successful in our work together, we should see signs

of improvement earlier rather than later. If what we're doing works, then we'll continue. If not, then I'll try to change or modify the treatment. If things still don't improve, then I'll work with you to find someone or someplace else for you to get the help you want. Does that make sense to you? (S. D. Miller & Bargmann, 2011; S. D. Miller & Duncan, 2004)

Here is an alternative way of introducing the ORS:

This scale is the Outcome Rating Scale or ORS. As you can see, the scale has four items: Individual, Interpersonal, Social, and Overall. These are the areas of your life that could show improvement if the work you and I do together is effective. I'd like you to score this form each time we meet, which will give me/us a sense of how things are progressing in your life. Today, when we are meeting for the first time, we need to get a "start score" that tells us how things have been in your life before you and I started meeting. I would like you to look back on the last week, including today, and rate how you have been feeling on each of the four items. Does that make sense to you?

If a client asks for clarification of one or more of the four subscales on the ORS, they can be explained in the following ways:

Individually: This scale refers to "how you see yourself feeling and doing individually," or "your personal functioning or well-being."

Interpersonally: This scale refers to "how things are with those who you are most close to in your life; it could include partner or family relationships."

Socially: This refers to "your life outside the home or in your community. It could include work, school, friends and acquaintances, or church."

Overall: This scale refers to "how things are going for you overall; given how you answered about specific areas of your life, how would you rate how things are in your life overall?"

It can also be helpful to let clients know they can score overall on the scale to suit their perceptions of their life. This can be done by saying:

For some, work is really important, so if their functioning is really good socially, that reflects on their overall sense of well-being. Others may see how they are doing individually as the most important area when scoring their overall sense of well-being. I'd like you to show me how these three areas of your life influence your overall sense of well-being.

Scoring the ORS

The ORS is scored immediately after the client has completed the form. To score the ORS, determine the distance in centimeters (to the nearest millimeter [e.g., 6.8]) between the left pole and the client's hash mark on each item. Add all four numbers to obtain the total score. A metric ruler can be used or a downloadable scoring overlay can be copied onto a transparency (available at www.scottdmiller.com). The transparency can be used as a full sheet with all four scales or cut into small "rulers" that can be used to score each scale individually. The score can be plotted on a paper graph (see Appendix for examples). Before using the ORS (and all the measures that follow) and making copies, check to be certain that the lines are 10 centimeters in length.

The graph shows how the client's score compares with the clinical cutoff. Low scores on the ORS correspond to low well-being (or high distress). Note that the average ORS intake score in outpatient mental healthcare treatment settings is between 18 and 19. The first step in interpreting an intake score is simply to describe to the client what the possible range of well-being is, what the clinical cutoff means, and how the client's score relates to these scores. Here is how a therapist might talk with a 26-year-old who has a total ORS score of 18.3 at the first session.

Example 4.1

I've plotted your score on the ORS on this graph, and as you can see there is a dotted line on 25. What we know is that, generally, people your age who score above the dotted line are more like a broad range of people who have not chosen to be in therapy. By comparison, people who score below the dotted line are more like people who seek therapy. They are more like people who are saying, "There are things in my life that I would like to change; things that are bothering me." Your score is 18.3 and it's below the dotted line. Does that make sense to you? (client nods) So it seems that coming here to see me . . . that you're feeling distressed. A score of 18.3 on a scale of 0 to 40 indicates that. Does that sound right? Does that match how you're feeling?"

Scores above the clinical cutoff are important to discuss because these clients are at higher risk for deterioration. The most common reason for a score above the clinical cutoff is that a client has come to therapy involuntarily (i.e., the client was mandated into services or therapy was initiated by a caregiver). In such cases, it can be helpful to also have a collateral rater (Bertolino, 2014, 2017). The idea of using collaterals will be discussed shortly.

Another common reason for scores falling above the clinical cutoff at intake is that the client wants help with a very specific problem—one that does not impact the overall quality of life or functioning but is troubling nonetheless. Given the heightened risk of deterioration for clients entering treatment above the clinical cutoff, therapists are advised against "exploratory" and "depth-oriented" work. The best approach, in such instances, is a cautious one, using the least invasive and intensive methods needed to resolve the problem at hand. This kind of approach will be discussed in Chapter 6.

Less frequent causes for high initial ORS scores include (a) high-functioning clients who want services for growth, self-actualization, and optimization of performance; and (b) clients who may have difficulties reading and writing or who have not understood the meaning or purpose of the measure. In the latter instance, time can be taken to explain the measure and build a "culture of feedback," or in the case of reading or language difficulties, the oral version can be administered. For high-functioning clients, caution is warranted. A strength-based, coaching-type approach focused on achieving specific, targeted, and measurable goals is likely to be most helpful while minimizing risks of deterioration.

The SRS

The SRS is a four-item, self-report alliance measure. Like the ORS, the SRS is a visual analogue scale that takes less than 1 minute to administer, score, and interpret. Items on the scale reflect the classical definition of the alliance first stated by Bordin (1979). The scale assesses the quality of the relational bond, the degree of agreement on the goals, the methods, and the overall approach of therapy. The SRS is available in an adult version (ages 13+), a children's version (CSRS) for children ages 6 to 12, and a version for children below 6 years (YCSRS). It is also available in a group therapy version (GSRS) and has been translated into more than 19 languages. As with the ORS, there is a script available for the oral administration of the SRS (www.scottdmiller.com). Samples of the SRS, CSRS, YCSRS, and GSRS are provided in the Appendix.

SRS Cutoff

The cutoff for an alliance measure is the point at which providers should be especially alert to the possibility of a failure of the working relationship. The alliance cutoff enables therapists to identify relationships that are at a statistically greater risk for client dropout or negative or null outcome from treatment. On the SRS, a score of 36 or below is considered cause for concern because fewer than 24% of cases score lower than 36 (S. D. Miller & Duncan, 2004).

Introducing the SRS

Client dropout, particularly after the first session, is commonly the result of alliance issues (S. D. Miller & Maeschalck, 2015). This speaks to the high importance of soliciting feedback regarding clients' experience before completing the first session. Therefore, the way the SRS is introduced plays a significant role in the quality of feedback received and in the strength of the alliance. Like the ORS, the SRS is designed not only to measure, but also to positively impact what it measures through careful use of the information it provides. The SRS is administered just before the end of each meeting or session, and it is important to frame the SRS by emphasizing the importance of the relationship in successful treatment and encouraging feedback.

Therapists often wonder about clients who may, for cultural reasons, find it difficult to give any kind of critical feedback to a professional whom they perceive to be in a position of authority. These therapists often suggest that clients feel uncomfortable and pressured by an invitation to provide critical feedback to somebody with whom they feel especially humble. A way to address this can be to frame the SRS introduction in a positive light. Instead of the client being asked, "What was wrong with the service I received?" we ask, "What could have made this service even more helpful to you?" We describe this process as our standard way of working with people, and clients may then feel they are being more cooperative if they give us the feedback that we say is critical to our doing our job well. The following is one example of how to introduce the SRS to clients:

> I'd like to ask you to fill out one additional form called the Session Rating Scale or SRS. This is a measure that you and I will use at each session to adjust and improve the way we work together. A great deal of research shows that your experience of our work together is a good predictor of whether we'll be successful. I want to emphasize that I'm not aiming for a perfect score. Life isn't perfect, and neither am I. What I'm aiming for is your feedback about even the smallest things—even if it seems unimportant—so that we can adjust our work and make sure we don't veer off course. Whatever your feedback might be, I promise I won't take it personally. I'm always learning and am curious about what I can learn from getting this feedback from you that will in time help me improve my skills. Does this make sense? (S. D. Miller & Bargmann, 2011; S. D. Miller & Duncan, 2004)

Here is a slightly different way to introduce the SRS:

> I'd like to ask that you complete one additional form called the Session Rating Scale or SRS. It is a measure that you and I will use at each session to adjust and improve the way we work together. Research shows that your experience of our work together/at our agency—whether you feel understood, whether we focus on what is important to you, whether the approach I'm taking makes sense and feels right—is a good predictor of whether we'll be successful. I want to emphasize that I'm not aiming for a perfect score. What I'm aiming for is your feedback—even if it seems small and unimportant—so we can adjust our work and make sure we don't steer off course. Whatever your feedback, I promise I won't take it personally. I am curious about what I can learn from your feedback that will both now and in the future help me improve my skills. Does this make sense?

Scoring the SRS

The SRS is scored in the same way as the ORS. The lines are 10 centimeters in length and are scored to the nearest millimeter between the left pole and the client's hash mark on each individual item. All four numbers are added together to obtain the total score. The score can be plotted on a paper graph. Both ORS and SRS scores are typically placed on the same graphs (see Appendix for examples of graphs).

A score of 36 is considered the cutoff for the SRS and is depicted by the dotted line on the graph. Research to date shows that about 75% of clients will score 36 or above on the SRS (Maeschalck & Barfknecht, 2017; S. D. Miller & Duncan, 2000). Conversely, client scores above 36 do not confirm a strong alliance. Although a high score may reflect a strong alliance, it can also indicate that at this point in services, the client does not feel comfortable enough to give negative feedback. Some clinicians argue that clients "will tell therapists what they want to hear," "won't want the therapist to feel bad," or "want to avoid tension." We are not testing the character of the client but instead the integrity of the client–therapist relationship. Although no evidence supports the notion that the presence of the therapist or the clients' knowledge that the therapist will observe scores leads to inflation of alliance scores (Reese et al., 2013), therapists can better serve clients by practicing ways to introduce the SRS, emphasizing the collaborative nature of therapy and the therapist as "learner" to attain useful feedback.

Scores that fall at or below 36 are considered cause for concern and should be discussed with clients prior to ending the session. Single-point declines in SRS scores from meeting to meeting have also been found to be associated with poorer outcomes at termination—even when the total score consistently falls above 36—and should also be discussed (Duncan et al., 2003). In sum, the SRS helps therapists identify problems in the alliance (e.g., misunderstandings, disagreement about goals and methods) early in services, thereby preventing dropout or deterioration.

Although low SRS scores necessitate a timely response by the therapist, the task of the therapist is to attain negative feedback. Negative feedback is part of an "error-centric" culture, which is instructive because it provides therapists with opportunities to learn firsthand from clients about what is not working (i.e., alliance ruptures; discussed in Chapter 7) and what needs improvement. In this way, "bad" scores are good! The key is for the alliance to improve over the course of therapy. Research suggests that improvements in the alliance (intake to termination) are associated with better outcomes and lower dropout rates (Duncan et al., 2010; Harmon et al., 2007; Lambert, 2010; Owen, Miller, Seidel, & Chow, 2016).

Regardless of the circumstance, openness and transparency are central to successfully eliciting meaningful feedback on the SRS. When the total score falls below 36, for example, the therapist can encourage discussion by saying:

Example 4.2

Your experience here is important to me. Filling out the SRS gives me a chance to check in, one last time, before we end today to make sure we are on the same page—that this is working for you. Thanks for the care you took in filling out the measure. Most of the time, about 75% actually, people score above 36. And today, your score is (a number 36 or lower), which can mean we need to consider making some changes in the way we are working together. Is it okay if I ask you a little more about your experience here today?

When a particular subscale on the SRS is lower compared with the others, the therapist can also inquire directly about that subscale regardless of whether the total score is above cutoff. A good starting place is to inquire about individual subscales that total eight or lower. Here is an example of how to do this:

Example 4.3

Thank you for completing the SRS. I want to do whatever I can to ensure that we are working together in a way that is right for you. Looking at the SRS gives me a chance to make sure I'm not missing something big or going in the wrong direction for you. I've noticed here (showing the completed form to the client) that your mark on the subscale about "approach and method" is lower compared with the others. What can you tell me about that?

When seeking feedback about the SRS, it can be helpful to frame follow-up questions in as "task-specific" a manner as possible. Research shows, for example, that people are more likely to provide feedback when it is not perceived as a criticism of one person or the other but is rather about specific behaviors (Ericsson, Charness, Feltovich, & Hoffman, 2006). For example, instead of inquiring generally about how a session went for a client, the therapist would frame questions in a way that elicits concrete, specific suggestions for altering the type, course, and delivery of services:

- Did we talk about the things that are most important to you today?
- What was the least helpful thing that happened today?
- Did my questions make sense to you?
- Did I fail to ask you about something you consider important or wanted to talk about but didn't?
- Was the meeting or session too short/long/just right for you?
- Did my responses make you feel like I understood what you were telling me, or do you need me to respond differently?
- Is there anything that happened (or did not happen) today that would cause you to not want to talk next time?

At times, clients may struggle with identifying specifics that led to giving a particular score on the SRS. In such instances, the therapist should remain patient and avoid an interrogational tone. One possibility is to say, "What was running through your mind just prior to giving your score?" If struggles continue invite the client to call if reminded of something after leaving. The same approach may be useful with clients who score above 36. We find it best to thank them for their feedback and to add that we would really appreciate if they would let us know if they think of something later on about the meeting or session that they would like for us to change a bit. In closing, if concerns remain, the therapist may want to ask, "How likely is your score (or overall experience) today to influence your decision about returning?" Doing so can help the therapist gauge the severity of the issue and in some cases, create an opportunity for further discussion.

Further Considerations With PCOMS

All outcome and alliance measures have benefits and drawbacks. It is therefore important that individual clinicians and agencies practice due diligence in making choices as to which measures best fit the practice philosophy and clientele served, are most feasible, and are affordable. In organizations, it is also a good idea to consider how outcomes and choices of measurement correspond with each other. For example, at my agency, Youth In Need (YIN), Inc., a Midwestern community-based nonprofit that serves a diverse population of children, youth, young adults, and families, the PCOMS measures (and FIT, which will be discussed further later in this chapter) are inextricably tied to the agency's strengths-based perspective and outcomes in outclient and school-based counseling, emergency shelter care, and transitional living programs (Bertolino, 2011, 2017). Taking the time to make good decisions up-front is likely to increase staff buy-in, result in smoother implementation, and result in well-thought-out data-management processes in the future. The topic of implementation will be explored further in the final chapter.

Remaining with the PCOMS as our example, what follows is a discussion of four additional points of consideration in using ROM. Each point involves a degree of choice to be made by individual clinicians or group of clinicians in a private or agency setting. By nuancing the use of ROM, we continue to work with clients in ways that are collaborative and transparent to improve the likelihood of success.

Specific Populations

The PCOMS are enhanced through FIT (which will be expanded on shortly), the cornerstone of which is collaboration. Therapists partner with clients to determine how to best meet the needs of clients, which requires understanding, respect, and flexibility, which are especially important with persons who have been disempowered and marginalized (Chesworth et al., 2017). Disempowered and marginalized populations include, but are not limited to, people:

- who identify as lesbian, gay, bisexual, transgender, and queer (LGBTQ)
- who have disabilities

- who are labeled as "severely and persistently mentally ill" (SPMI)
- who are in substance abuse treatment
- who experience partner violence
- who are mandated to therapy
- who experience marginalization because of their age, race, class, gender expression, sexual orientation, immigrant or refugee status, ability, religious or spiritual affiliation, ethnicity, or any combination of such identifiers (Tilsen, Maeschalck, Seidel, Robinson, & Miller, 2013)

When using the ORS and SRS measures with people who experience marginalization, therapists are encouraged to be curious and respectful about clients' caution, honoring it as an important act of resistance to their experience of oppression and/or an act of self-agency and critical thinking. In addition, it is a good practice to find what meaning clients make of measurement in general and of the ORS/SRS in particular. For example, a therapist might ask, "I'm really interested in your position on this and respect your caution. What kinds of experiences have you had with measures that lead you to question their use here?" or "What concerns in particular do you have about how this may be harmful to you or others?" We do not try to persuade, explain, justify, or convince. Instead, we ask questions that communicate openness, respect, and interest in the client's experience. For example, we ask, "It sounds really important that you take a stand on this. What do you need me to understand about your position on this so that we may work together?" Or, "Sounds like you have some really serious reasons for not trusting what this is about, is that right?" When misunderstandings occur, focus is on understanding what was experienced rather than clarifying what was intended (Tilsen et al., 2013).

If the alliance appears to be at risk, it's a good idea to set the measures aside. We can then explore ways to work together that fit with the client's values and ways of making meaning. The following questions can be helpful:

- What are some things we can do or ways we can talk that fit for you, respect your concerns, and help us work our best together?
- If we toss out the lines and the numbers, what ways would you suggest that we could use?
- How might we talk about and understand together how the concerns that have brought you here are impacting you and how our conversations are impacting those concerns?
- If we think of the lines and numbers on the forms as a kind of language, what language can we translate to that allows you to speak about your experience in a way that better fits for you?
- Is there a language of colors or shapes or images or . . . ?
- In your relationships, how do people talk about these things and work things out in ways that are helpful, respectful, and meaningful?

We aim to create a culture of feedback that helps to us work with clients in ways that are right for them. Chesworth et al. (2017) stated:

> Cultivating a culturally responsive practice is vital to creating a culture of feedback, the hallmark of FIT. Being culturally responsive requires, in part, that therapists engage in reflexive consideration of their own social locations and assumptions about the world and clinical practice. (p. 263)

As therapists, we know that people who seek therapy are in some state of vulnerability and distress. Amid that distress may be marginalization, shame, disempowerment, and pathological labeling. The PCOMS measures—which are intended to provide a way of working *with* clients to achieve the change they desire and live the lives they dream of—when used with compassion and sensitivity are well suited for clients of most, if not all, backgrounds, experiences, and heritages.

Switching Measures to Increase Client Fit

Both the ORS and SRS have been normed for specific age ranges (Bertolino & Miller, 2013). However, based on maturity, cognitive ability, or preference, it may be necessary to change the type of ORS and SRS measures used. For example, some 12-year-olds are more comfortable with the adult versions, and there may be 14-year-olds who prefer the child versions (i.e., CORS and CSRS). Scoring for all the measures is the same, so they are easily interchangeable. Accordingly, we want to be sure the language we use to describe the measures is understood by clients. Therapists are encouraged to practice ways of talking with clients so that the measures will be more easily understood. Next is an example of how to introduce the CORS that follows can serve as a guide.

Example 4.4

I'd like to ask you for your help with something. When I work with young people like yourself I want to make sure that they are feeling helped. So, I use these two short scales to keep track of things. The first one we use at the beginning each time we talk, and the second one we use at the end, after we are just about done talking. I'd like to ask for your help showing me how things have been this last week, before you came to you see me. Is that okay with you? This scale is the one we use to see how you have been feeling. As you can see it has four lines with faces at each side—happy smiley faces to the right and sad frowny faces to the left. And you can see that above each line it says "me," "family," "school," and "everything." All you have to do is think about the last week and how things have been in these four areas. Then make a mark on the line to show me how things are going. The closer to the happy smiley, the better things have been; the closer to the sad frowny, the worse or harder things have been. Does that make sense?

Using Collateral Raters

Earlier the idea of using additional raters was raised. Doing this can be helpful, particularly for clients who attend services at the request of a caregiver or an external entity (e.g., school personnel, court officials, family services). The key is to figure out whose ORS score will be the best measure of the progress of services. In other words, whose ratings will be most reliable in determining the outcome of services? One way to approach this is by talking with those who are involved in treatment, including clients and stakeholders. To further aid with that decision, it can be helpful to determine who has the authority to begin and end services and who you will be able to get scores from on a consistent basis. In other words, if a therapist is meeting with an adolescent and a parent but the parent is not present at every session, then it would be best to use the adolescent's scores. The parent could still be used as a collateral; however, without consistent ratings, the information is less likely to reflect the client's state of change in real time.

Sometimes, it is not possible for collaterals to be physically present for each session. In such cases, arrangements can be made for ORS data to be collected over the phone or through electronic means such as email. For example, in YIN's school-based counseling program, ORS forms are often left in teachers' school mailboxes. The ORS forms are completed and picked up by counselors who then plot, compare, and discuss the results with students. Again, planning is essential; with some thought and discussion, the logistics of how to apply ROM can be worked out.

Multiple raters or collaterals can be helpful in determining the benefit of services. Let's consider an example of a youth and parent who each complete a measure. Because youth often rate their situations differently than adults, having two or more ORSs can provide points of comparison. In such an instance, a therapist might say, "Reggie, I noticed that you have rated things currently at a solid 34. Your mom gave a rating of 19.1. Can you tell me about the difference between your and your mom's scores?" Differences in scores between youth and caregivers (or stakeholders) are very common. Discussion about differences can be invaluable in clarifying how the presenting issue is seen by both or all the involved parties. The progress as reported by both the youth and the collateral rater can be tracked and used as a reference point for the therapy, with the collateral rating being the most reliable indicator of progress.

Yet another way of using a collateral is with persons who attend involuntarily. For example, if an adult who was sent to therapy by his parole officer scored a 37.8 on the ORS, the therapist might say, "I'd like you to complete the ORS once more. But this time, I'd like you to please complete it as your parole officer. How would he complete an ORS about you?" This method can be used in any instance, with either adults or youth, in which a caregiver or external stakeholder is responsible for the client being in therapy.

An additional example of multiple raters is with couples. In such cases, the ratings of both members of the couple are considered. The therapist's role is to explore any differences in the couples' scores, which reflect each person's perception of the relationship, and work toward indicators of improvement that are acceptable to all parties involved (Robinson, 2017). Therapy is considered successful when each member of the couple reports a change that is both reliable and valid (Anker et al., 2009).

Outcomes Management Systems

The use of paper graphs, such as those provided in the Appendix, is the most commonly used method of tracking the results of therapy. Figure 4.1 provides an example of how a paper graph might appear. In Figure 4.1, the top circle is the SRS and the circle below is the ORS. When multiple raters are used, therapists can choose to put all scores on one graph by using different colors of ink or use separate graphs for each person.

An affordable means of compiling and managing data is through the creation of spreadsheets (e.g., Excel). A challenge with spreadsheets is to keep data accessible and user-friendly. In addition, spreadsheets also increase the probability of errors associated with documenting, aggregating, and analyzing data. It's best to sort out in advance how data will be managed.

Another option for completing the PCOMS measures, scoring, and reviewing the results is through an electronic outcomes management system (OMS) that is network-based, cloud-based, and/or through an app. Multiple options are available as stand-alone systems or as part of an electronic medical record (EMR). Some computerized OMSs also calculate statistics such as client target scores (based on national datasets and algorithms), expected treatment responses (ETRs), effect sizes, and percentages of clients who achieve a reliable change.

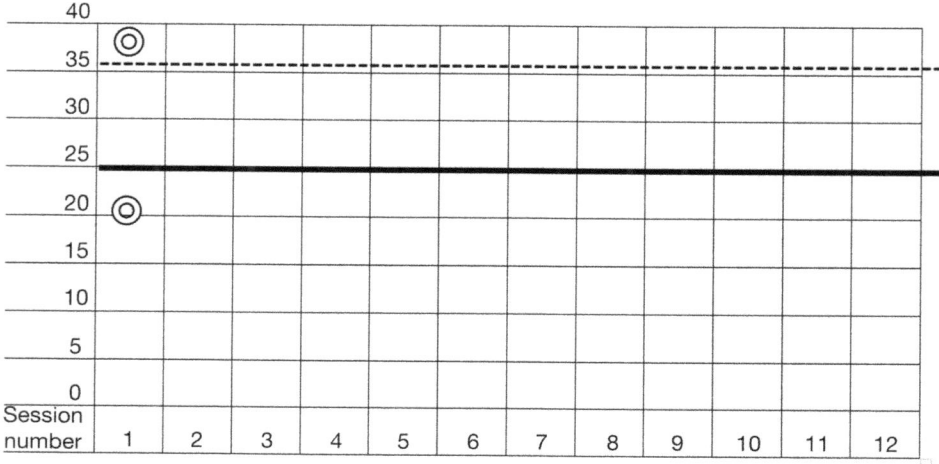

FIGURE 4.1 Example of paper graph.

The functionality of systems does vary. As with discussions about choices of measures, decisions about use of any OMS should be done with consideration of feasibility, cost, and the needs of the clinician or organization. Figure 4.2 is an electronic graph of an initial session created by YIN's proprietary OMS, Imagine, a cloud-based system used across services. In Figure 4.2, the circle near the top is the SRS and the circle below is the ORS. The shaded areas, beginning with the bottom of the chart ascending to the top, represent ranges within which the client is considered deteriorated (high risk), unimproved (moderate), or improved (low risk). The corresponding key in Figure 4.2 indicates the clinical cutoffs for the ORS and SRS, as well as other information for the therapist to review. Further illustrations with multiple session scores will be provided in upcoming chapters to demonstrate the use of ROM.

Graphing the results provides a vehicle for open conversations inclusive of clients' perspectives (and others who may be involved) about the course of therapy. Client feedback can help to ensure that the service is adjusted and tailored in response to the clients' feedback. Graphs also reveal patterns related to client progress and the alliance. Knowledge of specific patterns makes it possible for therapists to respond if there are signs of "threats" to service outcome or alliance (and risk for dropout), and can be used to inform the decision to seek consultation on a particular case. In this sense, the ORS and SRS can be viewed as quality assurance instruments. Chapter 7 will detail some of the most common client scoring patterns and describe the ways of responding to those patterns.

The ORS in Subsequent Sessions

Once clients are accustomed to completing the ORS, provisions can be made to have clients complete the measure as they wait for their sessions. In some

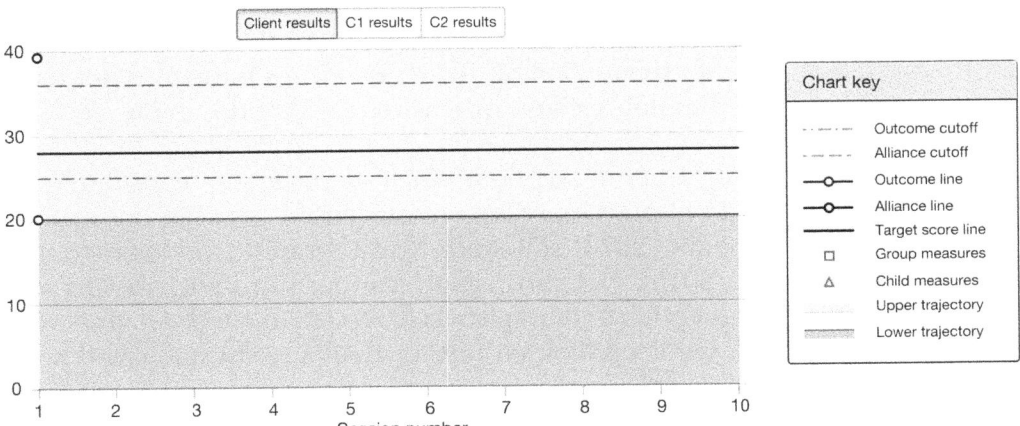

FIGURE 4.2 First session Outcome Rating Scale and Session Rating Scale scores from Imagine Outcomes Management Systems.

settings the measure is in a box or folder in a waiting room, and clients are instructed to fill it out prior to meeting with their therapist. In other settings, clients are given a computer tablet by agency staff or use a desktop computer to enter and complete the ORS while in the waiting room. In such instances clients are provided with unique user codes. The results are then sent to the therapist who can open the client's electronic record and have it ready from the start of the session.

From ROM to PCOMS to FIT: A Critical Step

For some clinicians, there are overarching beliefs that prevent them from fully embracing ROM as anything more than collecting data. According to Prescott (2017), reasons that clinicians avoid seeking feedback include the belief that it is somehow contrary to one's therapeutic modality, therapists are experts and know how treatment is progressing, therapists are already getting feedback (e.g., asking, "Are you feeling better," "How was this today?"), and using feedback processes will slow the pace of therapy or interfere with the therapist's protocols. Clinicians are hesitant about collecting feedback for many reasons. First, for decades, psychotherapy training has emphasized learning models as the way to best help clients. Despite evidence to the contrary, this practice remains a central focus of many graduate programs and training curriculums. A second reason is fear. Fear of change, fear of learning something that may run counter to what was learned, and perhaps most worrisome, the fear of possibly discovering that one is not as effective as one thought.

Consider the work of psychologist Paul Clement (2013), who studied his outcomes from 45 years in private practice. His review included 2,259 patients, of which he had outcome data on 1,599 cases. Following his review, Clement concluded, "Measured by percent improved per year, not only have I failed to improve across the years, my outcomes have gotten worse across time" (p. 41). By comparison, Clement's outcomes were actually on par with other therapists' in terms of average performance. What is refreshing is his willingness to share his findings in an open forum. Yet this is what is required of each of us if we are to improve. Clement (1994, 2008, 2013) reviewed his outcomes not once but three times! He did so not because he was required to do, so but because it mattered.

Whether out of fear, training, or theoretical ideology, the consequences of not using feedback to improve services are evident. A growing body of research supports Clement's (2013) self-study that therapists, on average, get worse (Goldberg et al., 2016). Not surprisingly, various third-party payers and funders are no longer accepting of therapists' self-reports of client progress void of clients' voices. Last, we need look no further than a well-established body of research into psychotherapy outcomes showing that therapists' reasons for not incorporating feedback mechanisms do not hold up under scrutiny. Simply, effective therapists express no hang-ups about feedback. In fact, it's quite the opposite. By and large, the most effective therapists are humble and sponge-like, continually observing, absorbing, and learning. Whereas therapists with average outcomes tend to overrate their performance, the most effective therapists see themselves as average compared to their peers (Lambert, 2010; Sapyta, Riemer, & Bickman, 2005; Walfish, McAlister, O'Donnell, & Lambert, 2012). Truly effective therapists recognize the value of client feedback and embrace its use in everyday practice. To this end, it can be said that therapy does not become feedback-informed until clinicians commit to not only using a system of ROM, such as the PCOMS, but also beginning to respond to client feedback to inform practice.

Earlier in this chapter, FIT was introduced. FIT is a pantheoretical approach involving the use of reliable and valid (empirically validated) outcomes and alliance measurements to monitor client progress and the therapeutic alliance in real time. The approach has been shown to reduce the rate of treatment failure and improve outcomes (Shimokawa, Lambert, & Smart, 2010). FIT provides guidance for how to elicit and respond to client feedback, establish baseline rates of effectiveness, create plans to improve from those baselines, and most important, improve the benefit of services to clients. In the coming chapters, we will explore specific ways that outcome and alliance data are used to inform services in ways that make the most of client contributions to change; strengthen the alliance; attend to clients' cultures, expectations, and preferences; and increase hope.

To assist and support clinicians in the use of FIT, the SONAR Session Feedback Checklist (SSFC) offers a structural process that includes areas to cover in each session (Bertolino, 2013, 2017). SONAR stands for:

SETUP

- (Intake/Initial Session) Introduce and discuss the role of real-time feedback.
- (Subsequent Sessions) Reorient to the role of real-time feedback.

OUTCOME

- Complete outcome measure(s).
- Score measure(s) and plot the results.
- Identify high/low scores and variations from previous scores (in subsequent sessions).

NOW

- Discuss outcome feedback.
- Collaborate and proceed.
- Continuously monitor.

ALLIANCE

- Complete alliance measure(s).
- Score measure(s) and plot results.
- Identify low scores.

RESPOND

- Discuss alliance feedback.
- Determine next steps.

The SONAR SFC helps to keep feedback at the forefront of therapy. At my agency, YIN, the SONAR SFC has contributed to a client outcome measurement completion rate of 98.2% (Bertolino, 2017). To further assist clinicians, a SONAR SFC wall-chart has been included in the Appendix. Collecting client feedback in each and every session is an important routine to adopt, particularly in the face of evidence suggesting that periodic (e.g., every third session, once a month) measurement is insufficient in tracking client progress (Warren et al., 2010).

We have now examined how to introduce ROM, thoughtfully choose measures, administer those measures, and consider how FIT can assist with responding to client feedback. By attending to clients' ratings of the outcome and alliance, we zero in on the 20% of information that is most valuable to increasing the benefit of services. Next, we explore how to gather further information about clients and their situations through interviewing.

PROCESS 2: INTERVIEWING FOR STRENGTHS

At this juncture and very early in the therapeutic interaction, the first collaboration key, "orient clients to information-gathering processes," has been accomplished. The therapist will want to have a good sense of the paperwork involved and when possible, have some of it completed. Accordingly, the therapist will have discussed the second collaboration key, "introduce routine and ongoing monitoring," given an overview of the ORS (perhaps from the examples offered earlier in this chapter), and have a completed initial ORS by the client. If the therapist hasn't already done so, it is a good idea to further normalize the process of gathering information. Here is one way to do this:

> I'd like to ask you some questions that I/we ask of everyone who come to see me/us. The information you give will help me/us to understand how things are going with you, including what you're concerned about and how that's affected you, what you'd like to see change, what has and hasn't worked for you in trying to manage your concerns, and how we can be of help to you. As we proceed, if you feel like or think I've/we've missed something, please be sure to let me/us know. I/We want to make sure that we fully understand what you need. How does that sound?

When information is gathered and FIT is used for guidance, a primary task of the therapist is to gain an understanding of the client's rating of distress and functioning from the ORS. The therapist endeavors to learn about the client's life. Doing so brings into play collaboration keys three through five which involve creating space and attending to the client's expectations and preferences. As we explore the meaning of the client's distress, inquire about any ideas the client might have about how therapy might be helpful and what is thought about the therapist's role in the change process. Our purpose is to work together with clients to achieve an improved outcome. This is consistent with the developers of motivational interviewing, W. R. Miller and Rollnick (2013), who described therapy as "something done *for* and *with* someone, not *on* and *to* them" (p. 24). This again speaks to the collaborative partnership between the therapist and the client.

In most settings, at least some form of information gathering is formal, structured, and/or "front-loaded" (Bertolino, 2010, 2014). The PCOMS, for example, is a form of structured measurement. Examples of formal, structured assessment practices include standardized forms and measures (i.e., behavior checklists, personality tests) used to identify risks and safety concerns. Many standardized methods are used just once, during an assessment or interview phase or in initial face-to-face contacts. Others are periodic or ongoing, most commonly to monitor improvement or the effects or services (e.g., ROM).

It is not uncommon for forms and questionnaires to be focused on pathology. Questions are aimed at gathering information about the details of problems and historical data. A reasonable question for a therapist is, How helpful is the information gathered from my forms during initial contacts and interviews (assessments)? We again refer back to the 80/20 rule. Are we collecting information that is purposeful and useful with this client? Of course, some therapists gather information that they know will not be particularly useful, but are required to do so for funders or organizational data-collection reasons. As discussed, a good practice is for therapists to learn their respective paperwork well, try to consolidate questions when possible, and have clients complete whatever they can prior to sessions.

An additional practice that therapists can use is to seek creative ways to intersperse strengths-based questioning in otherwise pathology-focused assessments. Doing so offers opportunities for therapists to explore client strengths. To do this, read the question and consider the ways it might be asked to learn how a client has persevered, coped with, or managed regarding to the question. For example, if a question is, "How bad has (the problem) gotten for you?" After the client answers, the therapist might follow with, "How were you able to make it here today (or keep your job, remain afloat, etc.) with (the problem) happening in your life?" Through strengths-based questions, we learn about the challenges in our clients' lives *and* the way that they manage those challenges in any way. Specifically, what strengths, resiliencies, and/or resources have they used to meet the challenges with their situations? The dichotomy between problems and strengths is one in which therapists continuously try to strike a balance. Although many forms of information gathering are negatively skewed, there are always opportunities to explore internal and external resources that may assist in resolving concerns and complaints.

Shortly, examples of strengths-based questions corresponding to specific content areas that are often part of formal assessment will be given. The questions offered are aimed at learning about client qualities, characteristics, capabilities, coping skills, resiliencies, exceptions to problems, and so forth. Neither the content areas nor the questions are exhaustive. A task of the therapist is to select the questions that best fit the client and to modify those questions as needed. In addition, therapists are encouraged to create their own questions and share them with others.

Strengths-Based Content-Area Questioning

The first content area relates to the client's concern overall. The ORS provides an opportunity to learn about the client's rating of distress, with follow-up questions serving as a means of gaining further details. We want to explore the client's life to understand when things are most difficult, how the client manages the difficulty, and when things go differently, even if just a little. Our aim is to elicit small exceptions. We search for the topography of problems to find the proverbial needle in a haystack or a ray of light in a dark sky. Exceptions not only represent opportunities to facilitate present and future change, but also increase hope. Next are examples of exception-oriented questions related to presenting problems/situations:

Problem/Situation

- When does the problem or concern that brought you here seem a little less noticeable (or happen less) to you?
- What is happening when things are a bit more manageable regarding the problem?
- What is it like when the problem is a little less dominating in your life?
- What's different about those times?
- What do you do differently?
- Tell me about a specific time recently when things went a little bit better for you in regard to the concern that brought you in.
- What was different?
- What did you do differently?
- What are others doing when the problem is a little less noticeable?
- What persons, places, or things were helpful to you?
- How will you know when things are better with the concern or problem you're facing?

- What will be different in your life?
- What keeps you going and from giving up?

Notice that these questions are subtle and don't ask about extreme differences. We don't ask, "When don't you have the problem?" That is too big a leap for most and can prove invalidating for those who may get the sense that therapists are glossing over problems, moving too quickly, or perhaps focusing too extensively on solutions. It is important to let clients know that we understand their pain. Using questions that elicit small differences can do this and can be enough to help move in the direction of positive change. We now explore some specific content areas to ask strengths-based questions.

Personal Characteristics/Qualities

- What qualities do you have that have been or could be of help to you in times of trouble?
- What is it about you that allows you to keep going?
- What is it about you that seems to come to the forefront when you're facing difficult situations/problems?
- What is it about you that you keep going despite all that you've faced?
- Who are you that you've been able to face up to the challenges that life has presented you?
- What would others say are the qualities that you have that keep you going?
- What have the qualities that you possess allowed you to do that you might not have otherwise done?
- Given the type of person that you are, what do you do on a regular basis to manage the challenges that you face?
- How have you managed, in the midst of all that's happened, to keep going? How have you done that?
- Tell me about a time when you were able to deal with something that could have stopped you from moving forward in life. What did you do?

Culture/Ethnicity/Gender Identity/Religion-Spirituality

- What is your current gender identity?
- How do you describe yourself in terms of your gender identity?
- Do you think of yourself as straight, gay or lesbian, bisexual, transgender, transsexual, gender nonconforming, or other?
- What does your gender identity say about you?

- How do you identify culturally?
- How does your culture influence your everyday life?
- In what ways, in any, does your nationality influence your everyday life?
- What does spirituality or religion or higher power mean to you?
- How do you experience spirituality or religion or higher power?
- What is most meaningful to you about your (culture, ethnic background, nationality, spiritual beliefs, etc.)?
- How has this been a resource for you?
- How do you maintain its presence in your life?

Family/Social Relationships

- Who are you closest to in your (group, life, family, etc.)?
- What do you appreciate most about this relationship?
- What would he/she/they say are your best qualities as a (friend, father/mother, caregiver, uncle/aunt, grandparent, peer, etc.)?
- How is it helpful for you to know that?
- What does it feel like to know that?
- Which relationships have been more challenging/difficult for you?
- How have you dealt with those challenges/difficulties?
- Who can you go to for help?
- Who has made a positive difference in your life?
- How so?
- What difference has that made for you?
- When are others most helpful to you?

Work/Employment/Career

- How would you describe your current employment status?
- (If applicable) Would you say your employment represents a job, a career, or both? How so?
- (If applicable) How did you get your current job?
- (If applicable) How did you get yourself into position to get the job?
- (If applicable) What do you think your employer saw in you that might have contributed to your being hired?

- (If applicable) What have you found to be most challenging or difficult about your job?
- (If applicable) How have you met or worked toward meeting those challenges/difficulties?
- (If applicable) What keeps you at your job?
- (If applicable) What skills and qualities do you think you employer sees in you?
- (If applicable) What qualities do you think you possess that are assets to the job?
- (if unemployed) What kind of employment would you like to see yourself involved with in the future?
- (if unemployed) What qualities and skills do you bring to a job?
- What would be a first step for you in moving toward the kind of career you desire?

Education/School/Vocational Training

- How would you describe your current educational status (i.e., active or inactive in an educational program)?
- How did you manage to make it to/through (a specific grade, middle school, high school, trade school, 2 years of college, etc.)?
- What qualities do you possess that made that happen?
- What did you like best about school?
- What did you find most challenging/difficult about school?
- How did you manage any difficulties that you may have encountered while in school (completing homework/assignments, tests, getting to school on time, moving from one grade to another, teacher/classmate relationships, sports, etc.)?
- In what ways did school prepare you for future challenges?
- Do you aspire to continue your education?
- What might that do for you to continue your education?
- What would it take for you to continue your education?

Hobbies/Interests

- What do you do for fun?
- What hobbies or interests do you have or have you had in the past?
- What kinds of activities are you drawn to?

- What kinds of activities would you rather not be involved with?
- What would you rather do instead?

Previous Therapy (or Behavioral Healthcare) Experiences
- What did you find helpful about being in therapy in the past?
- What did the therapist (or other mental health professional) do that was helpful?
- How did that make a difference for you?
- What wasn't so helpful?
- What is one thing your therapist (or other mental health professional) failed to understand about you?
- What do you hope for most from therapy?
- (If currently or previously on psychotropic medication) How is/was the medication helpful to you?
- What, if anything, did/does the medication allow you to do that you wouldn't otherwise be (been) able to do?
- What qualities do you possess so that you were/are able to work with the medication to improve things for yourself?

These questions are a starting point. Although information gathering or assessment begins with initial contacts, we want to continue with strengths-based questions until outcomes and goals are met and there is a measurable benefit of therapy to the client.

Strengths-Based Exploratory Questioning

Formal, content-area questions are but one pathway of learning about clients and their lives. A second and more common pathway for information gathering is through less formal, exploratory conversation. Informal, exploratory conversations allow for questions to create space for client narratives or stories to emerge. This form of conversation is what most therapists and clients consider *real therapy*. Two (or more) people have a conversation about a concern one has and the other attempts to learn about that concern and help to resolve it.

Exploratory conversations are designed to create space for clients to tell their stories, with questions serving more as a guide, unlike standardized methods, which are more structured. It can be said that there is more "room" for conversations to evolve. Still, exploratory conversations are also purposeful because they afford opportunities to gain valuable information. We learn more about clients' expectations and preferences and work together to develop a mutual understanding of the purpose of services. Therefore, active listening is critical to effective questioning.

A collaborative posture is central to gathering information, and we extend this posture to others (i.e., family members, social service workers, probation officers, teachers) who may be involved or have investment in therapy. Being collaborative does not mean never being directive. Therapists may need to become more or less directive depending on client preferences, context, and issues such as safety, particularly when it comes to risk of harm to self or others.

Consistent with content-area questioning, the 80/20 rule provides guidance. We ask, What kinds of information will be most beneficial in deepening our understanding of the clients' predicament and in achieving some measurable, beneficial change? To orient to these questions, we refer to the initial ORS score. How did the client score? Is the client at or above the clinical cutoff? How did the client respond to the therapist's summary of the results of the ORS? A lack of focus and structure can contribute to client frustration and, perhaps, dropout or negative outcome. It is also clear that lack of agreement on the focus of services can lead to the selection of misguided methods that are a poor fit for clients, which will be discussed later in this chapter and in Chapters 5 and 6.

One way to begin to gain focus is by summarizing the results of the ORS as a conversation lead-in. Here is an illustration of how to do this following Example 4.1 from earlier in the chapter:

Example 4.5

On the scale we did a few minutes ago, you scored 18.3. From what you said, that matches how things have been at work and home. It hasn't been too great. Would it be okay if I asked you some questions to better understand what is going on and how I might help?

In the event that there is more than one person present in therapy, such a family member or other collateral, we include their perspectives. Here is how to do this, based on an earlier in-text example:

Example 4.6

A few moments ago, we talked about the differences between the scores each of you gave. Reggie, you scored 34. Your mom rated things at a 19.1. If it's okay, I'd like to ask a few more questions to help me to better understand the concerns. Is that okay with each of you?

Therapy continues with exploratory questions to gather further information and deepen the understanding of the impact that the problem is having on the client's life. Examples of questions to be asked here include:

- What is most important for me to understand about your life as it is now?
- What is most important for me to know about the problem you've been facing?

- How has the problem affected you? Individually (personally)? Interpersonally (very close and intimate relationships)? Socially (friends, work, school, community)? [Note: Refer to the individual subscale scores on the ORS for guidance.]

- What have others failed to understand about the problem you've been up against or about your situation?

A consideration for therapists is to determine whether to use *content* and/or *process* questions. Both content and process questions can be useful in therapy, but they serve different purposes. *Content* questions are aimed at gathering specifics about a person or situation. For example, we may want to know more about "what" a client is talking about. We ask, "What is on your mind?" *Process* questions inquire about "how." We ask, "How did you arrive at that idea?" Most therapists use a combination of content and process questions.

We also want to remain purposeful in what is being asked of clients. Beyond content and process, certain forms of questions can open up or close down conversations. In my experience, 4WH questions are very useful. The acronym stands for who, what, when, where, and how. Questions that begin with 4WH are exploratory because they tend to orient clients toward details. We might ask, "Who was with you when you first started feeling anxious?" "What were you doing when the anxiety started?" "When did you first notice yourself becoming anxious?" "Where were you when the anxiety began?" "How did you make it until the anxiety subsided?" Such questions require thought on the part of the client but are rather straightforward. In contrast, "why" questions may be used to understand clients' motivations or rationales. A potential problem with "why" questions is they can put clients on the defensive because they typically require them to provide explanations. Asking, "Why did you get anxious?" is very different than asking, "What led to you becoming anxious?" The matter of what kinds of questions to ask is not an "either/or" proposition. Again, our aim is to be purposeful by using questions to gain information that is likely to be helpful in the resolution of client concerns.

As information is gathered, the therapist wants to avoid the tendency to assume that enough is known to use more advanced methods of intervention. It is understood that therapists start to develop ideas and strategies and want to try to bring clients relief and perhaps even resolve concerns right away. Without sufficient information, premature attempts at problem solving can prove costly. For example, clients may feel cut off from telling their stories, attempts may be made to solve problems that aren't really problems (i.e., clients have not had the space to fully reveal what they are experiencing before the therapist steps in), and suggestions may be made for things that have already been tried and failed. The result may be the client losing faith in therapy and the therapist, the therapist losing credibility in the client's view, the client dropping out of therapy, and outcomes being negative.

To be clear, any time that a therapist is in conversation with a client, therapy is interventive. Conversation in and of itself can be healing. In most cases, however, more details will be necessary to provide sound rationale for the use of more advanced methods and techniques (e.g., desensitization, exposure, the empty chair). We want to ensure a good *fit* between the client and such methods and techniques so that the desired *effect* is achieved. To remain attuned to clients and their situations and avoid premature and, perhaps, misguided attempts at intervention, therapists focus on four things:

1. Maintain awareness regarding the impact of both verbal and nonverbal language
2. Acknowledge and validate
3. Check in regularly with the alliance
4. Continue with exploratory questions

1) Maintain Awareness of Verbal and Nonverbal Language

Previous chapters have offered distinctions and examples between pathology and strengths-based language. In Chapter 3, we learned about correlations between language and physical health. Language can affect our immediate physiological states. Some words can cause negative physical experiences such as heaviness in the body, tiredness, and even somatic sensations (e.g., stomach upset, body tension). Other words can lead to feeling physically stronger and having an increase in energy. But as it turns out, the implications of language are more far-reaching.

Research suggests that under certain conditions (e.g., stress, threats, catastrophic events), the frontal cortex of the brain, which is responsible for thinking, speech, and language, becomes inhibited, thereby limiting one's ability to reason and articulate thoughts (Gottman, 1999; van der Kolk, 1994; van der Kolk, McFarlane, & Weisaeth, 1996). Concurrently, portions of the area around the brainstem, including the amygdala and hypothalamus that are responsible for physiological reactions, become increasingly active. This combination contributes to hyperarousal, affecting one's ability to regulate emotion and think clearly. One implication of this research is the notion that under perceived stress, clients may experience both physiological arousal and psychological shutdown. The result is that clients may experience difficulty to self-soothe, regulate emotion, and respond in calm ways when under distress.

Therapists can respond to the physiological arousal–psychological shutdown in several ways. The first is to pay close attention to both their own and clients' verbal and nonverbal communication such as voice tone, volume, pitch, rate of speech, and body posture. We can accomplish this through *matching*.

Matching Language

As discussed, therapists need to remain aware of both verbal and nonverbal communication. Clients often communicate in patterns that can go unrecognized and unattended. Recall that higher ratings of client satisfaction are significantly related to similarity in client–therapist linguistic style. Matching clients' language through using words and phrases, speed, intonation, and patterns can help practitioners create inroads to strengthen connections and initiate change. The following example from the work of Milton Erickson (1965) illustrates this idea:

> A 25-year-old man named George was picked up by the police for irrational behavior and committed to the state mental hospital. His only rational utterances were, "My name is George," "Good morning," and "Good night." All of his other verbal offerings were continuous word-salad—a mixture of made-up sounds, syllables, words, and incomplete phrases. On any given day George might be heard saying, "Bucket of lard," "Didn't pay up," "Sand on the beach," or irrelevant, mixed-up words that did not make sense.
>
> For a few years, George sat by himself and mumbled his word-salad. Psychiatrists, psychologists, social service workers, nurses, other personnel, and even other patients had tried to engage him in intelligible conversation but to no avail. George would simply continue his word-salad, in conversation with himself. Over time, George began to greet people who entered the ward with an outburst of word-salad. In between, he sat by himself, seeming to be mildly depressed. When approached he would typically spit out a few minutes of anger-laced word-salad.
>
> Erickson joined the hospital staff during the sixth year of George's stay. He quickly learned about George and found that both staff and patients could sit next to him without eliciting word-salad as long as they did not speak to him. Erickson tried on occasion to learn his name, but all he got was an outpouring of garbled language. Erickson enlisted his secretary to transcribe, in shorthand, George's word-salad. Although no meaning could be discovered from the transcriptions, Erickson found that he could make use of them.
>
> Erickson carefully studied and learned George's pattern of using word-salad. He then paraphrased the word-salads, but used words that were least likely to be found in George's rants. Erickson could then improvise a word-salad pattern that was similar to George's, but with a completely different vocabulary.
>
> Erickson began to sit alongside George on a hospital bench that the patient frequented. He did this in increasing amounts of time until he was able to sit with George for an hour. At that point, Erickson addressed the empty air and identified himself but gained no response from George. The next day, he again identified himself, but this time directly to George. To this, George responded with an angry offering of word-salad. In reply, Erickson voiced out an equal amount of carefully contrived word-salad. George seemed puzzled, and uttered a small amount of word-salad back with an inquiring intonation. Erickson responded in word-salad as if to answer the inquiry. After a few more interchanges, George lapsed into silence.
>
> At their next meeting, both exchanged greetings and then George launched into a long word-salad speech. Erickson replied. He continued to

visit with George on a regular basis and had word-salad conversations each time. Some of the conversations were long and taxing on Erickson.

One morning, after their usual greetings, and a few sentences of nonsense, George said to Erickson, "Talk sense, Doctor." "Certainly, I'd be glad to. What's your name?" asked Erickson. "O'Donovan, and it's about time somebody who knows how to talk asked. Over five years in this lousy joint. . . ." (to which a couple of sentences of word-salad were added), replied George. Erickson responded, "I'm glad to get your name, George. Five years is too long a time. . . ." (adding an equal amount of word-salad at the end).

The conversation continued with Erickson gaining a complete history from George that was sprinkled with word-salad. Each time Erickson responded, he interspersed the same amount of word-salad back. Although George was never completely free of word-salad, he spoke clearly with only an occasional offering of unintelligible mumbles. This led him to be discharged from the hospital within a year and become gainfully employed. George eventually moved to a distant city, where he informed Erickson of his satisfactory adjustments. He ended his last correspondence with Erickson by signing his name properly and adding a few jumbled syllables.

The case illustration draws on the significance of speaking the same language as clients and moving away from psychological jargon that often accompanies conversations. Although they often introduce subtle changes in language to open up possibilities, therapists continuously adjust to clients' ways of communicating rather than having clients make the adjustments. Changes occur at the nonverbal communication level, which can be particularly important when clients appear to be resistant, disagreeable, noncompliant, uncooperative, or overly quiet or are tuning the therapist out (Bertolino & O'Hanlon, 2002). Instead of attending to such communication as resistance or lack of cooperation, therapists should consider whether clients are responding to what is being done or are pushing for change too quickly and not doing enough acknowledging. The remedy in such cases is to change processes and try to communicate better with clients so that they will feel heard and understood. The following are respectful ways to use matching language.

1. *Match clients' rate and pace of speech*. Match clients' rate and pace of speech as a way to join them. When in sync with the client, the therapist can change the rate and/or pace, if necessary, to promote relaxation and calmness, to neutralize anxiety, and so on. Take care to not come across as mocking or mimicking, which can be invalidating.

Client: [Quickly] I sometimes struggle to find the words . . . . [pause] like now.

Therapist: [Mirroring the client's pace] Sometimes it's hard to find the words . . . [pause] and that's okay.

Client: I can't. . . . I can't believe . . . All of this is so confusing.

Therapist: It's hard to believe. . . . It just seems so confusing.

2. *Match clients' general use of language.* Listen to the words that clients use and use aspects of that language to strengthen the therapeutic relationship.

Client: I just don't get it, man.

Therapist: Yeah, man, it does seem confusing.

Client: She just needs to chill. It doesn't help when she's all ballistic.

Therapist: If she were to chill a bit, what difference would that make for you?

3. *Match clients' use of sensory-based language.* Listen for and match clients' use of sensory-based (visual, auditory, kinesthetic/tactile, gustatory, olfactory) language.

Client: No matter where I turn, the message is the same, . . . "you'll never amount to anything."

Therapist: It seems like you've been hearing the same message from different directions.

Client: The way I see it, he'll never change.

Therapist: I see, . . . that's the vision you've had of him.

The methods offered for matching language can be used independently or in combination with any of the others discussed throughout this chapter.

A second way is to impart strengths-based language into conversations. Examples of how to do this were provided in Chapter 3. A third way is to avoid the use of unnecessary labels that can minimally upset clients and, at worst, depersonalize, stigmatize, and harm. People are people, not disabilities. Our language needs to reflect this fact. A disability may be an aspect of a person's life but does not identify who that person is as a person. Last, we can practice and develop good attending and listening skills.

2) Acknowledge and Validate

A second consideration is to ensure attunement with clients through *empathy*, *positive regard*, and *congruence* as they share their experiences. *Empathy* is a person's ability to understand another's perspective or way to experience the world. Meta-analyses by Bohart, Elliott, Greenberg, and Watson (2002) and Orlinksy, Grawe, and Parks (1994) have found a positive correlation between empathy and outcome. *Positive regard* is usually described as a person's warmth and acceptance toward the self or another. Using the Division 29 Task Force standard (Ackerman et al., 2001) of 50% or more in a study demonstrating an element as positively correlated with outcome, it can be said that positive regard is a moderator of successful outcome. In addition, a meta-analysis of 18 studies examining positive regard and outcome found a significant relationship (Farber & Doolin, 2011). Still further, positive regard has been shown to increase treatment retention (Farber & Lane, 2002). *Congruence*, sometimes referred to as genuineness, has been characterized by the helper's personal involvement in a relationship and willingness to share this awareness through open and honest communication. According to the Division 29 Task Force standard, a preponderance of evidence has indicated a significant positive relationship between congruence and outcome (Klein, Kolden, Michels, & Chisolm-Stockard, 2002; Lafferty, Beutler, & Crago, 1989; Orlinsky et al., 1994; Orlinsky & Howard, 1986). Although empathy, positive regard, and congruence can seem mysterious, perhaps because they exist in the experience of those we endeavor to help, they underscore the importance of feedback to learn about clients' experiences of therapeutic interactions.

A good way to communicate understanding, warmth, and interest in the client is through *acknowledgment* and *validation*. *Acknowledgment* involves attending to what clients have communicated both verbally and nonverbally. Doing so lets them know that their experience, points of view, and actions have been heard and noted. It also serves as a prompt to encourage further communication. One way to acknowledge is to say, "Uh huh" or "I see." Another is to reflect back, without interpretation, what was said. A therapist might say, "You're frustrated" or "I heard you say you're worried." Acknowledgment can also be conveyed by attending to nonverbal behaviors. For example, a therapist might say, "I noticed you shiver when you mentioned being around your mom" or "I can see the tears."

Validation is an extension of, and is most often used in conjunction with, acknowledgment. It involves letting clients know that whatever they are experiencing is valid. We want to communicate to clients that they are not bad, crazy, sick, or weird for being who they are and experiencing whatever they may. Therapists can use validation to normalize or convey that others have experienced the same or similar things. Validation is often expressed through statements such as, "It's/That's okay" or "It's/That's all right." To combine acknowledgment with validation, add words or statements such as "It's/That's okay" or "It's all right" to what is being acknowledged. A therapist using acknowledgment and validation might say, "It's okay to be sad" or "It's all right if you're angry" or "I heard you say that you're nervous, and you can just let that be there." Acknowledgment and validation are responses that should be used in all interactions.

It can also be effective to use acknowledgment and validation as part of reflection, which involves restating back to clients their feelings and words. Two primary ways of reflecting are through paraphrasing and summarizing.

Paraphrasing involves reflecting back to the client to affirm what has been said in a condensed, nonjudgmental way. Paraphrasing shows that the therapist is listening and attempting to understand what the client has said. Let's explore how to do this through examples.

Example 4.7

Client: My boss thinks his way is the only way. "Do this, do that." "Look at me when I'm talking." He's like a drill sergeant. He never lets up. I'm sick of it.

Therapist: Your boss' way of approaching you seems relentless to you—you wish he would cut you some slack.

Example 4.8

Client: I'm really feeling pressure with how to deal with Joanne. I mean, it's just one thing after another with her at home.

Therapist: It sounds like you're feeling a lot of pressure about how to deal with what's going on at home with Joanne.

Summarizing offers a way to check out what has been said by pulling together what a client has said over a period of time (i.e., a few minutes of conversation or different segments from different points of a conversation). Summarizing provides a brief synopsis to acknowledge, clarify, and gain focus. Next are examples.

Example 4.9

Client: [End of a lengthy statement] . . . That's about it. That's what's going on.

Therapist: Let me see if I follow you. You mentioned several things that seem to be on your mind. One is the arguing between you and your husband. Another is that it seems to you that things aren't really panning out so far in terms of finding a job. Is that right?

Example 4.10

Client: . . . I feel like I could just keep talking about it, but it wouldn't get me anywhere. My life is going down the drain, and there isn't anything I can do about it.

Therapist: It certainly seems like you've been through a lot in a short period of time. First, you thought you were doing better in school than you were. And when you got your grades, you were shocked. And on top of that what I'm hearing is that two people who you've been close to and have supported you moved away.

In Chapter 5, we will explore a myriad of ways to more actively and deliberately use language to facilitate change. Early in therapy, it is important that the therapist stay attuned to the client's story and convey an understanding of what the client is thinking and feeling. Doing so helps to strengthen the alliance, which increases the likelihood that more sophisticated linguistic interventions will take root.

3) Check-in Regularly With the Alliance

Studies have shown that the modal number of sessions clients attend is one, indicating that many clients do not return after the first session (Connolly Gibbons et al., 2011). Dropout rates are nearly 50% for adult therapy and even higher for children and adolescents (Garcia & Weisz, 2002; Kazdin, 1996; Lambert et al., 2003; Wierzbicki & Pekarik, 1993). The majority of clients who do not return to therapy do so because of a problem in the alliance. The SRS, which is completed near the end of each session, is an excellent tool for gaining feedback from the client about the alliance. Since changes to the alliance can happen suddenly and without any prior indication, it is crucial that therapists become accustomed to checking in with clients periodically as sessions progress.

Earlier in the chapter, the SONAR SFC was introduced. The N in *SONAR* stands for "Now." In this case, "now" refers to an ongoing process in which therapists inquire about clients' experiences in therapy; in effect, they keep their fingers on the pulse of the therapeutic alliance. By checking in with clients, therapists can gain valuable information in terms of what to do more of, do less of, or change. In some cases, clients' statements and/or nonverbal reactions in therapy will signal to the therapist that something has changed with the alliance. The idea here is for therapists to be more active in eliciting feedback, thereby reducing the chance that an alliance rupture may have occurred without their knowledge.

In many ways, the process of checking in with clients is akin to what healthcare professionals practice during medical procedures. They ask, "How are you doing so far?" or "Are you comfortable?" or "Are you experiencing any pain?" Understanding the patient's experiences is difficult—if not impossible—without feedback. In healthcare, patients who are more comfortable (in other words, experience lower levels of pain) typically recover faster. This idea applies fully to psychotherapy as well.

Check-ins can and should occur any time therapists want to better gauge a conversation, if there is a change in the way a client is relating (e.g., becomes very quiet after talking freely), or if a reaction of a client suggests that something may be "off." The following questions can be used during meetings/sessions to check in:

- Have you felt heard and understood?
- Do you feel/think we're talking about what you want to talk about?
- Have we been working on what you want to work on?
- How has the session been for you so far?
- Are we moving in a direction that seems right for you?

- What has the conversation we've been having been like for you?
- What has been helpful or not helpful?
- Are there other things that you feel/think we should be discussing instead?
- Is there anything I should have asked that I haven't asked?
- How satisfied are you with how things are going so far on a scale from 1 to 10, with 10 meaning you are completely satisfied with things?
- Are there any changes we should make at this point?
- To what degree has what we've been doing met your expectations so far?

Feedback allows therapists to learn whether services are on track or adjustments need to be made. Therapists also need to keep in mind that even in strong alliances, trouble spots and strains can occur. In fact, evidence suggests that alliances with "tears and repairs" can be better predictors of subsequent improvement than those that were stable and grew linearly (Kivlighan, 2001). The point is that therapists must respond to feedback and continue this practice throughout each session.

We are reminded of cultural differences that could influence how clients might respond to our questions. If a feedback-oriented approach is inconsistent with clients' cultural backgrounds, then we respond accordingly. Our aim is to invite clients to share their experiences so that we can be as helpful as possible, not to judge clients' motives or the quality of feedback. Most clients, if not asked for feedback, typically do not volunteer it. Poor alliances are a primary reason for clients to end services. Simply eliciting and responding to feedback reduces the risk of premature dropout, helps to get relationships back on track, and increases the likelihood of positive outcome. Research makes it clear that the most effective therapists are very attuned to clients' experiences of the alliance. In fact, one study found that 97% of the differences in outcome between therapists was attributable to differences in their ability to form alliances with clients (Anderson, Ogles, Patterson, Lambert, & Vermeersch, 2009; Baldwin, Wampold, & Imel, 2007).

4) Continue Exploratory Questioning

A final consideration for remaining attuned to clients and their situations to avoid premature and perhaps misguided use of methods and advanced strategies is to continue with exploratory questions, particularly those that have subtle interventive qualities. Doing this can both assist with gathering information and drawing clients' attention to what may gone "unnoticed." We consider questions that require clients to consider alternatives regarding their lives, concerns, or situations and can help deconstruct problematic views that can lead clients to reposition themselves in relation to the problems that brought them to therapy. Our questions can be particularly effective when they are both exploratory (or investigative) and *generative* because they facilitate the construction of new meanings.

Tomm (1988) described four different categories of questions: lineal, circular, strategic, and reflexive. Lineal questions are investigative, straightforward ones intended to gather facts. They can be open or close-ended (e.g., answered with "yes" or "no") and are most frequently cause-and-effect driven. Examples of lineal questions include:

- What is most anxiety provoking for you?
- How long has it been going on?
- Who else knows about your situation?
- What do you think about that?
- When is it most noticeable?
- Where does it happen most?
- How do others usually react when that is happening?

Questions are considered circular when they are used to bring forth connections, such as those between persons, objects, perceptions, ideas, feelings, actions, and/or events (Tomm, 1988). Circular questions are primarily systemic: They are used to learn more about the relationship between things and are posed from a position of curiosity or conjecture in which therapists wonder about, rather than imply, associations. Circular questions are also 4WH questions, as discussed earlier in the chapter. Examples include:

- What do you do when she does that?
- How does that affect you?
- What does your partner do when she sees you doing that?
- Who else does it that seems to affect?

Strategic questions propose options for viewing situations differently. In most cases, these types of questions have been used predominantly as a means of instruction (i.e., when the therapist behaves more like a teacher or instructor). Sometimes strategic questions can be used to move a stuck system and are intended to directly introduce different viewpoints. These are examples:

- Wouldn't you rather feel less anxious and leave those thoughts behind?
- When are you going to take a stance against that?
- What would happen if you decided to take action?
- Is this habit you have something you are okay living with?

The therapist's intent shapes the manner in which the questions are asked. When strategic questions prove a good fit for clients, they typically elicit useful information and stimulate change. Therapists should use discretion when using strategic questions, however. Because these types of questions require clients to take a position on their actions or situations, they can seem intrusive, which can lead to ruptures in the therapeutic alliance.

A final category posed by Tomm (1988) is reflexive questions, which are used to facilitate self-healing by creating new meanings that emerge from pre-existing belief systems. Reflexive questions are often used to help clients create new meanings by viewing their lives and situations in a different light or from a previously unforeseen position. They also represent a more inquisitive and "curious" stance on the part of therapists. Because they are process oriented, these questions can be used to focus on the future, facilitate self-awareness, gather information, explore context, and so on. Examples of reflexive questions include:

- How do you think your life will be different when you've gained the upper hand with this concern?
- From where you stand, what might be a reasonable response to that situation?
- What else have you considered?
- Who is most likely to notice the change first?
- How do you think it would go if you were to take that step?
- What difference might it make if you were to do that?

Because therapy is an interactional process, the more comfortable and skilled therapists become with generating and asking questions, the better they will become at gathering information. A further benefit of devoting time to the practice of questioning is that therapists learn to become more purposeful with their questions. In this way, therapists develop focused ways of gathering information that is most critical to clients and their situations, spending less time on conversations that, although interesting, provide no clear benefit to clients and extend therapy beyond what is necessary.

In this chapter, we explored how ACE can be used to gather information about clients, their lives, and situations. We began by revisiting the 80/20 rule to better understand the importance of collecting purposeful information to build integrity in our relationships with clients and make therapy outcome-informed. From there, we delved into details of ROM and FIT before moving to a discussion about interviewing for client strengths. With all information-gathering processes, our aim is to be interventive. We work to facilitate change in each interaction. The next chapter brings increased focus to information gathering by examining ways to establish direction in therapy, using language in subtle ways to both acknowledge and introduce the element of possibility, and formulating goals.

REFERENCES

Ackerman, S. J., Benjamin, L. S., Beutler, L. E., Gelso, C. J., Goldfried, M. R., Hill, C., . . . Rainer, J. (2001). Empirically supported therapy relationships: Conclusions and recommendations of the Division 29 Task Force. *Psychotherapy, 38*(4), 495–497. doi:10.1037/0033-3204.38.4.495

Anderson, T., Ogles, B. M., Patterson, C. L., Lambert, M. J., & Vermeersch, D. A. (2009). Therapist effects: Facilitative interpersonal skills as a predictor of therapist effects. *Journal of Clinical Psychology, 65*(7), 755–768. doi:10.1002/jclp.20583

Anker, M. G., Duncan, B. L., & Sparks, J. A. (2009). Using client feedback to improve couple therapy outcomes: A randomized clinical trial in a naturalistic setting. *Journal of Consulting and Clinical Psychology, 77*(4), 693–704. doi:10.1037/a0016062

Baldwin, S. A., Wampold, B. E., & Imel, Z. E. (2007). Untangling the alliance-outcome correlation: Exploring the relative importance of therapist and patient variability in the alliance. *Journal of Consulting and Clinical Psychology, 75*(6), 842–852. doi:10.1037/0022-006X.75.6.842

Barkham, M., Mellor-Clark, J., Connell, J., & Cahill, J. (2006). A CORE approach to practice-based evidence: A brief history of the origins and applications CORE-OM and CORE System. *Counselling and Psychotherapy Research, 6*, 3–15. doi:10.1080/14733140600581218

Bertolino, B. (2010). *Strengths-based engagement and practice: Creating effective helping relationships.* Boston, MA: Allyn & Bacon.

Bertolino, B. (2011). Building a culture of excellence: Anatomy of a community agency that works. *Psychotherapy Networker, 35*(3), 32–39.

Bertolino, B. (2013). The SONAR Session Feedback Checklist (SSFC) (v1.5). Retrieved from https://www.bobbertolino.com/handouts

Bertolino, B. (2014). *Thriving on the front lines: Strengths-based youth care work.* New York, NY: Routledge.

Bertolino, B. (2017). Feedback-informed treatment in an agency serving, children, youth, and families. In D. S. Prescott, C. L. Maeschalck., & S. D. Miller (Eds.), *Feedback-informed treatment in clinical practice: Reaching for excellence* (pp. 187–209). Washington, DC: American Psychological Association.

Bertolino, B., Axsen, R., Maeschalck, C., Miller, S. D., & Babbins-Wagner, R. (2013). Manual 6: Implementing feedback-informed work in agencies and systems of care. Chicago, IL: International Center for Clinical Excellence. Retrieved from https://scott-d-miller-ph-d.myshopify.com/collections/fit-manuals/products/manual-6-implementing-feedback-informed-work-in-agencies-and-systems-of-care

Bertolino, B., & Miller, S. D. (Eds.). (2013). *The ICCE manuals of feedback informed treatment* (Vols. 1–6). Chicago, IL: International Center for Clinical Excellence. Retrieved from https://scott-d-miller-ph-d.myshopify.com/collections/fit-manuals/products/the-complete-set-of-all-6-fit-manuals

Bertolino, B., & O'Hanlon, B. (2002). *Collaborative, competency-based counseling and therapy.* Boston, MA: Allyn & Bacon.

Bohart, A. C., Elliott, R., Greenberg, L. S., & Watson, J. C. (2002). Empathy. In J. C. Norcross (Ed.), *Psychotherapy relationships that work: Therapist contributions and responsiveness to patients* (pp. 89–108). New York, NY: Oxford University Press.

Bordin, E. S. (1979). The generalizability of the psychoanalytic concept of the working alliance. *Psychotherapy: Theory, Research, and Practice, 16*, 252–260. doi: 10.1037/h0085885

Burlingame, G. B., Lambert, M. J., Reisinger, C. W., Neff, W. L., & Mosier, J. (1995). Pragmatics of tracking mental health outcomes in a managed care setting. *Journal of Mental Health Administration, 22*, 226–236. doi:10.1007/BF02521118

Burlingame, G. B., Mosier, J. L., Wells, M. G., Atkin, Q. G., Lambert, M. J., & Whoolery, M. (2001). Tracking the influence of mental health outcome. *Clinical Psychology and Psychotherapy, 8*, 361–379. doi:10.1002/cpp.315

Burlingame, G. B., Wells, M. G., & Lambert, M. J. (1996). *Youth Outcome Questionnaire.* Stevenson, MD: American Professional Credentialing Services.

Burlingame, G. B., Wells, M. G., Lambert, M. J., & Cox, J. (2004). Youth Outcome Questionnaire: Updated psychometric properties. In M. E. Maruish (Ed.), *The use of psychological testing for treatment planning and outcome assessment* (3rd ed., pp. 235–273). Mahwah, NJ: Lawrence Erlbaum.

Chesworth, B., Filipelli, A., Nylund, D., Tilsen, J., Minami, T., & Barranti, C. (2017). Feedback-informed treatment with LGBTQ clients: Social justice and evidence-based practice. In D. S. Prescott, C. L. Maeschalck, & S. D. Miller (Eds.), *Feedback-informed treatment in clinical practice: Reaching for excellence* (pp. 249–265). Washington, DC: American Psychological Association.

Clement, P. W. (1994). Quantitative evaluation of 26 years of private practice. *Professional Psychology: Research and Practice, 36*, 105–113. doi:10.1037/0735-7028.25.2.173

Clement, P. W. (2008). Outcomes from 40 years of psychotherapy in a private practice. *American Journal of Psychotherapy, 62*, 215–239. doi:10.1037/0735-7028.25.2.173

Clement, P. W. (2013). Practice-based evidence: 45 years of psychotherapy's effectiveness in private practice. *American Journal of Psychotherapy, 67*(1), 23–46.

Connolly Gibbons, M. B., Rothbard, A., Farris, K. D., Wiltsey Stirman, S., Thompson, S. M., Scott, K., . . . Crits-Christoph, C. (2011). Changes in psychotherapy utilization among consumers of services for major depressive disorder in the community mental health system. *Administration and Policy in Mental Health, 38*, 495–503. doi:10.1007/s10488-011-0336-1

Crits-Christoph, P., & Mintz, J. (1991). Implications of therapist effects for the design and analysis of comparative studies of psychotherapies. *Journal of Consulting and Clinical Psychology, 59*(1), 20–26.

Drapeau, M. (2012). The value of tracking in psychotherapy. *Integrating Science & Practice, 2*, 2–6.

Duncan, B. L., Miller, S. D., Sparks, J. A., Claud, D. A., Reynolds, L. R., Brown, J., & Johnson, L. D. (2003). The Session Rating Scale: Preliminary psychometric properties of a "working" alliance measure. *Journal of Brief Therapy, 3*(1), 3–12.

Duncan, B. L., Miller, S. D., Wampold, B. E., & Hubble, M. A. (Eds.). (2010). *The heart and soul of change: Delivering what works in therapy* (2nd ed.). Washington, DC: American Psychological Association.

Dunn, T. W., Burlingame, G. M., Walbridge, M., Smith, J., & Crum, M. J. (2005). Outcome assessment for children and adolescents: Psychometric validation of the Youth Outcome Questionnaire 30.1 (Y-OQ®-30.1). *Clinical Psychology and Psychotherapy, 12*, 388–401. doi:10.1002/cpp.461

Erickson, M. H. (1965). The use of symptoms as an integral part of hypnotherapy. *American Journal of Clinical Hypnosis, 8*, 57–65. doi:10.1080/00029157.1965.10402461

Ericsson, K. A., Charness, N., Feltovich, P. J., & Hoffman, R. R. (Eds.). (2006). *The Cambridge handbook of expertise and expert performance.* New York, NY: Cambridge University Press.

Evans, C., Connell, J., Barkham, M., Margison, E., McGrath, G., Mellor-Clark, J., & Audin K. (2002). Towards a standardized brief outcome measure: Psychometric properties and utility of the CORE-OM. *British Journal of Psychiatry, 180*, 51–60. doi:10.1192/bjp.180.1.51

Farber, B. A., & Doolin, E. M. (2011). Positive regard. *Psychotherapy, 48*, 58–64. doi:10.1037/a0022141

Farber, B. A., & Lane, J. S. (2002). Positive regard. In J. C. Norcross (Ed.), *Psychotherapy relationships that work: Therapist contributions and responsiveness to patients* (pp. 175–194). New York, NY: Oxford University Press.

Garcia, J. A., & Weisz, J. R. (2002). When youth mental health care stops: Therapeutic relationships problems and other reasons for ending youth outpatient treatment. *Journal of Consulting and Clinical Psychology, 70*(2), 439–443. doi:10.1037/0022-006X.70.2.439

Gladwell, M. (2005). *Blink: The power of thinking without thinking.* New York, NY: Little, Brown and Company.

Goldberg, S. B., Rousmaniere, T., Miller, S. D., Whipple, J., Nielsen, S. R., Hoyt, W. T., & Wampold, B. E. (2016). Do psychotherapists improve with time and experience? A longitudinal analysis of outcomes in a clinical setting. *Journal of Counseling Psychology, 63*(1), 1–11. doi:10.1037/cou0000131

Gottman, J. M. (1999). *The marriage clinic.* New York, NY: W. W. Norton.

Haas, E., Hill, R. D., Lambert, M. J., & Morrell, B. (2002). Do early responders to psychotherapy maintain treatment gains? *Journal of Clinical Psychology, 58*(9), 1157–1172. doi:10.1002/jclp.10044

Harmon, S. C., Lambert, M. J., Smart, D. M., Hawkins, E., Nielsen, S. L., Slade, K., & Lutz, W. (2007). Enhancing outcome for potential treatment failures: Therapist-client feedback and support tools. *Psychotherapy Research, 17*(4), 379–392. doi:10.1080/10503300600702331

Horvath, A. O., & Greenberg, L. S. (1989). Development and validation of the Working Alliance Inventory. *Journal of Counseling Psychology, 36*(2), 223–233. doi:10.1037/0022-0167.36.2.223

Jacobson, N. S., & Truax, P. (1991). Clinical significance: A statistical approach to defining meaningful change in psychotherapy research. *Journal of Consulting and Clinical Psychology, 59*(1), 12–19. doi:10.1037/0022-006X.59.1.12

Jennings, L., & Skovholt, T. M. (2016). *Expertise in counseling and psychotherapy: Master therapist studies from around the world.* New York, NY: Oxford University Press.

Kazdin, A. E. (1996). Dropping out of child psychotherapy: Issues for research and implications for practice. *Clinical Child Psychology and Psychiatry, 1*, 133–156. doi:10.1177/1359104596011012

Kivlighan, D. (2001). Patterns of working alliance development. *Journal of Consulting and Clinical Psychology, 47*, 362–371. doi:10.1037/0022-0167.47.3.362

Klein, M. H., Kolden, G. G., Michels, J. L., & Chisolm-Stockard, S. (2002). Congruence. In J. C. Norcross (Ed.), *Psychotherapy relationships that work: Therapist contributions and responsiveness to patients* (pp. 195–215). New York, NY: Oxford University Press.

Lafferty, P., Beutler, L. E., & Crago, M. (1989). Differences between more and less effective psychotherapists: A study of select therapist variables. *Journal of Consulting and Clinical Psychology, 57*, 76–80. doi:10.1037/0022-006X.57.1.76

Lambert, M. J. (2010). *Prevention of treatment failure: The use of measuring, monitoring, and feedback in clinical practice*. Washington, DC: American Psychological Association.

Lambert, M. J., & Burlingame, G. R. (1996). *Outcome Questionnaire 45.2*. Wilmington, DE: American Professional Credentialing Services.

Lambert, M. J., Burlingame, G. R., Umphress, V., Hansen, N. B., Vermeersch, D. A., Clouse, G. C., & Yanchar, S. C. (1996). The reliability and validity of the Outcome Questionnaire. *Clinical Psychology, 3*(4), 249–258. doi:10.1002/(SICI)1099-0879(199612)3:4249::AID-CPP1063.0.CO;2-S doi:10.1002/(SICI)1099-0879(199612)3:4249::AID-CPP1063.0.CO;2-S

Lambert, M. J., & Finch, A. E. (1999). The Outcome Questionnaire. In M. E. Maruish (Ed.), *The use of psychological testing for treatment planning and outcome assessment* (2nd ed., pp. 831–864). Mahwah, NJ: Lawrence Erlbaum.

Lambert, M. J., Whipple, J. L., Hawkins, E. J., Vermeersch, D. A., Nielsen, S. L., & Smart, D W. (2003). Is it time for clinicians routinely to track outcome? A meta-analysis. *Clinical Psychologist, 10*, 288–301. doi:10.1093/clipsy/bpg025

Lambert, M. J., Whipple, J. L., Smart, D. W., Vermeersch, D. A., Hawkins, E. J., Nielsen, S. L., & Hawkins, E. J. (2001). The effects of providing therapists with feedback on patient progress during psychotherapy: Are outcomes enhanced? *Psychotherapy Research, 11*, 49–68. doi:10.1080/713663852

Lambert, M. J., Whipple, J. L., Vermeersch, D. A., Smart, D. W., Hawkins, E. J., Nielsen, S. L., & Goates, M. (2002). Enhancing psychotherapy outcomes via providing feedback on client progress: A replication. *Clinical Psychology and Psychotherapy, 9*, 91–103. doi:10.1002/cpp.324

Luborsky, L., Barber, J. P., Siqueland, L., Johnson, S., Najavits, L. M., Frank, A., & Daley, D. (1996). The revised Helping Alliance Questionnaire (HAq-II): Psychometric properties. *The Journal of Psychotherapy: Practice and Research, 5*(3), 260–271.

Maeschalck, C. L., & Barfknecht, L. R. (2017). Using client feedback to inform treatment. In D. S. Prescott, C. L. Maeschalck., & S. D. Miller (Eds.), *Feedback-informed treatment in clinical practice: Reaching for excellence* (pp. 53–77). Washington, DC: American Psychological Association.

Miller, S. D., & Bargmann, S. (2011). Feedback-informed treatment (FIT): Improving outcome with male clients one man at a time. In J. A. Ashfield & M. Groth (Eds.), *Doing psychotherapy with men* (pp. 194–207). St. Peters, Australia: Australian Institute of Male Health Studies.

Miller, S. D., & Duncan, B. L. (2000). *The Outcome Rating Scale*. Chicago, IL: Author. Retrieved from http://scottdmiller.com/wp-content/uploads/documents/OutcomeRatingScale-JBTv2n2.pdf

Miller, S. D., & Duncan, B. L. (2004). *The Outcome and Session Rating Scales: Administration and scoring manual*. Chicago, IL: Institute for the Study of Therapeutic Change.

Miller, S. D., Duncan, B. L., Brown, J. S., Sorrell, R., & Chalk, M. B. (2006). Using formal client feedback to improve retention and outcome: Making ongoing, real-time assessment feasible. *Journal of Brief Therapy, 5*, 5–22.

Miller, S. D., Duncan, B. L., Brown, J. S., Sparks, J. A., & Claud, D. A. (2003). The Outcome Rating Scale: A preliminary study of the reliability, validity, and feasibility of a brief, visual, analog measure. *Journal of Brief Therapy, 2*, 91–100.

Miller, S. D., Duncan, B. L., & Hubble, M. A. (1997). *Escape from Babel: Toward a unifying language for psychotherapy practice*. New York, NY: W. W. Norton.

Miller, S. D., Duncan, B. L., & Hubble, M. A. (2004). Beyond integration: The triumph of outcome over process in clinical practice. *Psychotherapy in Australia, 10*, 2–19.

Miller, S. D., Duncan, B. L., Sorrell, R., & Brown, G. S. (2005). The Partners for Change Outcome Management System. *Journal of Clinical Psychology, 61*(2), 199–208. doi:10.1002/jclp.20111

Miller, S. D., & Maeschalck, C. L. (2015, November). Understanding outcome and alliance data [Webinar]. *Fall FIT Webinar Series*. Retrieved from http://www.centerforclinicalexcellence.com/training-and-consulting

Miller, W. R., & Rollnick, S. (2013). *Motivational interviewing: Helping people to change* (3rd ed.). New York, NY: Guilford Press.

Mohr, D. C. (1995). Negative outcome in psychotherapy: A critical review. *Clinical Psychology: Science and Practice, 2*(1), 1–27. doi:10.1111/j.1468-2850.1995.tb00022.x

Moss, R. K., & Mousavizadeh, V. (2017). Implementing feedback-informed treatment: Challenges and solutions. In D. S. Prescott, C. L. Maeschalck, & S. D. Miller (Eds.), *Feedback-informed treatment in clinical practice: Reaching for excellence* (pp. 101–121). Washington, DC: American Psychological Association.

Okiishi, J., Lambert, M. J., Nielsen, S. L., & Ogles, B. M. (2003). Waiting for supershrink: An empirical analysis of therapist effects. *Clinical Psychology and Psychotherapy, 10*(6), 361–373. doi:10.1002/cpp.383

Orlinsky, D. E., Grawe, K., & Parks, B. K. (1994). Process and outcome in psychotherapy—noch einmal. In A. E. Bergin & S. L. Garfield (Eds.), *Handbook of psychotherapy and behavior change* (4th ed., pp. 270–378). New York, NY: Wiley.

Orlinsky, D. E., & Howard, K. I. (1986). The psychological interior of psychotherapy: Explorations with the therapy session reports. In L. S. Greenberg & W. M. Pinsof (Eds.), *The psychotherapeutic process: A research handbook* (pp. 477–501). New York, NY: Guilford Press.

Owen, J., Miller, S. D., Seidel, J., & Chow, D. (2016). The working alliance in treatment of military adolescents. *Journal of Consulting and Clinical Psychology, 84*(3), 200–210. doi:10.1037/ccp0000035

Percevic, R., Lambert, M. J., & Kordy, H. (2006). What is the predictive value of responses to psychotherapy for its future course? Empirical explorations and consequences for outcome monitoring. *Psychotherapy Research, 16*(3), 364–273. doi: 10.1080/10503300500485524

Prescott, D. S. (2017). Feedback-informed treatment: An overview of the basics and core competencies. In D. S. Prescott, C. L. Maeschalck, & S. D. Miller (Eds.), *Feedback-informed treatment in clinical practice: Reaching for excellence* (pp. 37–52). Washington, DC: American Psychological Association.

Prescott, D. S., Maeschalck, C. L., & Miller, S. D. (Eds.). (2017). *Feedback-informed treatment in clinical practice: Reaching for excellence*. Washington, DC: American Psychological Association.

Reese, R. J., Gillaspy, J. A., Owen, J. J., Flora, K. L., Cunningham, L. C., Archie, D., & Marsden, T. M. (2013). The influence of demand characteristics and social desirability on clients' ratings of the therapeutic alliance. *Journal of Clinical Psychology, 69*(7), 696–709. doi:10.1002/jclp.21946

Reese, R. J., Norsworthy, L. A., & Rowlands, S. R. (2009). Does a continuous feedback system improve psychotherapy outcome? *Psychotherapy: Theory, Research, Practice, Training, 46*, 418–431. doi:10.1037/a0017901

Robinson, B. (2017). Feedback-informed treatment with couples. In D. S. Prescott, C. L. Maeschalck, & S. D. Miller (Eds.), *Feedback-informed treatment in clinical practice: Reaching for excellence* (pp. 13–35). Washington, DC: American Psychological Association.

Sapyta, J., Riemer, M., & Bickman, L. (2005). Feedback to clinicians: Theory, research, and practice. *Journal of Clinical Psychology, 61*(2), 145–153. doi:10.1002/jclp.20107

Schuckard, E., & Miller, S. D. (2016). Psychometrics of the ORS and SRS: Results from RCTs and meta-analyses of routine outcome monitoring and feedback. Retrieved from http://scottdmiller.com/wp-content/uploads/2016/09/Measures-and-Feedback-2016.pdf

Schuckard, E., Miller, S. D., & Hubble, M. A. (2017). Feedback-informed treatment: Historical and empirical foundations. In D. S. Prescott, C. L. Maeschalck, & S. D. Miller (Eds.), *Feedback-informed treatment in clinical practice: Reaching for excellence* (pp. 13–35). Washington, DC: American Psychological Association.

Shimokawa, K., Lambert, M. J., & Smart, D. W. (2010). Enhancing treatment outcome of patients at risk of treatment failure: Meta-analytic and mega-analytic review of a psychotherapy quality assurance program. *Journal of Consulting and Clinical Psychology, 78*(3), 298–311. doi:10.1037/a0019247

Tilsen, J., Maeschalck, C., Seidel, J., Robinson, B., & Miller, S. D. (2013). Manual 5: Feedback-informed clinical work: Specific populations and service settings. In B. Bertolino & S. D. Miller (Eds.), *The ICCE manuals of feedback informed treatment*. Chicago, IL: International Center for Clinical Excellence.

Tomm, K. (1988). Interventive interviewing: Part III: Intending to ask lineal, circular, strategic, or reflexive questions? *Family Process, 27*(1), 1–15. doi:10.1111/j.1545-5300.1988.00001.x

van der Kolk, B. A. (1994). The body keeps score: Memory and the emerging psychobiology of posttraumatic stress. *Harvard Review of Psychiatry, 1*, 253–265.

van der Kolk, B. A., McFarlane, A. C., & Weisaeth, L. (Eds.). (1996). *Traumatic stress: The effects of overwhelming experience on mind, body, and society*. New York, NY: Guilford Press.

Walfish, S., McAlister, B., O'Donnell, P., & Lambert, M. J. (2012). An assessment of self-assessment bias in mental health providers. *Psychological Reports, 110*(2), 639–644. doi:10.2466/02.07.17.PR0.110.2.639-644

Wampold, B. E., & Brown, G. S. (2005). Estimating variability in outcomes attributable to therapists: A naturalistic study of outcomes in managed care. *Journal of Consulting and Clinical Psychology, 73*(5), 914–923. doi:10.1037/0022-006X.73.5.914

Wampold, B. E., & Imel, Z. E. (2015). *The great psychotherapy debate: The evidence for what makes therapy work* (2nd ed.). New York, NY: Routledge.

Warren, J. S., Nelson, P. L., Mondragon, S. A., Baldwin, S. A., & Burlingame, G. A. (2010). Youth psychotherapy change trajectories and outcomes in usual care: Community mental health versus managed care settings. *Journal of Consulting and Clinical Psychology, 78*(2), 144–155.

Whipple, J. L., Lambert, M. J., Vermeersch, D. A., Smart, D. W., Nielsen, S. L., & Hawkins, E. J. (2003). Improving the effects of psychotherapy: The use of early identification of treatment and problem-solving strategies in routine practice. *Journal of Counseling Psychology, 50*(1), 59–68. doi:10.1037/0022-0167.50.1.59

Wierzbicki, M., & Pekarik, G. (1993). A meta-analysis of psychotherapy dropout. *Professional Psychology: Research and Practice, 24*(2), 190–195. doi:10.1037/0735-7028.24.2.190

CHAPTER 5

Therapeutic Conversations for Achieving Structure and Direction

In the previous chapter, we explored ways to gather preliminary information through outcome measurement and interviewing. In doing so, we also examined points at which to engage clients in conversations to facilitate change. In this way, information gathering is interventive. Our next task is to work with clients to better formulate a direction for therapy to inform treatment planning. We can accomplish this through strategic questioning and advanced methods of listening and attending skills that both acknowledge and open up possibilities for present and future change. Done effectively, client–therapist alliances are further strengthened and therapy becomes more goal- and outcome-driven. We can then begin to select and match more advanced interventions (i.e., methods, techniques) to fit clients and their situations, which is a focus of Chapter 6.

FUNNELING: BRINGING FOCUS TO THERAPEUTIC CONVERSATIONS

In Chapter 3, a distinction between strengths-based and non–strengths-based (pathology) conversations was provided. Recall that there is no evidence that using deficit-oriented language enhances the therapeutic alliance or yields better outcomes. Conversely, a growing body of research reveals the negative effects of deficit- and pathology-based language (see Chapter 3). Most clients will benefit from conversations aimed at change and growth. There are, however, exceptions, such as when using strengths-based language is at odds with a client's preferred way of communicating. Just as people respond to different forms of empathy, one-size-fits-all approaches do not account for individual client's experience. A task of the therapist is to create conditions that are safe and supportive, which more often than not will involve conversations that highlight hope, competency, and positive change.

As we continue with the information-gathering processes described in the previous chapter, we begin to introduce more structure and direction in therapy. We do not avoid client conversations that drift or lose direction. Instead, we reorient clients by paraphrasing and summarizing what has been said *and* follow with well-thought-out questions to gain agreement about the purpose of therapy. For example, a therapist might use summarization to reorient a client:

> You seem to have quite a lot on your mind. You've mentioned several things, and I want to make sure I understand their relevance in your life. How does what you've just said connect with the concern that brought you to therapy?

There are many reasons that conversations can begin to drift. Sometimes, clients just need space to air out whatever is on their minds. There is always a degree of subjectivity when it comes to how long a conversation should continue or how much should be said by a client before the therapist begins to impart more direction. Paraphrasing and summarizing are but two ways to refocus conversations.

Another way to develop direction in the therapeutic conversation is through funneling (Bertolino, 2014). *Funneling* involves moving from broad conversations to focused ones. The following questions may be useful in developing further focus:

- How can our conversation help me to better understand what you are most concerned about right now?
- Based on what you have told me so far, what is most important for me to understand about you or your situation?
- What can you tell me that would really help me to understand how you want things to be like for you in the near future?
- What would you like to have different with your situation/life?
- What would you like to see change?
- What are your best hopes?
- What did you hope would be different as a result of coming here?
- How would you know that the problem that brought you here is no longer a problem?
- What would have to be minimally different to consider working with me/us a success?

Questions such as the ones above are meant to help clients in the creation of well-articulated, preferred futures. Some clients will need more encouragement to help them to imagine what is possible and how their futures can be different and better than the past. The result of asking questions that begin to orient clients toward the future and a more concentrated sense of direction will lead most of them to respond in one of two ways. They could describe what they do not want, which is useful information because it can help therapists to understand more about clients' concerns and problems. The other way clients typically respond is by conveying what they do want. Whether describing what they do or do not want, clients commonly respond with statements such as, "I want to be happy," "I just want some peace," "I want to get rid of anxiety," "I don't want to be depressed," or "I don't want him to be so argumentative." The problem with these statements is they are vague and not descriptive.

Vague words and ambiguous statements can activate therapists' beliefs, biases, and theoretical opinions and lead them to assume that they know what clients mean. Imagine, for example, a client says that he is "anxious." By not taking time to find out what he means by this, the therapist is at risk of relying on personal experience and understandings of anxiety to guide change processes. Although experience working with clients who have reported "anxiety" in the past may be an asset, the problem is ambiguous without a description of the client's experience and could lead to misguided attempts at problem resolution. To guard against this, it is important for the therapist to elicit clear descriptions of clients' concerns. *Action-talk* provides a way of clarifying unclear, vague descriptions.

Action-Talk: Clarifying Client Concerns

One of the places that therapy can go off track is when there is a lack of understanding about client concerns. The quest for clarity involves questions that help to translate vague, ambiguous client statements into behaviorally based descriptions. These kinds of questions also assist with understanding the impact of the problem on the client's functioning, which incorporates the Outcome Rating Scale (ORS) and its subscales (i.e., individual, interpersonal, and social). To gain clear descriptions, therapists use action-talk (Bertolino & O'Hanlon, 2002). Action-talk involves determining how clients "do" their problem concerns and subsequently, what they will be doing when positive change has occurred and/or goals have been met.

To use action-talk, when clients use vague, non–sensory-based words, phrases, statements, or labels, therapists follow up with questions to turn elicit action- or interaction-based (i.e., involving two or more people) descriptions. For example, if a client says, "I'm depressed," the therapist is likely to begin with a question most are trained to ask, "Could you tell me what you mean by 'depressed?'" How the client answers this question may or may not lead to clarification. In fact, it could lead to further ambiguity if the client replies, "I feel down in the dumps. You know, general malaise."

Action-talk is reliant on a different kind of questioning. We want to understand *how* the client *does* depression. We ask, "Can you describe for me what you do or don't do when you are depressed?" or "How would I know by watching you each day that you were depressed? What would I see?" The idea is to learn specifics such as, does the client oversleep? Miss work? Eat too much or not enough? Our aim is to use action-talk to clarify—to understand more about how "depression," in this case, is expressed in the client's life.

There are five forms of action-talk, the first of which applies to understanding client concerns:

1. *Action problems:* Descriptions of a person does not like or is unhappy with about life.
2. *Action complaints:* Communication to others about what they have done or are doing that is disliked, undesirable, or problematic. The communication should be clear and descriptive (what can be seen or heard) and void of explanations or interpretations about other's motives, intentions, or character.
3. *Action change:* Descriptions of what a person would like to have change and/or improve in life.
4. *Action requests:* Descriptions of what actions are being requested of others in the present and future, again void of interpretations, characterizations, and vagueness.
5. *Action praise:* Statements to others about what has been or is being done that the person likes, appreciates, or values and would like to have continue.

As mentioned, client problem descriptions can be compared to ORS scores. Is the client's description of the problem consistent with the ORS? Does the problem description help with understanding which area or areas of the client's life are most affected? Returning to the previous example, is the client's description of depression reflected in a low score on the "interpersonal" subscale. Are other subscales influenced as well? The therapist might align the client's action-talk description and ORS scores in the following way:

Dialogue Example 5.1: Aligning Action-Talk and the ORS

Therapist: Can you describe what you do or don't do that would help me to better understand what you mean by being depressed?

Client: Mostly I think negative things—like, I'm not good at anything. And that my life hasn't gone the way I thought it would.

Therapist: Okay. You think negative things about yourself. And is it a few periodic thoughts or does it seem like you have quite a few negative ones?

Client: Oh, I have those negative thoughts a lot. Don't get me wrong, it's not like I want to die. I'm just unhappy and keep thinking these negative things.

Therapist: And how have those negative thoughts affected you?

Client: I don't take care of myself like I should. I don't eat well or work out anymore. I eat junk I never used to eat and don't go running anymore. I used to love to run.

Therapist: I think I understand. If I were a friend of yours and saw you, I might be able to tell you were depressed because you would be eating things not typical for you and maybe not running, which you've enjoyed in the past.

Client: Exactly.

Therapist: Your ORS score is 21.2, which is consistent with others who are also struggling with something and seeking the help of someone like me. And the first subscale, the "individual" scale, is at a 4.5, which is right in line with what you've just told me. I also see that the second subscale, the "interpersonal" scale, is at 4.8. Can you say more about that?

Client: Well, how I'm feeling has affected my love life. I haven't had a date in months. So, there's just not much happening there.

Therapist: Let me see if I understand the whole picture for you. You've been having some negative thoughts that have affected how you view your life and your self-care. And those thoughts have gotten in the way of you having the love life you'd like to have. Does that capture what you mean by being depressed?

Client: Yes, it does.

Therapist: Okay. Now, the third subscale, the "social" scale is just a shade higher at 6.3. Tell me about that.

Client: You know, work isn't too bad and I've got some good friends. I mean, I'd like to go out more but I'm a little more optimistic about that part of my life.

Therapist: Is it fair to say that that twinge of optimism you have about work and your friends has influenced the score of 5.6 you gave on the "overall" subscale?

Client: Yeah, my work and friends have kept me going.

The better the description, the more clarity we can have in terms of what the problems look like in clients' lives and how they are affecting their lives. The following questions can assist with gaining such clarity:

- When you are experiencing (concern or problem), what specifically is happening or not happening?
- What do you do or are you doing when you are in the throes of (concern or problem)?
- How do you experience (concern or problem)? [Listen for experiential, cognitive, behavioral, interactional, neurobiological, or some combination of these descriptors.]

In addition to understanding the effects of the problem, as in the previous dialogue example, we can also use ORS scores for comparison to determine consistency or differences to be explored. Last, action descriptions can also reveal strengths and exceptions to problems. We learned through the client illustration that there are resources in the client's life that may be helpful in achieving an improved outcome.

A variation of action-talk is *video-talk*, which involves using action-talk to describe the problem as if it could be seen or heard on video. We ask, "If I were to watch a video of you being/experiencing (concern/problem) what would I see you doing that would indicate to me that you were being/experiencing (concern/problem)?" If ambiguity persists, the therapist requests further clarification. Although it is not necessary to use clever language to engage clients in action-talk, adding an element of creativity can stimulate conversation and in some cases, provide a better fit for a client. In the next section, we will explore this idea further.

The use of action-talk is not limited to problem descriptions. It can be useful at any point in therapy in which clarification is needed. Next, we will learn how action-talk can be used to establish agreement on the meaning and purpose of therapy.

Goal Consensus: Agreement on the Meaning or Purpose of Treatment

In addition to gaining vivid problem descriptions, a second reason action-talk is so valuable is that it provides a means of identifying what clients would like to have change as a result of therapy. The focus becomes one of *action change*, which relates to the goals of therapy. By goals, we mean agreement on what the client hopes will be different as a result of therapy. Establishing an understanding of what clients want and what tasks appropriately fit those wants is crucial to successful therapy.

We first distinguish between goals and outcomes, the latter of which has been discussed at different points in this book. To recap, *outcomes* refer to the client's rating of the impact (benefit) of treatment on well-being and functioning (i.e., individual, interpersonal, social). In contrast, *goals* are clearly defined, observable, and measurable descriptions of what clients (and others involved) would like to have different in their lives. Most therapists are familiar with goals as they are part of treatment planning. Still, the concept of goals may be off-putting to some clients and even some therapists (Bertolino, 2010, 2015). Clients will say, "I don't really think that way" or "I don't really have goals, just things I want to be better." We strive to use the language of our clients, understanding that the point is to collaborate with clients to achieve a clear vision of the purpose of services.

To form agreement about the purposes of therapy, we ask clients (and others who may be involved), "How will you know therapy has been successful?" Our aim is to be clear as to what they believe needs to happen for services to be deemed effective or beneficial. In this sense, goals should be achievable in the context of therapy. There are two characteristics of achievable goals. They are (a) collaborative, agreed-upon by all parties involved; and (b) defined in clear, descriptive terms.

Earlier, it was mentioned that when asked about what clients' hopes for change are, they will respond in one of two ways. First, they will say what they do not want. For example, a client may say, "I don't want to be depressed," "I don't want to be so angry all the time," or "I want to stop arguing with my wife." A second kind of client response is to describe change in ambiguous ways. Clients will say, "I want to be satisfied with my life," "I want to have a better relationship," or "I want to have more energy." In the case of the former, we work with clients to describe what they would like to have happen *instead* of the problem. We say, "Instead of being depressed, how would you like things to be in your life?" When client responses are vague, we again turn to action-talk. We inquire, "What will be happening in your life when you are feeling more satisfied with it?" If a client provides another nondescriptive statement, the therapist requests clarification. For example, a therapist might say, "I have an idea of what feeling satisfied with life looks like for me. Help me to understand what it means to you. If I were to see you in six months and I could clearly tell that you were more satisfied with life, what would I see you doing?" The therapist might follow with, "And how would it be different from the way things are now?"

We are reminded that vague descriptions of both problems and goals can lead to misguided attempts at intervention, the repercussions of which can include loss of faith in therapy, loss of therapist credibility, frustration, negative outcome, and dropout. Our aim, then, is to engage clients in conversations about what they want to be different in their lives or situations so that we can spend less time on ambiguous descriptors (i.e., anxiety, depression) and more on changing actions and behaviors. The questions below can assist with using action-talk to gain perspective on client goals:

- How will you know when the problem is no longer a problem? What will be different?
- When you feel that you have turned the corner and are doing better, what will you be doing differently? What difference will that make for you?
- How will you know therapy has been successful?
- How will you know when you no longer need to come and see me for therapy? What will be different?

To better understand how to conceptualize goals, we revisit Case Example 5.1 from earlier in the chapter:

Case Example 5.1 (continued)

Therapist: I think I have a pretty good idea of what you mean by being depressed and the effect it's had on you. You mentioned that your negative thoughts have affected your care of yourself and have been a hurdle to the love life you'd like to have. Is that right?

Client: That's right.

Therapist: Now, I'd like to see if I can get a sense of how you'd like things to be moving forward. Let's fast forward ahead in time . . . just a few short months from now. Imagine you're three months down the road, and things have improved for you with the concerns that brought you to see me. If I were to run in to you on the street, how would I know that things were looking up?

Client: For one, I'd be smiling. That doesn't happen much these days. I might also be with a girlfriend or at least someone I was interested in. You never know!

Therapist: That's right, you never know! And what would you be smiling about?

Client: Probably the girlfriend! But I think I'd just be more satisfied about things.

Therapist: Say more about that. . . .

Client: Well, I'd like to be in a relationship but more I think about that, the more I realize that it will come when I am happier with myself. . . . More satisfied with myself.

Therapist: That's a really good observation. Sounds wise. I'm curious about being more satisfied. How so?

Client: Well, I wouldn't be so down on myself. You know, having those negative thoughts.

Therapist: What kind of thoughts would you be having instead?

Client: I'd be thinking more about what I could be doing rather than what I haven't done. And even if I had a setback, I'd say to myself, "No big deal. Everyone has ups and downs." I might even be a little inspired about something.

Therapist: So, your thoughts would be more about what you might be doing and perhaps even feeling some inspiration. . . . And it sounds like a big difference is you would be putting any challenges in context by saying to yourself, "Everyone faces challenges—ups and downs."

Client: That's exactly it.

Therapist: And how would I know you were inspired by something?

Client: I'd probably tell you about something I was interested in. . . . I'm not sure, maybe a work project, a relationship, or maybe even a trip I was taking.

Therapist: All good things! So, there would be a little inspiration there.

Client: For sure.

Therapist: And as a result of the new thoughts you were having, what would you be doing self-care wise?

Client: Definitely eating better—making better choices about that and going to the gym regularly.

Therapist: So maybe once in a while you might have something out of the ordinary but mostly you'd be making better food choices for yourself. . . . And when you say going to the gym regularly, how often would you say?

Client: At least four times a week.

Therapist: I see. Anything else that you would be doing that would let me know just how different things were for you?

Client: I think the main thing is I would be taking care of myself.

Therapist: By taking care of yourself you mean you'd be consistently making better choices about food, hitting the gym on average four times a week, and your thoughts would be more on what you want to pursue moving forward in life and maybe even feeling inspired by something. And that could be related to having something fun planned for yourself or something else in your life.

Client: Yeah. That pretty much sums it up.

Therapist: It also sounds like I heard you say that you were handling challenges better. If you faced a hurdle you'd put it in context and move from it.

Client: Absolutely.

Therapist: Got it. So how will you know you no longer need to come and see me?

Client: When I am able to eat well and work out at least three times for two consecutive weeks. Because that would mean I'm no longer falling into negative thinking.

Therapist: Right, even if you had negative thoughts, they wouldn't last, and you'd tune right back into life because you'd say to yourself, "Everyone has ups and downs."

Clients: Totally. That's exactly it.

For the client in the case example, there would be several goals. A first would be to improve care of self by making better choices about food and going to the gym on average four times a week. Next would be focusing his thoughts more on what he wants to pursue moving forward in life (which may provide some inspiration). Notice that the client initially talked about the effects of how he was feeling on his love life and that he had not had a date in a while. The interpersonal subscale score on his ORS corroborated how he was feeling. But as the conversation progressed, the client appeared to come to a new realization—that it might be better to focus on himself at this time. Therefore, no goal was developed around having a relationship at this point in therapy.

A further consideration with this example relates to client outcome scores. If we were to look at any full-scale ORS score or subscale void of client feedback, we might easily misunderstand the client and/or begin to assume things that may be false and derail therapy. Scores from outcome measures are only numbers. It is up to therapists to ask questions to understand the meanings of scores.

There are two additional considerations with determining goals. First, at times, clients will express a desire to change something that is simply not possible. For example, it is reasonable for a client who has lost someone close to want that person to return. Often, what a client requests symbolizes something else. In this case, it may be possible for the client to experience a caring relationship with another person, if that is what is hoped for. By acknowledging clients' internal experiences and views, therapists can neutralize many unrealistic expectations and cocreate a realistic goal, as illustrated in the following example.

Client: My aunt died last year. I wish she were still here. I really miss her. That's really what I want . . . her to be back. I know that sounds ridiculous, but I really miss her.

Therapist: I'm very sorry about your loss. And it's not ridiculous to want her back. I can hear much you miss her. She must have been very important to you. What do you miss most about her?

Client: She used to listen to me . . . really listen to me.

Therapist: How did you know when she was really listening to you?

Client: She would look me in the eyes and not judge me.

Therapist: What did she do to let you know that she wasn't judging you?

Client: Well, she didn't make comments like, "You should have . . ." or "That was stupid to do that."

Therapist: I see. And how did that help you?

Client: I knew she valued me and I haven't had that since.

Therapist: Is that something you would like to experience again in a relationship with someone—that sense of being listened to, not judged, and valued?

Client: I would love to have that again.

Therapist: What would be different for you as a result of having that again?

Client: I'd feel great. I'd feel better about going through each day knowing that I could talk with somebody who understood me.

When clients propose changes that are unrealistic we want to be sure we are listening carefully to what they are expressing. In most situations, we can help clients achieve some variation of their goals or what their goals symbolize. In other cases, acknowledgment will assist with filling emotional voids, allowing for both clients and therapists to regroup and work together to find something to work toward (Bertolino, 2014).

A second consideration is when a client has multiple concerns. In such cases, it can be helpful to summarize and acknowledge each concern and inquire as to which ones are most pressing. If all concerns are of equal weight to the client, we work to determine which concerns should be addressed first. One way to do this is to say,

> It seems that you have several concerns, all of which are important. I want you to know that we'll address them all. To get us started, please tell me which one or two of the concerns you mentioned rise to the top and should be looked at first.

It is well established that having agreement about the meaning or purpose of therapy is essential to outcome. Such agreement hinges on the therapist having a clear idea of the concern and the definition of improvement from the client's vantage point. In addition to asking straightforward questions about what clients want to change in their lives, a host of creative methods have been developed to intensify the focus of therapy and determine goals. Let us turn our attention to a few examples.

The Question

Alfred Adler (1956), the creator of individual psychology, maintained a present-to-future focus in his work and developed what became known as "the question." Rudolf Dreikurs (1954) later developed this frequently overlooked method. "The question" is, "Let us imagine I gave you a pill and you would be completely well as soon as you left this office. What would be different in your life, what would you do differently than before?" (p. 132). This method is considered by some as a precursor to the miracle question, which will be discussed next.

The Miracle Question

In the 1980s, Steve de Shazer (1988) and colleagues at the Brief Family Therapy Center (BFTC) developed the miracle question, which has since become synonymous with solution-focused brief therapy (SFBT). This method is used to help clients envision their lives in futures when their problems have been solved. The miracle question is generally set up by the therapist, encouraging the client to use his or her imagination. The therapist then asks, "Suppose you were to go home tonight, and while you were asleep, a miracle happened and this problem was solved. How will you know the miracle happened? What will be different?" (p. 5). This question is followed up in detail with questions about the miracle scenario given.

The Crystal Ball (Pseudo-orientation in Time)

Milton Erickson's (1954) "pseudo-orientation in time" is also considered a precursor to the miracle question. Erickson used this method hypnotically by having his patients positively hallucinate (i.e., see something that isn't really there) three crystal balls—one each representing the past, present, and future. He would have his patients peer into the crystal ball of the future and suggest that they could see what their lives would look like without the problems that brought them to therapy. Erickson would then have his patients describe, in detail, how their problems were resolved. Later, he would prescribe the remedies provided by his patients. Clinicians can use the same process without the hypnosis by having clients look out a window, at a blank wall, or at a piece of paper onto which they can imagine (or act as if they are seeing a movie) a future in which their problems are resolved (or alleviated to the degree that they no longer need to come to therapy) and describe that future as clearly as possible. The therapist uses action-talk to follow up with questions to have clients describe how their problems were resolved. A last part of the process is to have clients identify steps to make their future visions reality.

The Time Machine

A method that also involves some imagination and can be particularly useful for children and adolescents is the time machine (Bertolino, 1999). It is a way to help your clients envision a future where things work out. The time machine is introduced as follows:

Imagine there is a time machine sitting here in the office. You climb in and it propels you into the future, to a time when things are going the way you want them to go. After arriving at your future destination, the first thing you notice is that the problems that brought you to therapy have disappeared during the time travel.

The therapist follows with questions such as:

- Where are you?
- Who is with you?
- What is happening?

- What are you doing?
- How is your life different than before?
- Where did your problems go?
- How did they go away?
- Who, if anyone, helped you?
- How do you feel now that your problems have gone away?
- What can you do now?

Create Your World

For some clients, particularly children and youth, physical props (such as pictures, drawings) will help with developing a future-focus. For example, young people could be asked to create the future they would like by drawing a picture or using cutouts from magazines. The idea is to use what fits for the child or youth. Whether using basic questions or creative methods, therapists want to help clients to gain clarity and answer the rudimentary question, "How will you know when things are better?" Once what the client wants is clear, the therapist can begin to work with on steps to make those positive changes occur.

In each case, therapists keep in mind that methods and techniques are merely means to learning what clients want but contribute little to the overall variance in outcome. It is not the method that matters, but what the methods help to achieve with clients. Too much reliance on methods can lead to therapy that is "one-size-fits-all."

Goal-Setting With Multiple Clients and Outside Helpers

When working with multiple clients as with a couple or family, the therapist attends to each person's preferences, and goals, and ideas about therapy. There are likely to be different views expressed from persons involved, yet most often there are common threads among the complaints and identified goals. In searching for commonality, we coordinate complaints and goals by using three processes—acknowledgment, tracking, and linking (Bertolino, 2010). The therapist acknowledges and restates each person's perspective in the least inflammatory way possible while acknowledging and imparting the intended feeling and meaning. Statements that do so are linked by the word *and* because doing so builds on a common concern between all involved. Case Example 5.2 illustrates how to use acknowledgment, tracking, and linking.

Case Example 5.2: Setting Multiple Goals

Clarence (father): I just want her to return to school. It's ridiculous for her to be out. And besides, if she doesn't go, she'll never get the kind of job she wants.

Therapist: You're concerned because your sense is that there's really no reason for a 16-year-old to be out of school and that it could negatively affect her future.

Clarence: Right.

Alexis (daughter): What's the point? I can't stand school. Besides, if you're gonna continue to be on my case, then I'll never go back!

Eddie: See, that's what I get every day!

Therapist: I can see that it's been rough on both of you. And for you Clarence, you haven't found a reason to go to school and to tolerate it yet.

Alexis: Yeah. School is boring and if he doesn't back off . . . then, forget it.

Therapist: And what do you mean by your dad being "on your case"?

Alexis: He constantly says, "You better go. You better go. You can't miss another day!" It's like he thinks that I don't have a clue! I know that I need to graduate to get a good job. Duh!

Therapist: Okay, and the ways that he's tried so far to get you to go haven't work so well for you?

Alexis: Nope.

Therapist: Let me see if I'm following the two of you. Clarence, you'd really like Alexis return to school, finish her education, and have a better chance of reaching her dreams. And Alexis, you seem to have some dreams for yourself, and even though I haven't heard about them yet, perhaps school is a part of that in some way. So, you'd like to find a way to tolerate school so that you can graduate and work toward the career you want. And maybe there are other ways that your dad can be helpful to you with that—ways that don't involve him telling you to go, because you already know that—but ways that you see as being supportive with school.

Maintaining a collaborative posture, we work to create consensus among those involved through acknowledgment, tracking, and linking. *Acknowledgment* assists by letting each person involved know personal concerns have been heard and are valid. *Tracking* allows the therapist to log and follow each concern, and *linking* provides the thread that weaves each concern together to create mutually agreeable goals. Whether families or other multiple-client variations, clients are free to clarify any misperceptions or areas of discomfort until agreement emerges.

Similarly, when outside helpers (i.e., stakeholders) are involved, we maintain a collaborative posture. In doing so, we engage in conversations to learn about outside helpers' expectations and goals, keeping in mind that those who have stakes in the lives of clients often carry some level of responsibility and ability to alter the course of or end treatment. A good starting point is to first create consensus as to "what" needs to change or be different before exploring "how" best to accomplish those goals. Case Example 5.3 offers a way to work collaboratively with an outside entity.

Case Example 5.3: Goal-Setting and Outside Helpers

Therapist: Can you tell me what you hope to have addressed in therapy with Shane?

Probation Officer (PO): Shane's attitude. He seems to think that probation is a joke.

Therapist: What has happened that's given you that idea?

PO: He's stolen, and he keeps thinking that the next time he won't get caught even though he has [been caught] many times.

Therapist: You're concerned about Shane's history of stealing and that he might do it again.

PO: Yes. I think he will do it again.

Therapist: What might you see happening with Shane that would really lead you to wonder if he had changed his ways?

PO: It's very simple. He'd have to quit stealing. And I'd add that Shane would also have to be more respectful to me.

Therapist: And what would he be doing that would indicate that he was being more respectful toward you?

PO: He would talk calmly to me and agree to do what I ask him to do.

Therapist: Shane, what do you think about what your PO is saying?

Shane: Same old song and dance.

PO: That's exactly what I'm talking about. He's always sarcastic. . . .

Therapist: So, the sarcasm would drop out . . . and what would you see as a respectful way to responding to you?

PO: "Yes, sir" would be great. Heck, I'd settle for "okay." But the flip attitude has to go. It's flat-out disrespectful.

Therapist: Shane?

Shane: Fine.

Therapist: So, one thing is how Shane responds to you. The other is for Shane to not steal anymore and instead make positive choices about his life.

PO: Yes.

Therapist: What do think about that, Shane?

Shane: It's fine. I know that's what I'm supposed to do.

Therapist: Okay, but does it sound reasonable to you?

Shane: Of course.

PO: There's the sarcasm again.

Therapist: How do you differentiate between what's Shane just being Shane and what's cutting, disrespectful sarcasm?

PO: I get your point. It just seems unnecessary to act like that.

Therapist: Sure. And I'll bet you hear your share of sarcasm.

PO: Yeah, and it wears on you after a while.

Therapist: I can see why.

PO: But as long as he doesn't swear at me and acknowledges what I expect of him, I can let the rest slide.

Therapist: How does that sound, Shane?

Shane: I can live with that.

Therapist (to PO): What, then, might you see Shane do that would at least make you wonder a little if he's turned the corner with stealing and is ready for a probation-free life?

PO: If he went six months with no further incidents of stealing—well, any violations, other than a parking ticket, for that matter. But I can't see that happening. He's never gone more than a month before.

Therapist: So you would be surprised?

PO: That's putting it mildly. I'd be shocked.

Shane: Now that's sarcastic.

Therapist: From what I can tell, you both have a flair for sarcasm!

PO: That's for sure.

Therapist: Okay, well, for the sake of clarity, when Shane has gone six months without any major violations, what will that mean?

PO: I'll advocate for his release from probation.

Therapist: What do you think of that, Shane?

Shane: Wow. I didn't expect to hear that. I'm cool with that.

Being collaborative does not mean that everything is equal. Power differentials in therapy are particularly evident when clients attend therapy involuntarily. However, we can neutralize much of the inequity in such situations by ensuring that clients' voices are heard, respected, and included to create goal consensus.

In situations in which therapists do not have access to external stakeholders, an indirect way of bringing their presence into sessions is to ask clients, "Did [name of outside helper] tell you what [he or she] expects us to focus on here?" If the client can answer this question, the therapist proceeds by incorporating those goals or directions into the services. If the client does not know, speculation can be helpful: "What do you think [he/she] will say when I talk with [him/her]?" Therapists should invite all parties involved to share their perceptions and understandings of what may have been conveyed to them (Bertolino, 2003). If what the client shares is at odds with the stakeholder's concern, the therapist can gently say, "My understanding after talking with (stakeholder's name) is that he/she will have the sense that you're moving in the right direction when you're [list action(s)]." The therapist follows with, "How does that sound to you?" Similar to working with multiple clients, the therapist acknowledges both the client's and the stakeholder's perspective and searches for some agreement in goals.

Identifying Progress Toward Goals: Signposts of Change

With a sense of purpose in therapy and goals set, therapy becomes more focused. The benefit of this focus will become more apparent in the next chapter, when we explore ways of selecting and matching therapeutic strategies with clients. Before moving into that conversation, there is one additional, often-understated area related to goal setting to mention.

There are times that clients will see the gap between the problems that brought them to therapy and the goals they hope to attain as insurmountable. Clients will think or say, "I'll never get to that point" or "I am so far away from reaching that (goal)." Even well-constructed goals can seem unattainable, especially to very distressed clients. The result can be frustration, loss of hope, and in some cases, an increase in the intensity of problems. Even worse, these reactions put clients at greater risk of both dropout and negative outcome.

An effective way to both reduce the likelihood of client frustration and neutralize its effects, if it occurs, is to orient clients toward the indicators of forward movement. Doing so involves identifying indicators or signs that progress is being made toward the established goals. Here are some questions to assist with this process:

- What will be the first sign or indication that things have begun to turn the corner with your problem?
- What's one thing that might indicate to you that things are on the upswing?
- What will be the first sign or indication to you that you have taken a solid step on the road to improvement even though you might not yet be out of the woods?
- What will you see happening when things are beginning to go more the way you'd like them to go?
- What would have to happen that would indicate to you that things are changing in the direction you'd like them to change?
- What is happening right now with your situation that you would like to have continue?

The idea of identifying indicators of progress is not exclusive to psychotherapy. It is relative to many facets of life such as health, education, business, sports, and learning new skills. When people do not have the sense that they are making progress, motivation wanes, frustration sets in, and in some cases, they give up. In contrast, when people are engaged and sense that they are moving and making progress toward their destinations, they are more likely to remain engaged. As therapists, our task is to orient clients toward signposts of progress between the problem and the vision of an improved future. Action-talk remains an integral process of conversation about signposts of progress. We want to identify what specifically will be different, including, for example, how those things happen, when they happen, and who is involved. We aren't seeking explanations; rather we are seeking the "4WHs"—the who, what, when, where, and how—of progress.

Clarifying Problems, Goals, and Progress Through Scaling

For clinicians and clients who are more pragmatic in their approach to determining concerns, goals, and progress, using questions that focus on quantitative change can be helpful. One way to do this is to use scaling questions (de Shazer, 1991). To use scaling questions, the therapist first establishes a continuum using a scale, most commonly from 1 to 10. Each number represents a rating of how the client views life at different junctures (e.g., the present and later points). The therapist introduces the idea of scaling by saying, "On a scale of 1 to 10, with 1 being the worst this problem has ever been, and 10 being the best things could be, how would you rate things today?" Once a number has been given, the therapist uses action-talk to ensure that what the number represents is clear. For example, if a client rates the situation at a 4, the therapist asks, "What specifically is happening to indicate to you that it is a 4?"

The next step is to ask the client what number would indicate that the goals of therapy have been met, that services have been successful, or that sufficient improvement has occurred. If the client stated that an 8 would indicate sufficient change, the therapist would then ask for a description of what specifically will be happening when an 8 is reached. Again, action-talk is used to clarify.

The final part of scaling used in this way is for the therapist to explore with the client what will indicate in-between change and progress. The therapist might ask, "You mentioned that things are at a 4 now and 8 is where you would like to be. What will it take for your situation to edge forward a little, from a 4 to a 4.5?" We want to make sure the change we are looking for is not too big a leap for the client. For many clients, asking what it would take to move from a 4 to a 7 will seem overwhelming. Although it is possible for clients to make significant gains very quickly, it is usually a better idea to focus on movement that increases the likelihood of success.

To summarize, goals should reflect and match the motivational level of the client and others who may be involved. We do this by learning what clients view as presenting concerns, what they feel needs to improve, and what will indicate progress toward the desired change. As we will learn in Chapter 6, this information assists in matching methods with the client's level of motivation as a means of increasing the chance of a successful outcome.

ADVANCED LISTENING AND ATTENDING SKILLS: USING LANGUAGE TO STRENGTHEN THE ALLIANCE AND CREATE POSSIBILITIES

Therapy unfolds word by word, sentence by sentence, conversation by conversation. Because language is the most influential means we have of facilitating change, we want to become skilled in using it as a vehicle to acknowledge and validate, strengthen the alliance, empower, and develop possibilities for clients to experience greater well-being and functioning. As therapy progresses, we listen closely for opportunities to convey our understanding and move conversations forward, moment by moment. In this section, we explore various ways to accomplish this by using "linguistic subtlety." In other words, we use small changes and variations with words and phrases to introduce possibilities in otherwise closed-down situations.

A first task of the therapist is to develop familiarity and comfort with these other subtle methods of facilitating change. Second, the therapist must determine when to use such methods. One way to improve one's sense of awareness of language is to recognize words that are either invalidating, are jarring, or close down possibilities for change. Consider making a list of words that are intrusive or off-putting to you personally. Then make a note of the client's reactions to words you use in therapy. When a client's verbal or nonverbal response gives you reason to pause, check in with the client. Say, "I noticed that your facial expression changed and you looked away when just now. Can you tell me what you experienced in that moment?" Sometimes a client may be triggered into thought, but often it's our words that led to a specific reaction. The only way to understand the relative impact of those words is by asking. Through feedback, adjustments can be made, if necessary.

Another way of determining when to use the methods in this section is when clients make statements that suggest *blame*, *invalidation*, *nonaccountability*, or *impossibility* (Bertolino & O'Hanlon, 2002). *Blame* occurs when individuals or others label individuals as having bad intentions or bad personality traits. Clients will say things such as, "It's my fault that he hit me" or "I'm bad because I was sexually abused." They either perceive themselves as damaged goods or attribute bad intentions to themselves. Others can also convey these stories through statements such as, "He's always playing head games and is never serious about anything." *Invalidation* is when clients or others consider clients to be abnormal or wrong in some way or give clients the message that they can't trust their perceptions. Oftentimes, this occurs when the internal experience or knowledge of clients is undermined by others. Many clients will feel invalidated by others who say they are wrong, are making things up, are making too much of something, or should just move on and forget about things. Clients or others will say, "I know I shouldn't feel that way," "He just needs to learn to let it go," or "I'm too emotional."

Nonaccountability (or determinism) involves clients not accepting responsibility for themselves and their actions. Clients will say things such as, "He made me do it," "I was drunk," or "I can't help it." People are accountable for their actions (what they do with their bodies). This is very different from times when people have no choice and are intruded on without their consent. Then the person who committed the intrusive act is accountable. Finally, *impossibility* involves ideas maintaining that clients are unable to or are incapable of change. Clients will say things such as, "I'll never change," "She's just like her father," or "He can't help it, he's ADD."

When clients provide statements consistent with these examples, the therapist must determine how to best respond in a way that both acknowledges what has been said and subtly moves the conversation forward. As with all else in this book, the methods offered in this section are not the province of any one therapeutic modality. Similarly, they are not meant to serve as pre-established, planned interventions (e.g., thought stopping, exposure, the miracle question) associated with the popular models of today. Instead, their effectiveness relies solely on the therapist responding, in the moment, to what the client has just said as way of creating a new inroad in the conversation.

The hope is that these methods, as well as the many others not mentioned here, become part of every effective therapist's repertoire. Last, although the strategies proposed here have and can be used singularly (i.e., one at time), more often than not, multiple methods are used in the same conversation. Because therapy is conversational, there are likely to be many opportunities to impart possibility—and that really is a primary goal of the therapist. We invite clients into conversations in which they can experience and see the world anew. What follows is a series of unique and specific ways to use language in the service of change.

Using Person-First Language: Working With People, Not Labels

At several junctures, we have examined the influence of pathology-based language and conversations on optimism and health. Further concerns with such language, particularly in the area of diagnostic labeling, include depersonalization and nondescriptiveness. In addition to examples already used (i.e., anxiety, depression), common labels include attention deficit hyperactivity disorder (ADHD), bipolar disorder (BPD), and obsessive-compulsive disorder (OCD), sourced from the *Diagnostic and Statistical Manual of Mental Disorders* (5th ed.; *DSM-5;* (American Psychiatric Association [APA], 2013). Broader but still frequently used categories of mental health labels include serious and persistent mental illness (SPMI) and severely emotionally disturbed (SED). Beyond mental health labels, which largely address emotional disability, are those used for persons with physical, intellectual, learning, speech and language, sensory, or brain-based disabilities. It is understood that in many cases a diagnosis must be assigned for clients to qualify for services that are reimbursed by third-party payers.

The issue of diagnosis is complex. Although empirical evidence supports diagnosis as necessary for psychotherapy, some clients may expect diagnosis to be part of assessment and in fact find empowerment through medicalized explanations. Similarly, clients may find diagnostic labels meaningful. Labels can defuse blame regarding conditions/situations that clients or others have placed on them. Simply having a diagnosis can bring about relief, letting people know they are not to blame or alone. In some cases, having a name for something—a diagnosis—has led to research to expand knowledge and to find effective treatment approaches. In each of these instances, labeling serves a purpose and can benefit clients.

Concerns with diagnostic labels and the *DSM*, in particular, are well documented. The public nomenclature provides daily examples of people being labeled and objectified. Examples are when a person is referred to as "bulimic" or "schizophrenic." These sorts of references are so commonplace that the persons who use such language seldom recognize that they are depersonalizing others. Unfortunately, many mental health professionals continue to use labels when referring to their clients and patients, setting a poor example for others.

The issue is far-reaching. Pathology-based labeling is so pervasive that some people use depersonalizing language when referring to themselves. They say, "I'm bipolar" or "That's what us manics do." What seems to happen in these cases is that clients lose their sense of self and develop identities consistent with the label. In turn, others see only the symptoms associated with the label, losing sight of the client as a person. In such cases, the diagnosis or label often becomes the focal point of services. Therapists then try to resolve BPD, for example, instead of concentrating efforts on trying to understand and support the unique individual whose behaviors fit a specific set of diagnostic criteria.

The unnecessary assignment of labels can stigmatize clients and subject them to prejudices and biases and, in extreme cases, ostracize them from life activities.

Therapists have a responsibility to consider the potential depersonalizing and stigmatizing effects that the identification of pathology can cause. A risk is that clients are seen as their diagnoses rather than as people. Psychiatrist Jerome Frank (1973) once observed that psychotherapy might be the only treatment that creates the illness it treats.

There are three ways to counter the use of labels and depersonalizing statements: (a) person-first language, (b) elimination of stigmatizing words, and (c) action-talk. First and most important, clients are people, not disorders or disabilities. Our language should reflect this fact. A disorder or disability may be an aspect of a client's life but certainly does not identify who the person is. To learn about clients and who they are as people, it is imperative that we attend closely to how we see others and what words we use to describe their situations.

To use person-first language first, we take the "-ic" out of the equation. Rather than saying "Curtis is schizophrenic," we say, "Curtis has been diagnosed with schizophrenia." Person-first language is consistent with the view of disability along a continuum of health (Olkin, 1999). To eliminate stigmatizing words, we avoid terms such as "suffers," "confined," and "requires." These words are unnecessary. Some disabilities present hurdles with a person's functioning in some, but not all, circumstances. Other disabilities have few or no effects on general health. It is therefore important to understand the effects of the disability on the range of functions faced by the individual. Psychologist Laura Brown (2008) echoed this point:

> What is true is that people with disabilities have some (or several) aspects of their bodies that function differently than those of a majority of other humans. Frequently, however, the challenges for these individuals lie not in those physical differences but in the barriers created to fullest possible function by cultural institutions and practice (p. 29).

A third response to labeling is to use action-talk—as described throughout this chapter—to counter the ambiguity and vagueness that often accompany labels. Next are examples of each response by placing the focus of therapy on the person, rather than on the disorder or disability.

1. *Use person-first language.* State the person's name prior to any label, diagnosis, or name of a disorder. Next, be sure to take "-ic" out of the label used.

Statement: Phillip is dyslexic.

Restatement: Phillip has dyslexia.

Professional: Schizophrenics like Katherine do strange things.

Therapist: Katherine, who has been diagnosed with schizophrenia, sometimes exhibits behaviors that are consistent with her diagnosis.

2. *Eliminate unnecessary and stigmatizing terms.* Consider whether particular words are necessary to describing another person, paying close attention to those that may hinder, blame, or negatively characterize another.

Statement: Alissa is confined to a wheelchair.

Restatement: Alissa uses a wheelchair.

Statement: Ty requires glasses due to his poor vision.

Restatement: Ty wears glasses.

3. *Use action-talk to translate vague labels.* Take the label, diagnosis, or name of a disorder and translate it into a clear, descriptive action.

Parent: Jamie is working on her ADHD.

Therapist: Jamie is working on completing her assignments on time.

Client: I'm bipolar and predisposed to negative thinking, which makes me scattered at work.

Therapist: You'd like to stay on task and organized when you have negative thoughts at work.

Diagnosis and labels are part of the landscape of healthcare and behavioral healthcare and in some ways, reflect societal discourses, which tend to be seeped in negativity. Language is a powerful medium that can lead to alienation, marginalization, and depersonalization. Language can also be used to empower and strengthen. In this section, we take this idea a step further as we consider numerous ways of using language to acknowledge and create possibilities for change in the present and future.

Extend Permission

Of all the methods described in the section, none may be as straightforward yet misunderstood as *giving permission*. At first glance, it is reasonable for a therapist to wonder, "Why would I need to extend permission to a client about anything? It is, after all, the client's life." If the people who surround clients and the voices of society would concur, such a response would be warranted. One of the reasons people seek therapy is for acknowledgment and validation. Too often, at their own suggestions or the opinions of others, they have arrived at the idea that they are bad or terrible because of their experiences or thoughts. A fundamental response is to extend clients permission to experience whatever is going on with them internally (i.e., feelings, sensory experiences, thoughts) to let them know that they are not bad, crazy, or weird and that others have felt the same way. Extending permission for internal experience does not mean giving permission for action. Internal experiences are quite different from the actions. Therapists do not give permission for actions or behaviors that pose risk to the client or others. Instead, therapists let clients know that whatever they are experiencing is acceptable *and* that they are responsible for their actions. There are three kinds of permission: "To," "not to have to," and "to and not to have to" (both). What follows are examples of each.

1. *Give permission "to."* Give clients permission for experiences, feelings, thoughts, and fantasies.

> *Client:* I just feel like quitting my job. I'm really a bad person for just wanting to walk out in it.
>
> *Therapist:* It's okay to feel like quitting your job, and that doesn't make you a bad person.
>
> *Client:* Every time I get depressed, I start cutting on my arms with whatever I can get my hands on.
>
> *Therapist:* It's okay to feel so depressed that you feel like cutting on yourself, but it's not okay to cut on yourself.

2. *Give permission "not to have to."* Give clients permission not to have to have experience, think, or do things that do not fit with them.

> *Client:* People keep telling me that I need to go through the anger stage of grieving. But I just don't feel angry. There must be something wrong with me.
>
> *Therapist:* Each person goes through grief in his or her own way. Some will experience anger and some won't. You can take your own path to healing.
>
> *Client:* I'm not really the kind of person who is emotionally expressive. I've been criticized for that.
>
> *Therapist:* It's okay not to have to express yourself in ways that aren't right for you.

3. *Give permission "to" and "not to have to."* Include both permissions at the same time.

> *Client:* Sometimes, I'm angry and sometimes I'm not. I must be crazy.
>
> *Therapist:* You can be angry and not angry about it, and that doesn't make you crazy.
>
> *Client:* I'm really hurt about what that says about me but not about what actually happened. Do you think that's weird?
>
> *Therapist:* It's okay to feel hurt about what you think it says about you and not about the event itself and that doesn't mean you're weird.

For some clients, extending permission will provide relief by serving as messages that there are right and wrong ways to feel or be. At the same time, if therapists give only one type of permission, some clients may feel pressured to experience just one part of the equation or may find the other side emerging in a more compelling or disturbing way (B. O'Hanlon & Bertolino, 1998, 2002). For example, if a therapist only says, "It's okay to be angry," the client might say, "But I don't want to be angry!" The therapist can counter this response by giving permission "to" and "not to have to": "It's okay to be angry and you don't have to be angry." Last, as discussed, therapists should exercise caution regarding actions for which they extend permission. A therapist would not say, "It's okay to cut yourself and you don't have to cut yourself." Permission is never extended for harmful, destructive, or illegal behavior.

Normalize Experience

Another way of acknowledging and extending permission to clients is through normalizing. One of the reasons people share their experiences with one another is to see how others respond. Of course, the negative reactions of others can lead to a host of negative feelings and thoughts. On the other hand, having someone say, "I've felt that way too," can release a person from negativity. In therapy, when clients know that they are not crazy or weird for feeling the way they do, they may experience deeper degrees of empathy and self-acceptance. In turn, this can lead to greater awareness and introspection. To normalize, therapists acknowledge clients' experiences by using some form of anecdote or analogy. Anecdotes, analogies, and stories have been used historically as well-thought-out interventions in many different therapies. The idea here, however, is to normalize the client's experience through very brief statements. For example, Carl Rogers would often say to his clients, "I've felt that way before too." Particularly in early interactions, as we create space for the client's story and strengthen the alliance, we want to encourage conversation through pointed, focused responses. For many clients, just knowing that others have had similar experiences can be liberating and open them to new perspectives. Next are four different ways to normalize clients' experiences.

1. *Use everyday examples*. Reflect that the concern or problem is within the realm of normal human experience and is not bad, terrible, weird, bizarre, or otherwise.

Client: How many people would let something like what happened to me at work weigh on them the way I have?

Therapist: Given what you've been through at work, especially in recent days, I think most people would expect it to weigh on you.

Client: Sometimes I just want to wring his neck. I know I've only been his stepmother for three months, but he still needs to listen. It's so frustrating!

Therapist: I understand that it has been frustrating for you. One of the things I've heard from other stepparents is that sometimes it takes a little time before kids start to tune in and really listen the way you need them to. I'm wondering if that's a possibility here.

2. *Use self-disclosure.* Use personal experience to normalize others' concerns or problems.

Client: I really struggle with math. I just don't think that way.

Therapist: I can relate, having struggled with math as well. What specifically have you found challenging about it?

Client: I get down on myself when things don't go right—like when I fail to meet deadlines.

Therapist: I think I follow you. I used to get down on myself when I set goals for myself and then didn't reach them. I'd go and wallow. What have you done when things haven't gone right for you?

3. *Use metaphor.* Metaphor is an implied comparison between two dissimilar things. It can play multiple roles in therapy. It is important to recognize metaphors and use attending and listening to acknowledge, match language, and promote hope.

Client: I don't like it when people talk about me when I walk by.

Therapist: You mentioned that you really love music, and sometimes it's a matter of tuning in what you want and tuning out the rest.

Client: I feel like I'm treading in rough waters and the waves are splashing in my eyes.

Therapist: Sometimes, the waves can be rough and choppy. And, if you're able to look just below the surface, you might notice that it's calmer and easier to see things more clearly.

4. *Go with it.* When clients have difficulty coming up with answers or respond with "I don't know," first acknowledge, then reflect back the hesitation, worry, discomfort, or other feeling or thought behind the response. Next are two variations—the first is in regard to clients who struggle with coming up with responses or do not want to talk.

Client: (Silence)

Therapist: Sometimes it's hard to think of what to say. That's okay.

Client: (Shrugs shoulders and looks down)

Therapist: It's okay to not have an answer. There are times when I either don't have anything to say or just don't want to talk. And if that's true for you, you perhaps you'll feel differently a little later in the session.

Next, are two examples of how to respond when clients say, "I don't know."

Client: I don't know.

Therapist: At this moment, you are really stumped as you search for an answer.

Client: I have no idea. I don't know.

Therapist: It's difficult to come up with something right now.

When asked about their experiences in therapy, clients routinely report greater connection with their therapists when they feel heard, understood, acknowledged, and accepted. Normalizing provides an effective way to let clients know that they are not alone, are respected, and have experiences that are valid and that do not make them crazy, weird, or abnormal.

Installation of Hope: Acknowledgment and Possibility

Rogers (1957) expounded on the importance of acknowledging and validating clients' internal experience. At the same time, if practitioners only reflect back these experiences and views, many clients will continue to use words that close down possibilities for change. In essence, they will paint themselves into corners through words and phrases by describing their views of themselves, others, and situations that imply impossibility. To counter this, the therapist combines acknowledgment with various forms of subtle changes in language, each of which provides a doorway to different or new view of a potentially closed-down client account. This can be done adding a twist to pure reflection in three different ways (Bertolino & O'Hanlon, 2002).

1. *Use the past tense.* Repeat clients' statements or problem reports in the past tense to create subtle openings in their perspectives. If only acknowledgment is used, clients may remain stuck. If only a search for possibilities occurs, some clients will feel invalidated. Using the past tense helps clients to feel understood but suggests that things can be different now or in the future.

Client: My situation isn't getting any better.

Therapist: Your situation hasn't gotten any better.

Client: Our problems are constant.

Therapist: The problems you've experienced have been constant.

Using the past tense to reflect the problem when the client uses the present tense can offer the possibility of a different present or future. We are both acknowledging and introducing possibility into the conversation. This can be especially helpful knowing that for many clients, straight acknowledgment will be insufficient. In fact, many will continue to describe situations as impossible and/or unchangeable. The combination of acknowledgment and possibility suggested by using the past tense offers a way to dissolve present-tense problem talk by introducing possibilities into otherwise closed-down statements and conversations.

2. *Translate client statements into partial statements*. Respond to clients' global all or nothing statements of "everything," "everybody," "always," and "never" by introducing qualifiers related to time (e.g., some things, somebody, sometimes, and much of the time), intensity (e.g., a lot, a bit less, somewhat more), or partiality (e.g., a lot, some, most, many). Therapists should take care not to minimize or invalidate clients' experiences.

Client: I'm always in trouble.

Therapist: You've been in trouble a lot.

Client: It just gets worse day after day.

Therapist: Lately, it seems like it's been getting worse.

Global (e.g., all or nothing, this or that) statements can impede change, but combining qualifiers with acknowledgment—going from global to partial—can help to introduce the element of possibility into otherwise closed-down statements. At the same time, if clients feel that their experiences are being minimized or they are being pushed to move on, they will likely respond with a statement such as, "Not a lot—always." If a client reacts in such a manner, the therapist must make sure the client feels heard and understood by validating further while keeping an eye on possibilities. For example, a therapist might respond to the previous client statement by saying, "Okay. The way you see it, you're always in trouble."

3. *Translate into perceptual statements*. Take clients' statements of truth or reality—the way they explain things for themselves—and translate them into perceptual statements or subjective realities (e.g., "In your eyes," "Your sense is," "From where you stand," "You've gotten the idea").

Client: Things will never change.

Therapist: Your sense is that things will never change.

Client: I'm a not a good person.

Therapist: You've gotten the idea that you've not been a good person.

Clients' statements reflecting their perceptions of events, situations, or themselves, as discussed previously, are stories—powerful and influential—but they are social constructions, not the way things are. When reflecting back clients' statements as their perceptions, therapists acknowledge such points of view without subscribing to the idea of impossibility.

Several of the previous examples used a combination of different methods of changing language; for example, "You've been in trouble a lot" uses past tense/partial statement, and "You've gotten the idea that you've not been a good person" uses perceptual statement/past tense. The more therapists practice with such changes in language, the more comfortable and consistent they become in identifying and attending to words, phrases, and statements that suggest impossibility.

We do not want to lose focus on the importance of acknowledging clients' experiences by echoing the voices of society that suggest what clients are experiencing is in some way wrong or that they must "move on" or "get over it" (Bertolino & O'Hanlon, 2002). Clients have often heard enough of such talk, which generally translates into invalidation and blame. We do not coerce clients but instead invite them into different perspectives by infusing hope. Offering the idea that even though things have been difficult, painful, or overwhelming lets clients know that their suffering, concerns, felt experiences, and points of view have been heard and understood. O'Hanlon and Bertolino (1998) commented on a hoped-for result of changing clients' basic language: "When acknowledgement and validation are combined with language of change and possibility in ongoing therapist reflections, clients begin to shift their self-perceptions. This process continues throughout the therapy. In time, clients can develop a more possibility-oriented sense of themselves" (p. 49).

Future-Talk: Acknowledgment and a Vision for the Future

In their distress and suffering, clients will sometimes describe their situations in ways that reflect little hope for the future. In these instances, language can work like the moving walkways in airports. We can use language to move clients in the direction of possibilities without them actually having to take steps toward their goals. Here are four ways to do this.

1. *Assume future change and/or solutions.* Assume the possibility that clients can find solutions by using words such as "yet" and "so far." These words presuppose that even though things feel stuck or unchangeable in the present, they will change sometime in the future.

Client: Things will never go right for me.

Therapist: So far things haven't gone right for you.

Client: My life is going downhill.

Therapist: Your life hasn't headed in a direction you'd like yet.

Through small changes in language, therapists are introducing the possibility that change can occur in the future. This seemingly simple shift gently challenges closed-down views and can open doorways to other, more significant changes.

2. *Turn problem statements into preferences or goals.* Take clients' problem statements and change them into statements or questions about a preference, preferred future, or goal.

> *Client:* It just seems like we argue all of the time.
>
> *Therapist:* Is finding alternatives to arguing one of the things you'd like to have happen?
>
> *Client:* Work is driving me crazy.
>
> *Therapist:* Would it be helpful for you to spend some time on how work might be better for you?

As we have learned, one of the four parts of the therapeutic alliance is agreement on the goals, meaning, or purpose of therapy. It's not uncommon for there to be some back and forth when it comes to the focus of therapy. A subtle way of acknowledging and clarifying is by inquiring about the significance of clients' statements as they relate to the goals of therapy. In a previous publication, my colleague, Bill O'Hanlon, and I wrote that this particular way of responding to clients serves several purposes:

> First . . . it offers a way to acknowledging clients. A second purpose relates to situations that therapists often find themselves in. In the course of listening to the client's story it can become difficult to discern which problem concerns the client the most. Therapists must routinely make decisions regarding which client words, phrases, comments, and remarks should gain more or less attention. By turning problem statements into goals, therapists can acknowledge clients' statements and simultaneously clarify which problems are most important to them. (Bertolino & O'Hanlon, 2002, p. 42)

Because clients have so much going on, it is common, especially early in interactions, for them to speak about what is foremost in their minds. In many cases, what clients mention "off the cuff" is not intended to be part of the ongoing conversation. Some will just want to update therapists on recent events, whereas others have things they want to get off their chests. The therapist cannot know this. As discussed, without soliciting client feedback, therapists are subject to their own interpretations, which are often incorrect. By turning problem statements into goals, therapists can get feedback as to which points clients would like to focus on.

> *Client:* Everything is a mess. Work is awful. I don't have any friends—no social life at all. I also want to eat everything in sight. I do that when I'm bored.
>
> *Therapist:* It sounds as if you've got a lot going on. And if I'm hearing you right, some of the things that we could focus on here are work, improving

your social life and friendships, and the feeling of wanting to eat more than you would prefer.

Client: Yeah, I think so. Well, I mean, I do want a better social life. I also want to talk about eating less at some point. But really, the most important thing to me is work. It's a nightmare and what really made me decide to come here.

In addition to clarifying what clients are more or less concerned about, this method assists with prioritizing concerns (particularly when there are several). We want to understand which issues clients view as most concerning as opposed to therapists' ideas about what should or should not be the focus.

3. *Presuppose changes and progress.* Assume changes and progress toward goals and preferred futures by using words such as "when" and "will."

Client: No one wants to be friends with me. I don't have anyone to hang out with and do stuff with.

Therapist: When you've started to hang out with people you consider friends, I'm curious about what other kinds of changes you'll notice in your life.

Client: I'm always getting angry and then saying things I shouldn't say.

Therapist: When you're better able to manage and express your anger, how do you suppose your life will be different than the way it is now?

Psychiatrist Milton Erickson used presupposition in hypnosis to link his patients' outward movements with the suggestion of internal, automatic changes. For example, Erickson might say, "When your hand begins to lift, I wonder what changes you'll make within yourself?" In a nonhypnotic way, presupposition offers a way to orient clients toward future changes by linking one change with another. Its use helps to shift clients' attention toward change in general and to tap into the "ripple effect." Therapists work with clients to notice that like a stone landing in a pool of water, ripples or additional changes can result with the first splash.

There are two ways to use presupposition. The first involves responding with a statement such as the therapist responses under the first method: *Assume future change and/or solutions.* A second is to frame the response as a question, as in the second entry. Adding the use of conjecture, wonderment, or speculation, whether in a statement or a question, can be helpful. Doing so offers speculation or inquiry concerning how future changes will make a difference for the client. To use conjecture, simply add "I wonder" or "I'm curious." Examples of this can found with the third method: *Presuppose changes and progress.*

4. *Use contingent linking.* Connect together two or more thoughts and feelings to presuppose a future change. Contingent linking involves combining the words "more" and "less" in ways that convey either an increase or a decrease of

some desired experience or pattern of thinking. There are four possible combinations for contingent linking: "The more this, the more that," The more this, the less that," The less this, the less that," and "The less this, the more that." Here are two examples.

Client: I'll never have the career I want with all these distractions in my life.

Therapist: The more you focus on your career and focus on what you want, the less the distractions in your life can be to you.

Client: I can't remember the last time I fixed or repaired anything with my house. And now I can't imagine anything changing with that.

Therapist: The less you focus on what you haven't done with your house in the past the more time you can spend wondering how you will change things going forward.

Contingent linking is purposeful in two ways. First, it presupposes future change. Next, it can serve as a form of *inclusion*, which is the next method to be discussed. In the case of the latter, contingent linking includes aspects of experience that the client sees as incompatible. In the client's view, one thing cannot happen without the other. Our communication to the client is that not only can the two aspects coexist, but one can positively influence the other.

Future-focused language can be especially valuable with clients experiencing hopelessness, pain, and fear because a lack of a vision for the future often exacerbates these forms of emotional reaction. If clients have the sense that the pain or suffering that they are experiencing now will somehow be alleviated or dissipated altogether, they are better able to keep moving. As discussed in Chapter 3, a growing body of literature indicates that people who have a sense of hope, which is reflected in their use of language, are less prone to physical disease. Presuppositional language provides a respectful response to clients' verbalization of problems or concerns without minimizing them and the suffering they are currently experiencing.

Inclusion

As therapists become more attuned to clients' use of language, it can be helpful to use more advanced ways of both acknowledging experience and opening up possibilities for change. One overarching way to accomplish the two is through *inclusion*, which involves including aspects of a client's experience that may be left out or seen as a barrier. Inclusion can be particularly useful when clients think or feel as if they are in binds and experience opposite or contradictory experiences that seem to present conflict. We include any parts, objections, feelings, aspects of self, or concerns that might have been left out or seen as barriers to the therapy or goals. Our aim is in accordance with F. Scott Fitzgerald, who once said, "The test of a first rate intelligence is the ability to hold two opposed ideas in the mind at the same time and still retain the ability to function." When clients are able to include what may have been left out, devalued, or seen as irreconcilable opposites, they will often experience a sense of acknowledgment and hope. The method calls for the use and linking of client experiences. Five ways to do this follow.

1. *Include opposite or contradictory feelings and emotions.* Link seemingly opposite or contradictory feelings and emotions.

Client: Sometimes, when I'm under pressure, I'm bombarded by emotion to the point that I don't know what to feel. It's like I get frustrated and scared and nervous. . . . It's hard to know which one is my true feeling.

Therapist: At times, when you're under pressure, you feel frustrated, scared, nervous . . . and maybe others as well, and there's enough room within you for all those emotions.

Client: I really can't stand my job.

Therapist: You really can't stand your job and, as you've mentioned before, it can be very rewarding.

2. *Include opposite or contradictory aspects of self or others.* Link seemingly opposite or contradictory aspects of self or others.

Client: I constantly procrastinate.

Therapist: Yes, and you told me that yesterday you completed your page-long "to do" list on time. It seems you both procrastinate and get things done.

Client: I feel anxious whenever I start new classes.

Therapist: You've experienced anxiety at the start of your classes and have somehow managed to get straight As your first three semesters. It seems you have found a way to allow anxiety to exist in just the right amount so that you can excel in school.

3. *Use oxymoron.* Include the opposite side of a situation or experience in a phrase to create an oxymoron (a combination of contradictory or incongruous words or phrases) to include different feelings and aspects.

Client: I get so nervous that I feel like I need to get through things quickly, but I also know it's better for me to slow down.

Therapist: You slowly run through things in a way that is right for you.

Client: My friends told me I did well, but I think my performance was awful.

Therapist: You can be awfully pleased with your performance.

4. *Use apposition of opposite.* Include the opposite side of a situation or experience, but extend the tension throughout the sentence.

>   *Client:* I just feel like it's time to put an end to that part of my life, but I don't where to start.
>
>   *Therapist:* Perhaps by talking about it you are beginning to put an end to that part of your life.
>
>   *Client:* I'm ready to put that part of my life behind me.
>
>   *Therapist:* It sounds like you're open to closing the door on that part of your life.

5. *Use the opposite possibility.* Include the possibility of the opposite happening regarding a statement by highlighting the possibility that something positive can occur, as well as drawing attention to an unrealistic expectation or goal.

>   *Client:* The next time I see him, I'm sure we'll argue, as usual.
>
>   *Therapist:* That could happen, but perhaps it will go better than expected.
>
>   *Client:* I know I'll do just as poorly on the next exam as I did on the last one.
>
>   *Therapist:* That's a possibility, yet you might surprise yourself.

6. *Use splitting to draw distinctions.* Take aspects of a client's life or situation and create separation between them. There are numerous combinations such as distinguishing between the past and present, the present and future, then and now, this and that, the conscious and unconscious, and inside and outside.

>   *Client:* Sometimes, I really want to just get rid of those thoughts—the ones I have about my past relationship—but not always.
>
>   *Therapist:* I was wondering, how about keeping the thoughts about your past relationship that are good for you and you like but ridding yourself of the ones that aren't good for you and you don't like?
>
>   *Client:* I just keep repeating the same things over and over from the past.
>
>   *Therapist:* It seems that some things from the past have repeated for you. And I'm curious, what have you noticed that is different between the way you were then and the way you are now?

The idea with splitting is for clients to notice the differences between different aspects of themselves, their lives, and situations. We are not asking clients to forget or dismiss any of these aspects. It's quite the opposite. We acknowledge and include all aspects of clients and their lives while making the distinction that some aspects, depending on the situation or context, may not always be useful. By noticing subtle differences, clients may be able to begin moving forward from an outdated or no-longer-useful viewpoint. Splitting, as with each form of inclusion, offers a different response to helping clients to accept parts of the self and life circumstances in a constructive way.

Utilization

The final method in this section is arguably one of the most important yet challenging to master. Recall our discussion in Chapter 1 about personal philosophy (worldview). Our perspectives as therapists are critical to how we think about our clients and their capacities, our role as a therapist, the purpose of therapy, the ways that change occurs, and so on. Therapists help to create conditions in which clients are more likely to achieve positive change and success in the future. A specific way to create conditions for positive change is through utilization, a method that involves using what clients bring to therapy to help bring about change. Often, what is utilized is something that has gone unnoticed in the client's life and/or is no long being used as an active resource. In other instances, the therapist utilizes something that a client wants to get rid of, sees as negative, or devalues. Because clients are the ultimate engineers of their destinies, their strengths and resources provide the fodder for change. The task of the therapist is to identify, elicit, and utilize whatever the client presents to facilitate change in the client's perspective or action:

> A previous patient approached Dr. Erickson seeking his help with an aunt he had in Milwaukee. The man's aunt had become seriously depressed and there was concern that she may be suicidal. The patient asked Dr. Erickson if he would check in with his aunt while his was in the area to give a lecture. Dr. Erickson agreed.
> The woman was secure financially, lived alone in a mansion, having never married. Over the years she had lost most of her close friends and relatives who formed her support network. She was now in her 60s and had developed medical problems that led to her use of a wheelchair. As a result, the once vibrant, active woman had become increasingly socially reclusive.
> Following his lecture, as promised, Dr. Erickson arrived at the woman's house. She was expecting him. Following introductions, the woman offered Dr. Erickson a tour of her home. And while the home had been updated to make it more wheelchair accessible, it was evident from its décor that few other updates had been made since it was built in the late 1800s. The house was dark with its curtains drawn and air filled with a scent of musk. What was once a majestic old home full of joy had over time become a place of sadness.
> As the tour came to a close, the woman led Dr. Erickson to one final area of the spacious home. It was a magnificent greenhouse nursery. The woman's face lit with joy as she talked about the many tireless, happy hours she spent growing her plants. And in the midst of the many beautiful plants

was her newest endeavor. She was using clippings of African violet plants to grow new ones.

As Dr. Erickson and the woman continued their conversation, he learned that although she was now fairly isolated, her life wasn't always that way. She had in fact been active in her community and in particular, her church. That changed when she began using a wheelchair. She was did not want to get in anyone's way and had become more self-conscious, limiting her church attendance to Sunday services. The woman had hired the handyman who worked on things with her home to take her to and from church. The handyman would physically lift her in and out of the church, which was not wheelchair accessible. Because of her concerns about getting in others' way and blocking foot traffic, she would arrive late and leave early.

Dr. Erickson took in the tour of the home and listened intently to the woman's story. He added to their conversation that her nephew was very worried about her. He was aware of how depressed she had become which is why he requested that Dr. Erickson visit. The woman agreed that the situation was serious and that she was depressed. Then Dr. Erickson did a curious thing. He told the woman that he did not see depression as the problem. The woman listened intently as Dr. Erickson continued. Rather, he believed her condition to be the result of not been being a very good Christian. Taken aback by his comment, the woman was left to wonder what he meant and why he would say such a thing.

Then, Dr. Erickson explained, "Here you are with all this money, time on your hands, and a green thumb. And it's all going to waste. What I recommend is that you get a copy of the church directory and then look in the latest church bulletin. You'll find announcements of births, deaths, graduations, engagements, and marriages in there—all the happy and sad events in the lives of people in your congregation. Make a number of African violet cuttings and get them well-established. Then repot them into gift pots and have your handyman drive you to the homes of people who are affected by these happy or sad events. Bring them a plant and your congratulations or condolences and comfort, whichever is appropriate to the situation" (Bertolino, 2015, pp. 34–35).

The woman listened to Dr. Erickson and agreed that maybe she had fallen short of her responsibilities as a a Christian. She also agreed that she could do more. About a decade later the Milwaukee Sentinel newspaper published an article with the headline, "African Violet Queen of Milwaukee Dies, Mourned by Thousands." The piece described how the woman had touched many lives in times of sadness and joy with her trademark flowers and charitable work in her community. (adapted from Bertolino, 2015)

Dr. Erickson utilized the woman's compassion for others, commitment to her church, and skill in growing plants to help her re-engage in the community. Her depression lifted, she gained a new sense of purpose, and others became affectionate toward her. In fact, she came to be loved by those around her. Erickson remarked that she became "too busy to be depressed." The story illustrates how Erickson invited the woman to change by utilizing what mattered her.

As a therapist early in my career, familiar with Dr. Erickson's work, I knew the story well (Zeig, 1980). However, it wasn't until I spent time with one of my mentors, Bill O'Hanlon, that I truly understood the concept of utilization. Bill had been a student of Dr. Erickson and spent much time writing about his work (W. H. O'Hanlon, 1987; W. H. O'Hanlon & Hexum, 1990). A short time after I met Bill, he recounted how Dr. Erickson had told him the story of the "African Violet Queen." Since I had gained so much from it, I told Bill how excited I was to hear the story in person. Bill told it in much the same way as I had read it, with one exception.

He recounted that after Dr. Erickson finished telling the story, Bill said, "I don't get it. It's a good story, but that's not how we are trained. As therapists, we're trained to focus on depression and problems. Why did you talk about flowers?" Dr. Erickson replied, "As I walked through the house the only sign of life I saw was the African violet plants and the nursery. I thought it would be much easier to grow the African violet part of her life than to weed out the depression." When Bill revealed Erickson's response, it all came together for me. I understood utilization and also realized just how ahead of his time Dr. Erikson was. He was a strengths-based practitioner.

What Erickson taught a generation of therapists is to utilize what clients bring to therapy—no matter how small, strange, or negative the behavior or idea seems—to open possibilities for change. This process directly contrasts with more traditional approaches that often view what clients bring as symptoms or liabilities. Two ways to utilize client behaviors and ideas as vehicles for change follow.

1. *Use what is brought to services as resources to initiate change.* No matter how small, strange, or negative an idea or behavior may seem, use it to open possibilities for change.

> *Client:* He spends hours tinkering with electronic gadgets. I have no idea why he does it.
>
> *Therapist:* It sounds like he's found something that really grabs his attention, . . . something that he's interested in.
>
> *Client:* I don't like sports. I'm terrible at them anyway.
>
> *Therapist:* You've ruled out sports, at least for now, so what else might you focus your efforts on?

The idea is to take behaviors and ideas that are typically seen as deficits, inabilities, symptoms, or negative in general and turn them into assets. It can be a helpful way to get clients moving in the direction of the change they are seeking if they are not already doing so. In doing so, therapists are not dismissive of others' points of view, which might suggest that an idea or behavior is in some way negative. One way to avoid causing clients to feel invalidated is by first acknowledging their perspectives. With the previous example, the therapist might say, "I can see why his interest in electronics might lead you to wonder what he gets out of it. How do you think we might help him to use that interest in a way that can help with what you're concerned about?" Acknowledgment of one perspective should not be dismissive of another.

There are many methods associated with cognitive therapies, for example, that are used to more directly and deliberately help clients to change their perspectives. That is not the aim of the methods described in this section. Instead, each method is purposeful in two ways. First, we want to acknowledge clients' experiences. People are far more likely to make necessary efforts to change when they feel heard and understood. So again, our aim to build strong alliances. Second, we try to introduce the idea of possibility. We accomplish this through short, focused responses. Although spontaneous change is always possible, these methods serve a different purpose by creating a context for change through small openings.

It is hoped that, by now, you are convinced of the influence of language. The use of language is an important skill set for therapists to develop. The methods outlined to this point in this book are but a small example of how language can serve as a vehicle for change. Thirteenth-century poet Rumi once said, "Raise your words, not your voice. It is rain that grows flowers, not thunder." Confucius observed, "Without knowing the force of words, it is impossible to know more." Language is a virus—a good kind.

In this chapter, we explored multiple processes for strengthening the alliance and bringing structure and direction to therapeutic conversations. The clearer we are about what clients' concerns are, what they hope to achieve in therapy, and how they will know they are making progress, the greater the likelihood that our attempts to help them to change will be a good fit. Information about problems, goals, and progress represents part of the 20% of the 80/20 rule described in earlier chapters. As discussed in Chapter 4, we continue to check in with clients to ensure that we are on track, making any adjustments that are necessary to keep them engaged and verify that we are having the kinds of conversations that are most useful to them. In the next chapter, we add another layer of information gathering to assist with selecting and matching interventions. We then review classes of intervention.

REFERENCES

Adler, A. (1956). *The individual psychology of Alfred Adler: A systematic presentation in selections from his writings* [H. L. Ansbacher & R. R. Ansbacher, Trans.]. New York, NY: HarperCollins.

American Psychiatric Association. (2013). *Diagnostic and statistical manual of mental disorders* (5th ed.). Arlington, VA: American Psychiatric Publishing.

Bertolino, B. (1999). *Therapy with troubled teenagers: Rewriting young lives in progress*. New York, NY: Wiley.

Bertolino, B. (2003). *Change-oriented psychotherapy with adolescents and young adults: The next generation of respectful and effective therapeutic processes and practices.* New York, NY: W. W. Norton.

Bertolino, B. (2010). *Strengths-based engagement and practice: Creating effective helping relationships.* Boston, MA: Allyn & Bacon.

Bertolino, B. (2015). *Working with children and adolescents in residential care: A strengths-based approach.* New York, NY: Routledge.

Bertolino, B., & O'Hanlon, B. (2002). *Collaborative, competency-based counseling and therapy.* Boston, MA: Allyn & Bacon.

Brown, L. S. (2008). *Cultural competence in trauma therapy: Beyond the flashback.* Washington, DC: American Psychological Association.

de Shazer, S. (1988). *Clues: Investigating solutions in brief therapy.* New York, NY: W. W. Norton.

de Shazer, S. (1991). *Putting difference to work.* New York, NY: W. W. Norton.

Dreikurs, R. (1954). The psychological interview in medicine. *American Journal of Individual Psychology, 10,* 99–122.

Erickson, M. H. (1954). Pseudo-orientation in time as a hypnotherapeutic procedure. *Journal of Clinical and Experiential Hypnosis, 2,* 261–283. doi:10.1080/00207145408410117

Frank, J. D. (1973). *Persuasion and healing.* Baltimore, MD: Johns Hopkins University Press.

O'Hanlon, B., & Bertolino, B. (1998). *Even from a broken web: Brief, respectful solution-oriented therapy for sexual abuse and trauma.* New York, NY: Wiley.

O'Hanlon, B., & Bertolino, B. (2002). *Even from a broken web: Brief, respectful solution-oriented therapy for sexual abuse and trauma.* New York, NY: W. W. Norton.

O'Hanlon, W. H. (1987). *Taproots: Underlying principles of Milton Erickson's therapy and hypnosis.* New York, NY: W. W. Norton.

O'Hanlon, W. H., & Hexum, A. (1990). *An uncommon casebook: The complete clinical work of Milton H. Erickson.* New York, NY: Norton.

Olkin, R. (1999). *What psychotherapists should know about disability.* New York, NY: Guilford Press.

Rogers, C. R. (1957). The necessary and sufficient conditions of therapeutic personality change. *Journal of Consulting Psychology, 21,* 95–103. doi:10.1037/0033-3204.44.3.240

Zeig, J. K. (Ed.). (1980). *A teaching seminar with Milton H. Erickson.* New York, NY: Brunner/Mazel.

CHAPTER 6

Matching and Classes of Intervention

In the first part of this chapter, we explore how to match and select strategies to help clients reach their goals and achieve successful outcomes. This process is a form of "mapping." The second part of this chapter is a discussion of classes of intervention (COI). COI include specific methods selected and used by therapists to promote affective, cognitive, and behavioral/interactional change. Each class or domain will be described in brief to orient readers toward categories of intervention based on information gathered during client interactions and described over the first five chapters of this book.

THE I-AM APPROACH TO CLIENT ORIENTATIONS

As we delve deeper into each client's world, we keep in mind just how quickly therapists' biases are activated. The *more* therapists become interested in their own theories about clients and their situations, the *less* therapists are attuned to conversations happening in real time. We are reminded that there is no solid evidence to support the idea that therapist-derived explanations regarding the roots of dysfunction help clients to change (Beutler, 1989; Held, 1991, 1995). Truly, as therapists learn more about clients, they will begin to formulate ideas that may provide a match. However, client orientations—their expectations, preferences, ideas, problems, and potential solutions, as well as what feels right—should remain the primary driver of therapy. To remain attuned to clients' orientations, we *invite, acknowledge*, and *match* (I-AM) (Bertolino, 2010).

To *invite*, therapists encourage clients to share their ideas about therapy as they relate to the development of problems and solutions. Therapists continue to collaborate with clients, inviting clients into conversations that may help therapists to better understand their lives and situations. Therapists combine this information with what has been gathered through any routine outcome monitoring (ROM) and interviewing. As we have learned, therapists *acknowledge* by listening carefully to clients' ideas and extend respect for their points of view.

We do not have to agree with clients but instead convey that their perspectives are valid. We want to let clients know that they are not weird, crazy, bizarre, or seen as having bad intentions. The final part of the I-AM approach is to *match*. Matching refers to therapists' use of processes and practices that are respectful of and consistent with clients' ideas about their concerns and problems, possibilities for attaining positive change, and methods for achieving those desired changes.

MATCHING: INCREASING THE FACTOR OF FIT

As we have learned, a task of the therapist is to identify and employ strategies that provide the best *fit* for clients, and then monitor the *effect* of such strategies. Said differently, we aim to *match* our choices of interventions with clients to achieve desired goals and improved outcomes. Such an approach stands in contrast to the empirically supported treatment (EST) approach detailed in Chapters 1 and 2, which is reliant on the identification of the best treatment for a particular disorder with little or no consideration of the uniqueness of the individual client. We have a different idea. Instead, therapists focus on fit and effect to determine whether a given course of therapy works for an individual client. This approach has been referred to as *practice-based evidence* (PBE) (Barkham, Hardy, & Mellor-Clark, 2010; Duncan, Miller, Wampold, & Hubble, 2010; Lambert, 2010). Burlingame and Beecher (2008) stated, "Practice-based evidence consists of real-time patient outcomes being delivered to clinicians immediately before treatment sessions so that they can make decisions about effective interventions based on current patient status. The burning question guiding this EBP model is as follows: "Is this treatment working for this client?" (p. 1200). To recap, as described in Chapter 2, when talking about *fit we* ask: Is the intervention consistent with a client's worldview, culture, and ideas about change? *Effect* translates to outcome. We ask: Did the intervention benefit the client in some measurable way (i.e., individually, relationally, and/or socially) and contribute to improvement in functioning?

Building on information from initial client interactions, therapists hone in on two specific areas to better match interventions by learning about the client's:

1. theory of change and
2. readiness to change

Before examining each method of matching we revisit the 80/20 rule. Not all information is equal nor is it helpful. We want to be selective and gather information that will assist with resolving problems and moving things forward. The better we are at gathering information and responding to client feedback, the more we can reduce guesswork and provide more of an empirical basis for choosing methods to increase both the fit of interventions and ultimately increase the benefit of therapy.

The Client's Theory of Change

Clients often have ideas about how change might occur with their situations or lives. These ideas arise out of past life experiences, interactions with other professionals, and expectations about therapy and have been referred to as the *client's theory of change* (Duncan, Miller, & Sparks, 2004). Through focused questions, therapists can learn about clients' ideas, attitudes, and speculations regarding how they situate themselves in relation to problems, at what rate and when change might occur, who might be involved, and what factors could play a role in facilitating change. Duncan et al. (2004) discussed the importance of the client's theory:

> Honoring the client's theory occurs when a given therapeutic procedure fits or complements the client's preexisting beliefs about his or her problems and the change process. We, therefore, simply listen and then amplify stories, experiences, and interpretations that clients offer about their problems, as well as their thoughts, feelings, and ideas about how those problems might be best addressed. As the client's theory evolves, we implement the client's identified solutions or seek an approach that both fits the client's theory and provides possibilities for change. (p. 84)

A starting point is to begin by asking general questions about how change usually occurs in clients' lives and what factors are most responsible for those changes. The following questions can be helpful in learning about clients' experiences with change:

- How do things usually change in your life?
- What prompts or initiates change for you?
- What does change involve?
- What have you done in the past to address concerns/problems?
- How have the things you've tried worked?
- How do you expect things to change in therapy?

Information from the previous questions may be enough for therapists to ask more problem-specific questions. It may also be necessary to use more deliberate questions to shift from general ideas about change to those that relate to the problem(s) brought to therapy. In such cases the questions that follow can be useful:

- What ideas do you have about how change might happen with your concern/problem/situation?
- If someone you know had this concern/problem/situation, what would you suggest he or she do to resolve it?

- What do you believe needs to happen before the change you are seeking can occur?
- At what rate (i.e., slow or fast, over days or months, etc.) do you think change will occur?
- Will change likely be in big amounts, small amounts, incrementally, and so on?
- Do you expect change to occur by seeing things differently? By doing something different? By others doing something different? (Listen for experiential, cognitive, behavioral, interactional, neurobiological, or some combination of these descriptors.)
- What thoughts or ideas have you been considering about how this problem has come about and what might put it to rest?
- Given your ideas about the problem, what do you think would be the first step in addressing it?
- What might you do differently as a result of the thoughts or ideas you've developed?
- What have you considered trying that is consistent with your ideas about what's influencing this problem?
- If you had this thought/idea/theory about someone else, what would you suggest that he or she do to resolve it?

Clients do not usually have well-formulated "theories"; instead, they have ideas that can greatly influence the outcome of therapy. Through careful listening and questioning, therapists invite clients into conversations from which emerge details about how they feel and think their problems developed, what they have tried to resolve them (and to what degree those efforts have or have not been successful), what they have considered but have not tried, and what they might consider in the future to attain the change they desire (Bertolino, 2010). It is usually not necessary to ask more than a question or two to get a sense of what has worked (to any degree) or could work in the future. Once a client replies, the therapist follows up with questions to flesh out further details.

Occasionally clients will respond, "I don't know." This kind of response is to be expected as questions are invitations to share information, not inquisitions (Bertolino, 2014). If a client struggles to respond, the therapist says, "Please let me know if anything comes to mind." Explorations of previous successes are part of a larger perspective. When combined with knowledge of a client's relationship to a particular problem and coping style (which will be discussed shortly), previous successes assist with gaining a clearer idea of what kinds of methods will provide a good fit with this client, with this problem, in this situation.

Culture

An essential part of understanding our clients' theories of change is culture. In Chapter 2, the American Psychological Association's (APA) definition of evidence-based practice (EBP) was provided. The last line of the definition refers to "patient characteristics, culture, and preferences." Similarly, Principle 4 of a strengths-based approach is "Culture influences and shapes all aspects of human life." Madsen (2007) stated, "Just as anthropologists (or more accurately ethnographers) immerse themselves in a foreign culture to learn about it, therapy from an anthropological stance can begin with immersing ourselves in a family's phenomenological reality in order to fully understand their experience" (p. 26). Throughout this book we have explored ways of focusing on and enhancing those factors most responsible for change, and considering how to best help clients achieve their goals and outcomes. At the center of these conversations is culture. Decisions about therapeutic methods should be done in collaboration with clients and respect to their cultural heritages.

As described in Chapter 2, culture is inclusive of many factors. We begin by viewing clients as teachers and with a commitment to learn about cultures that differ from our own. We listen to how clients describe themselves, their lives, challenges, and ideas about change. Clients are motivated more by what they believe influences their problems and possible solutions than by therapist's theories. It's not that clients enter therapy with clear-cut theories of causation, but they do often have general ideas about the nature of or influences on their concerns. Often these ideas are embedded in their language and can be cultivated through careful listening. It is the therapist's job to ferret out these influences through conversation. The questions that follow can assist with ascertaining clients' cultural sensibilities regarding change. With each question, the words *ethnicity*, *age*, *gender*, *sexual orientation*, *spirituality/religion*, *relationships*, *community*, *disability*, *indigenous heritage*, *national origin*, and so on, can be used to better understand specific aspects of each client's culture.

- Who are you as a person?
- How do you describe yourself to others?
- What is most important for me to know about you and the things that most influence your life?
- What can you tell me about _____ that will help me to better understand you and your current life/situation?
- What has it been like for you to live with _____ as part of who you are as a person?
- What, if any, part of how you describe yourself relates to the problem that brought you to therapy?
- What do you see as being most significantly influencing in the problem that brought you to therapy?

- How have those influences affected you?
- How have they been helpful to you? Unhelpful?
- How might that/those influence(s) be a resource to you?
- In what ways has your _____ presented a challenge for you? How have you dealt with that challenge thus far?
- In what ways has your _____ been a strength for you? How could it be in the future?
- Given how you live life, what makes most sense to you in terms of how you expect change to happen moving forward?
- What other ideas have you considered, even if you're not fully convinced of them?

Aspects of culture do not cause people to do things; rather, they influence. Next is a case example of how a client's background can serve as an influence with a life circumstance.

Case Example 6.1: The Opinions of Others

A mother of two young children came to therapy with concern over the behavior of her son. She stated that her 5-year-old had been "having tantrums." By this she meant he would "kick and scream" when he did not "get his way." When invited to share how she had addressed her son's behavior in the past, the client remarked, "I never used to spank my child, but people told me that I better get a hold of him or he would become a terror and end up in jail. I don't like spanking, but I got worried." When asked to clarify who the "people" were who offered their advice, she described two close friends whose advice she valued. I acknowledged the woman's experiences and her perspective. I then said, "It sounds like sometimes you really get frustrated." The woman was tearful.

When the client was ready, I asked her several specific questions that focused on two areas: (a) What most influenced her idea about how to raise children and (b) What currently influenced her decisions around raising her children. With the former, the mother related that she was "hit" (she did not use the word *abuse*) as a child by her father, who claimed that "discipline is a requirement" in raising children. The client stated that she took her father's statement to mean that "hitting is the only way to discipline." However, the client had not followed her father's opinion about raising children until her friends spoke up. The client stated, "I would never hit my son hard. I just thought a spank would work. It did on me." I asked the client, "How did you discipline your son prior to your friends' comments?" The client replied, "I just handled each situation as it came up. I wasn't really worried until they said something."

I next asked the client about current influences on her decisions about raising her child. She immediately identified her friends. I asked if her father's past influence was still present. She replied, "A little bit but not as much. I really ignored what he thought until my friends made that comment." I followed, "You realized that maybe your father's advice was not right for you. Then at some point, perhaps because you were fearful and didn't know what to do, you decided to follow his advice. But you've had regrets about it and again realized that spanking is not an approach that you agree with." She replied, 'That's right.' I next asked a series of questions, "How often do you act on the opinions of others who are close to you?" "When people close to you share or give you their opinions, how do you figure out what fits with you and what doesn't?" and "How do you determine what to keep and use and how to cast aside what doesn't and say, 'That's just someone else's opinion and it's not right for me'?"

The client answered each question, and after reflecting on the final one, she replied, "I never really thought about that. It makes sense though. I don't agree with everything that my friends tell me, but sometimes I don't think about it enough. This is one of those times." With information from our conversation I was able to learn more about what most influenced the client's decisions with parenting, and as it turned out, with her relationships as well. I then used the knowledge gained as a factor in selecting an approach to help her more actively and deliberately reflect on others' opinions to determine which ones did and did not fit for her, particularly with critical life issues such as raising her child and relationships. And because the client already had sound ideas about how to raise her son and discipline without any form of spanking or punishment, we did not explore the topic any further.

In this case example, there were factors in the client's life that directly influenced her choices as to how she raised her son. There were sure some ideas she had internalized that worked well for her. However, several of the opinions she had adopted from others were troublesome. As therapists, we want to understand the topography of each client's life. One way to think about this is to consider what it would be like to play the role of your client in a movie. What would be most important for you to know to accurately portray your client? When we immerse ourselves in the lives of others our knowledge of their cultures grows accordingly. Things that did not previously make sense now have a context, and hopefully, our empathy deepens.

A strengths-based approach is not based on normative theory. We do not search for adherence to, or deviation from, cultural norms, which inherently leads to oppression. Therapists do, however, remain subject to blind spots that reflect cultural and personal assumptions and values. We counter these biases and blind spots through careful listening and attending to clients. Each client is a conglomeration of many different influences that separate her or him, however microscopically, from the next. Therefore, although everyone carries some general understandings and beliefs in relation to cultural influences, clinicians learn from clients what it is like to be them. With information gleaned from questions about clients' cultures, therapists can be more informed in selecting and matching methods, making sure to check in with clients to understand their experiences in therapy. To this end, therapists consider the best research evidence related to each particular client, in terms of treatment, problems, and social context.

There is an additional point to be made about culture as it relates to Case Example 6.1. I have shown part of a session with this client at various seminars in the United States and abroad. The reactions to the young mother's statement about spanking her child vary dramatically. For example, in the United States, mental health professionals, who certainly have personal opinions about corporal punishment, tend to focus on the client's presenting concern. In other parts of the world—for example, Scandinavia—audiences have responded to the issue of corporal punishment as it pertains to the treatment of human beings (see the Universal Declaration of Human Rights; United Nations, 1948). Principle 4 of a strengths-based perspective is, "Culture influences and shapes all aspects of human life." As clinicians, we consider that culture is always part of an individual's personal, interpersonal, and/or social distress and healing. But as we know, culture is much bigger than any individual. Psychiatrist Bessel van der Kolk (2014) astutely observed, "Our capacity to destroy one another is matched by our capacity to heal one another. . . . Restoring relationships and community is central to restoring well-being" (p. 38). Our efforts are therefore to achieve a multilevel understanding of culture as it relates to each individual client.

Readiness to Change

Even when self-reports of distress on a measure such as the Outcome Rating Scale (ORS) are within the clinical (i.e., distressed) range and there are well-defined goals, clients will express varying degrees of readiness to engage in activities associated with achieving the change they desire. This is because clients will have different ideas about how involved they are with problems (e.g., a client may believe that another person is responsible for his predicament), the nature of problems (whether problems are due to thinking, actions, etc.), how to best approach problems (change their thinking, take medication, etc.), how motivated they are to address a specific problem, and other closely related factors. To increase the fit between method or methods chosen, we explore each client's readiness to change. What follows is a discussion of three areas that can be explored in brief with clients to better inform choices of intervention and, in doing so, match the client's state of readiness. The three areas include coping style, relationship to concerns and problems, and perceptions and meaning of change.

Coping Style

A first way to hone in on clients' readiness to change is through their coping styles. A client's coping style indicates whether he or she tends to internalize or externalize when encountering stress and adversity. Beutler and Harwood (2000) stated, "People cope by activating behaviors that range from and combine those that allow direct escape or avoidance of the feared environment (externalization) and those that allow one to passively and indirectly control internal experience such as anxiety (internalization)" (p. 80). Therefore, clients who tend to be self-critical and cope by internalizing problems may benefit most from indirect, interpersonal, and insight-oriented approaches. By comparison, clients with externalized coping styles are likely to respond better to approaches that focus on symptom reduction, skill-building, and action (Beutler, Harwood, Kimpara, Verdirame, & Blau, 2010). Therapists can learn about clients' propensities to internalize or externalize by reviewing their histories of problem solving, as discussed earlier with "the client's theory of change." The following questions can also be helpful in ascertaining clients' preferred methods of coping:

- What first comes to mind when you think about how to approach problems you face in life?
- When you've experienced difficulties or problems in the past, what have you done to try to reduce the severity of those problems or resolve them altogether?
- What are you least inclined to do when facing problems in life?
- What kinds of problems in life are you more likely to try and solve yourself?
- What kinds of problems in life are you more likely to seek the help of others?

Coping style is relatively constant in people's lives. In other words, people who typically try to solve problems themselves do not usually seek the help of others as a first response. Nonetheless, because problems differ in type, seriousness, and importance to clients, we cannot assume that clients will also react the same way. In addition, coping style is also related to emotional, intellectual, and physical ability. We therefore consider factors that might affect a client's comprehension and ability to respond to an intervention.

Relationship to Concerns and Problems

A common mistake of therapists is attempting to intervene without a clear sense of how clients perceive their situations. Clients begin therapy for many reasons such as by their own accord, involuntarily, as part of a couple or family, and so on. As such, they will assume varying degrees of accountability to problems. For example, some clients will declare responsibility for the entirety of problems with statements such as, "It's on me, I'm the one who drove drunk" or "I know I need to change." Other clients will decline involvement and may even pass on responsibility to others for concerns or problems stating, "It's his fault" or "I wouldn't be here if they would've just left me alone." Still others will align themselves with some portion of a problem stating, "We both are responsible for what happened" or "I certainly have a part in all of this." A task of the therapist is to increase his or her understanding of how clients see themselves in relationship to their problems. It is not a question of whether clients are motivated, but rather what they are motivated for. In this case, we are interested in the aspects of problems with which clients express willingness to be involved. Duncan, Hubble, and Miller (1997) stated, "An unproductive and futile therapy can come about by mistaking or overlooking what the client wants to accomplish, misapprehending the client's readiness for change, or pursuing a personal motivation" (p. 11).

A way to further our understanding of the associations clients have with presenting problems is through careful attention to the use of pronouns such as, "I," "me," "mine," "my," "we," "us," "our," "you," "he/she," "him/her," and "they/them." Some pronouns, in this case the first seven listed here, typically indicate that clients are accepting some level of involvement with presenting problems and, perhaps, in being part of solutions to those problems. In contrast, the use of pronouns such as you/he/she/they/them often indicates that clients are removing or distancing themselves from involvement with problems. Because they are culture-specific—different pronouns mean different things in different cultures (e.g., the use of "you" by some Hispanic clients may include themselves: "When you get to work in the morning, you need to get the job done")—we follow up with questions to clarify what clients mean. We can also use one or more of the following questions to assist with exploring how clients situate themselves in relationship to presenting concerns:

- Who would you say is involved with this concern or problem?
- What's your role, if any, in the problem that led you to therapy (or to see me)?
- On a scale of 1 to 10, with 1 being "not at all" and 10 being "completely," how involved would you say you are with the concern or problem?
- Who else do you think is most involved with concern or problem?

How closely clients align themselves with presenting influences how therapists go about choosing methods of intervention. For instance, clients who see themselves as having little or no role problems are unlikely to do anything different to change their situations. Interventions should therefore be aimed at helping such clients to change their views or perspectives. In contrast, clients who closely align themselves with problems are likely to be more amenable to taking action to change their behavior or in their interactions with others. With these clients, therapists can employ interventions that emphasize changing views *and/or* encourage action. We will revisit this point shortly in our discussion of the stages of change (SOC) model.

Perceptions and Meaning of Change

A third aspect of readiness to change is clients' perceptions of change and the meaning change carries for them. Here we consider the client's perspective on the disadvantages and advantages of change, optimism, and intentions to change. Although change is constant and unavoidable, clients will vary in terms of the meaning of change and their level of interest to engage in change processes. It is common for clients to express some degree of ambivalence about change. As such, W. R. Miller and Rollnick's (2013) *Motivational Interviewing* provides excellent guidance for engaging clients in conversations about the prospects of change in their lives. Next are four areas with a series of questions to help tune into a client's perceptions of change.

Disadvantages of the Status Quo

- What concerns/worries you about your current situation? How has that affected you?
- What hardships has your current situation contributed to?
- How has that been troublesome for you?
- In what ways does that concern you?
- How might it be a concern for you if you decided to leave your situation alone?
- What do you think will happen if you decide not to change anything with your situation?

Advantages/Benefits of Change

- How would you like things to be different?
- What might it be like for you with your situation improved?
- Looking a few days/weeks/months/years into the future to a time when things are improved with your current situation, what might your life be like?
- What would be some of the advantages/benefits of things changing with your current situation?
- What would be advantages/benefits in your taking action to make changes?
- How might others benefit from changes you made?

Optimism About Change

- What affects your sense of optimism that you can make changes with your current situation?
- What makes you think that, should you decide to, you can make the changes you want?
- What encourages you or gives you hope that you can achieve the change you want?

- How confident are you that you can make changes with your situation?
- What experience in making changes can you draw on that might be helpful to you with your current situation?
- What strengths might be helpful to you in making this change?
- What external resources (people, relationships, support systems) might be helpful to you in making this change?

Intention to Change

- What is your stance on your concern?
- What are your thoughts about it?
- What are your intentions about it?
- How important is it for you for things to change with your current situation?
- What factors are currently influencing what you might do?
- What might you be willing to try?
- Of the possibilities discussed so far, which one(s) are most appealing to you?
- What would it take for you to begin to take a step toward changing your situation?

Increased understanding of how clients perceive change provides therapists with an additional layer of information, particularly in relation to clients' motivation. Therapists do not want to overlook the importance of evaluating each client's readiness to change. Decisions about methods without such consideration increase the likelihood of clients feeling misunderstood and in mismatches between therapists' and clients' ideas about change. These kinds of alliance ruptures, which are discussed in Chapter 7, can contribute to premature dropout and negative outcome. To increase attunement to clients' readiness to change and identify potential threats to the alliance, as described in earlier chapters, therapists are encouraged to use a measure such as the Session Rating Scale (SRS) and routinely check in with clients. In addition, for those interested in a more structured approach for matching interventions with clients' readiness to change, the SOC model offers further guidance. The SOC is discussed next.

Stages of Change

The SOC, also referred to as the transtheoretical model, is a framework both for gauging each client's readiness to change and selecting interventions that provide the best fit (Prochaska & DiClemente, 2005; Prochaska, DiClemente, & Norcross, 1992; Prochaska & Norcross, 2013). Through their studies of both people who went through self-change processes (without therapy) and those who attended therapy, Prochaska and colleagues found that individuals tend to move through "stages" and different degrees of motivation and willingness to respond to those concerns. These findings suggest that for each stage of change, certain methods of intervention are a better fit. The result of better matching is clients are more likely to move from one stage to the next, and subsequently, to the maintenance stage, the ideal outcome of treatment. The SOC has been found to be a better predictor of outcome than variables such as age, socioeconomic status, problem severity and duration, self-efficacy, or social supports (S. D. Miller, Duncan, & Hubble, 1997). The Division 29 Task Force of the APA concluded that consideration of a client's stage of change in assigning insight or behaviorally oriented therapies provides a promising means for enhancing the factor of fit (Ackerman et al., 2001). The SOC framework provides therapists with guidance about matching change facilitation methods based on client feedback.

Precontemplation

Most clients at this stage are typically unaware that problems exist and, in particular, that their behavior is problematic or produces negative consequences. To a lesser extent, some clients will acknowledge the presence of problems but will not see themselves as contributing to those problems and be unwilling to take action in the direction of positive change. Clients at the precontemplation stage often begin therapy involuntarily and are quick to reject responsibility. They may appear disinterested in discussing presenting concerns (which are often raised by those who initiated therapy), uncommitted and pressured to be in therapy, avoidant, and unaware of problems.

Consistent with earlier discussion regarding how clients view themselves in relationship to concerns/problems, precontemplative clients use pronouns (he, she, they) that deflect ownership. Instead, they point to external factors (e.g., other people, events, medication) to blame for problems. A task of the therapist is to align with such clients by creating environments in which clients feel heard and understood. Of critical importance is the alliance. Although clients at this stage may not have initiated therapy, evidence suggests that clients who have been mandated to therapy do as well as those who attend voluntarily as long as they feel connected with and understood by their therapists (Tohn & Oshlag, 1996). This finding supports clients' ratings of the relationship and alliance as being the most consistent process predictor of outcome (Bachelor & Horvath, 1999; Baldwin, Wampold, & Imel, 2007; Horvath & Bedi, 2002; Orlinsky, Grawe, & Parks, 1994; Orlinsky, Rønnestad, & Willutzki, 2004). Better alliances also increase expectancy and hope, which is especially important in early therapy interactions when clients are at high risk of dropout. We again turn to the use of formal alliance measurement and routine check-ins to assist with determining clients' interpretations of the therapeutic alliance.

Contemplation

This second stage is characterized by the acknowledgment of problems and recognition that change is necessary. Clients are more thoughtful about the pros and cons of changing their behaviors with equal emphasis placed on both. One way to further engage in conversations about pros and cons is to consider the disadvantages of the status quo and advantages/benefits of change, which were described under the section *Perceptions and Meaning of Change* earlier in this chapter. At this stage, clients often have ideas about goals for therapy and may even know how to reach those goals; however, they have ambivalence as to whether they believe the costs in terms of time, effort, and energy are worth putting in to achieve their goals (S. D. Miller et al., 1997). Therapists can help clients to determine where they stand through guided evaluation of their circumstances to understand their actions, thoughts about change, the pros and cons of their actions and the benefits and drawbacks of making changes, and by thinking about when they made attempts to change in the past.

At both the precontemplation and contemplation stages, it is important to be patient with clients and not push them to change. It may even be useful to join clients' ambivalence about change by suggesting that they go slowly or by discussing the "dangers of change" (Fisch, Weakland, & Segal, 1982). The latter is paradoxical and meant to match clients' teeter-tottering about change. By providing a supportive context, therapists can help clients at this stage to go at their own pace, thereby accommodating their varying states of readiness for change. Encouraging clients to think and observe change as opposed to suggesting that they take action to initiate it can also be helpful.

Preparation

The third stage represents a major step forward for most clients. At this point they are less delicate, less ambivalent, and more open to divulging the details of their lives and accepting responsibility. The therapist is an active participant during the preparation stage, helping clients identify the change they desire and consider realistic strategies for attaining that change. Indicators of being at this stage include clients expressing intentions to change their behavior, being on the verge of action in the direction of positive change, or having conversations as to how to bring about change. By this time clients are ready to take action within the next 30 days. Because clients are truly preparing to be more deliberate through action, many will have experimented—tried different methods of attaining change—to determine the results. Therapists utilize clients' drive to help them identify past successes and problem-solving strategies in exploring treatment options and taking small steps toward behavior change. In preparing clients for change, we communicate to clients that there are multiple pathways to achieving their goals and improved outcomes.

Action

The fourth stage is marked by client commitment to do something to create positive change and reach established goals. At the action stage, therapists collaborate with clients to identify and implement strategies that provide a good fit. In this way, therapists continue to be mindful of clients' contributions to change, taking care to remain client-, not theory-driven. Therapists also help clients to follow through, modifying, altering, and changing strategies based on the results achieved. Clients typically remain in the action stage for around 6 months, with intentions to keep moving forward with their behavior changes. It is noteworthy that many clients move back and forth between preparing to take action and actually doing so. Therapists work with clients by continuing to evaluate their readiness to change, which includes using the processes outlined in this chapter and ROM.

Maintenance

The fifth, and what some consider the final, stage of the SOC model is maintenance. At this stage clients have sustained their behavior change for around 6 months, depending on the client and situation, and intend to continue such change going forward. Therapists collaborate with clients to help them maintain the changes and gains that they have made and extend them into the future. As such, considerable attention is given to preventing slips and lapses. Clients will often express anxiety about and/or fear of setbacks. Therapists can help clients by anticipating possible hurdles or obstacles that might occur "down the road" and developing prevention strategies or plans to "hold the course." Another task of therapists is to help clients to extend changes that have been made to other areas of their lives, thereby improving overall well-being.

In the original SOC model, a sixth stage, *termination*, was outlined. There are likely to be cases in which clients' problems are fully resolved, never to surface again. In the self-change literature, for example, many people who have overcome smoking never return to that behavior again. In fact, a percentage of such persons would say they have no cravings or inclination to smoke again. In these cases, it is reasonable to say that the problem has been terminated and such persons have complete confidence that they will not engage in the old behavior again.

In psychotherapy, it appears that the majority of clients will not consider themselves as having reached the termination stage. S. D. Miller et al. (1997) note that the termination stage is more an ideal than a realistic or achievable state of change. Most clients remain in the maintenance stage and will "continue to be mindful of possible threats to their desired change and monitor what they need to do to keep the change in place" (p. 104). In accordance, clients appear to move through various SOC in one of two ways. Some advance in a linear fashion, passing from one stage to another. More often, however, people go a second route: They progress, have setbacks, progress, have setbacks, and move through the stages in a "three-steps-forward, two-steps-back" process. For the majority of clients, change is a process that unfolds over time.

In situations with uncomplicated client concerns (fear of riding elevators, anxiety over work performance, etc.), where there are no other identifiable, complicating factors, several systems have been developed for matching therapy methods with clients. These systems are consistent with the SOC and are designed to offer suggestions and guidance, not to serve as manualized protocols (Beutler & Harwood, 2000; Seligman & Reichenberg, 2017).

For many clients, their concerns will be multifaceted. That is, there are multiple concerns that are usually interrelated. In such cases, part of a situation may improve while other areas remain unchanged. It is recommended that therapists bring forth information gathered from ROM, interviewing, and from each of the areas outlined in this chapter to determine which methods are likely to provide the best fit. To this end, the use of a well-being/functioning index such as the ORS is vital as it will assist with understanding how clients rate themselves individually, interpersonally, socially, and overall. With ROM therapists will remain attuned to clients' experiences in therapy and maintain the flexibility to switch out of specific modalities and/or abandon them completely, as necessary. In sum, the purpose of the SOC is to help guide therapists in discussions with clients to learn about their motivations, ideas about change, and in selecting and matching interventions that provide the best possible fit and contribute to desired outcomes.

THE PATH TO MODELS: A BRIEF SUMMARY

To this point of the book we have explored research, principles, and practices that collectively reflect the best available research, clinical expertise, and client characteristics, culture, and preferences—the three cornerstones of EBP. Collectively, what has been discussed brings us to the point of selecting methods and interventions. Let's briefly summarize what we've learned that informs the selection process. First is Table 6.1, "8-Key Checklist for Method Selection" (8-KCMS), which outlines areas for therapists to incorporate into sessions. Second is a summary of questions that can provide further guidance for increasing the factor of fit:

- How does the client describe the concerns/problems (e.g., experientially, cognitively, in action or interactional terms, or in some combination)?
- What are the client's ideas about change (i.e., how and under what conditions does the client expect change to occur)?
- What cultural influences might affect the client's perceptions about change?
- How does the client describe her/his relationships to concerns/problems (in other words, how involved does she or he see herself or himself with the concerns raised)?
- What is the client's primary coping style?
- In general, at what stage of change does the client appear to be?

Among the many choices to be made in therapy, determining what approach creates the best fit for an individual, couple, or family is one of the most crucial. A poor fit between the client's perspective and the therapist and his or her approach leads to ruptures in the therapeutic alliance and ultimately results

TABLE 6.1

8-KEY CHECKLIST FOR METHOD SELECTION (8-KCMS)

Expectancy and hope are catalysts for change. Begin every therapeutic encounter with the expectation that therapy can help clients to improve their well-being and functioning. Inquire as to how the client has experienced change in his or her life, including methods of coping, and his or her readiness to change.

Client contributions are the most significant contributors in outcome. Identify, evoke, and utilize each client's range of strengths and resources in the service of change.

Client participation is essential. Engage clients by: tuning into the client's view of the relationship; establishing agreement on the goals, meaning, or purpose of the treatment; collaborating on the means and methods used in treatment; and accommodating the client's preferences.

Culture influences all aspects of human life. Create a culturally safe climate by learning about clients' lives and experiences, being responsive to and respectful of clients' views about therapy and all therapeutic processes.

Therapy is future-focused. Emphasize growth, development, well-being, and functioning.

Language and interaction are the primary vehicles for change. Use both verbal and nonverbal language and interaction to strengthen relationships, clarify problems and goal descriptions, and create possibilities for change.

Information-gathering processes provide multiple opportunities to learn about clients. Explore the impact of clients' problems on their lives, learn about their strengths and resources, establish goals and what they would like to have change in their lives, and to intervene in subtle ways that lead to larger, more substantial changes. Be mindful of the 80/20 rule, focusing on the 20% of information that accounts most for successful therapeutic outcomes.

ROM is critical to the fit and effect of therapy. ROM is comprised of both outcome and alliance measurement. With fit we ask: Does the method or intervention fit the client's worldview, culture, and ideas about change? With effect we ask: Did the intervention, at minimum, provide some benefit to the client (e.g., individually, relationally, and/or socially), and at best lead to a positive, measurable improvement in functioning? Begin using ROM with the first interaction and continue throughout the course of therapy. In addition to formal measurement, routinely check in with clients to learn their perceptions and respond to any threats to the alliance.

ROM, routine outcome monitoring.

---

in dropout or negative outcome. Choosing an approach may appear to be a complex, daunting task. However, clarity can be gleaned by incorporating the checklist and questions provided in Table 6.1.

FROM PHILOSOPHY TO THEORY TO PRACTICE

The therapist's personal philosophy is fundamental to the choice of models. In the opening chapter, a three-level system was described as a way of conceptualizing how therapy begins with the clinician and his or her fundamental beliefs about clients, change processes, and the proposed outcomes of therapy that inform theoretical frameworks and specific practices or interventions to stimulate client change (Bertolino, 2014; Madsen, 2007). Here is the system previously outlined:

Personal Philosophies	➡	Theory/Models	➡	Practices
"How we are"		"How we think"		"What we do"

The therapist's personal philosophy is influential in the choice of model and corresponding methods. A critical aspect of therapists' personal philosophies (see Chapter 1) is how they believe change occurs with clients. For example, some therapists hold that changes in thinking must precede changes in actions (behaviors or interactions). Other therapists believe that clients will need to express emotion or have cathartic experiences in therapy to resolve the problems that brought them to therapy. Theories are social constructions and do not represent reality. As such, a therapist's task is twofold. First, therapists remain attuned to their personal perspectives and work to reconcile any incongruences between those beliefs and clients' perspectives, should there be any. In cases in which a therapist cannot do this, he or she should seek supervision and if necessary, make an appropriate referral. A second task of the therapist is to work in ways that are consistent with clients' ideas about change.

The Model-Outcome Contradiction

We now come full circle, returning to the issue of methods, models, and techniques that were discussed in detail in the opening chapter. Recall that research indicates that therapy models account for only about 1% of the variance in outcome (Duncan et al., 2010). It is reasonable to then ask: Why learn therapy models? To reconcile what may appear a contradiction, let's consider just why models are critical to outcome. We begin with Jerome Frank (Frank & Frank, 1991), who remarked:

> My position is not that technique is irrelevant to outcome. Rather, I maintain that, as developed in the text, the success of all techniques depends on the patient's sense of alliance with an actual or symbolic healer. This implies that ideally therapists should select for each patient the therapy that accords, or can be brought to accord, with the patient's personal characteristics and view of the problem. Also implied is that therapists should seek to learn as many approaches as they find congenial and convincing. (p. xv)

Research makes it clear that therapy is more effective when there is a clear focus (often in the form of a treatment plan) and coherent articulation of an approach that fits with the client. Focus and model articulation put clients at the front and center of therapy as collaborators, which also builds expectancy because there is a clear rationale for therapists' choice of methods. In other words, clients understand why a particular model is recommended by a therapist, including benefits and drawbacks, extending full choice (i.e., informed consent) to clients. Clients are partners we work *with*, not *on*.

To practice in this way, therapists use a different framework. While there is a distinct lack of evidence to support the medical model perspective subscribed to by many therapists which states, "_____ (name of model) is the best model for _____ (name of problem)," there is very good evidence to support the ideology, "_____ (name of model) as delivered by _____ (name of the therapist) for _____ (name of the client) is effective." The latter statement makes therapy individualized, taking into account the unique characteristics of each client and information that factors into the choice of a specific model. Doing so, as we have learned, increases the fit between the client and the approach. In addition, the second ideology draws attention to the importance of *effect*. We want to know: Is this model, delivered by this particular therapist, working for this particular client, with this particular problem?

The choice of models requires thought and reflection on the part of the therapist, which unfortunately is not part of every therapist's practice. McAuliffe and Eriksen (2000) estimated that up to 50% of all mental health practitioners appear unreflective in selecting intervention strategies, which the authors defined as "adherence to a single technique, and/or maintenance of the status quo when more inclusive and socially critical interventions are needed" (p. 199). Therapists typically fall into one of three categories in terms of models. The first, which parallels the aforementioned quote, is to establish allegiance to one particular model and use that model with all clients. Second is therapists who know a couple, perhaps three models, and switch between those models. A third category is therapists who describe themselves as "eclectic," claiming to borrow from a multitude of approaches. But one can only be eclectic if he or she truly knows a wide range of approaches in detail. Lazarus (1992) wrote, "The technical eclectic uses procedures drawn from different sources without necessarily subscribing to the theories or disciplines that spawned them" (p. 323). But the average therapist knows only two or three theories, which is insufficient to consider oneself eclectic. Therefore, it's not that these therapists are practicing eclecticism; rather, they are using what they know.

While it is both unreasonable and unnecessary to know and practice a large number of approaches, there is inherent risk associated with too small of a knowledge base. Abraham Maslow (1966) famously stated, "I suppose it is tempting, if the only tool you have is a hammer, to treat everything as if it were a nail" (p. 15). Imagine if your doctor used such an approach to treatment. This is a troubling way to practice therapy.

We can address the issue of what therapists ought to know in terms of models in three ways. First, we can narrow the landscape of models by using only those considered bona fide. Recall that bona fide models are ones actually used in everyday practice and deemed viable by the psychotherapeutic community, delivered by trained therapists, and contain ingredients common to all legitimate psychotherapies (Bertolino, Bargmann, & Miller, 2013). Of the more than 400 models of psychotherapy described in more than 55,000 books, less than 10% meet the criteria for being a bona fide treatment. As a result, the choice for models is reduced substantially. A second way is to further narrow the choices of bona fide models even further by following the 8-KCMS. The checklist reflects the five principles of a strengths-based approach, which also provides a foundation of practice, which is absent to those who claim to be "eclectic," since eclecticism is not based on principles, only methods. Last is to learn three to five bona fide approaches that stimulate change in at least two of the four "classes." Classes include specific areas in which both represent areas that clients experience problems in and are the target of psychotherapy interventions. These classes will be discussed in the next section. Careful attention to these three ways can provide immediate direction and guidance for selection of therapy models. It is not a matter of achieving a perfect fit but rather using approaches that are both respectful of clients and provide the best possibilities for successful outcome. Through the use of ROM and close attention to the client's stage of change, we can adjust the approach based on the benefit, or lack thereof, to the client. This will be discussed further in Chapter 7.

CLASSES OF PROBLEMS/CLASSES OF INTERVENTION: SELECTING MODELS

Clients primarily experience and express problems in one or more of four areas or "classes." We'll refer to these as "Classes of Problems." These are *experiential and affective*, *cognition and views*, *action and interaction* (behavioral and systemic), and/or *neurobiological*. The *experiential and affective* class includes feelings, sense of self, bodily sensations, and automatic fantasies and thoughts. The second class, *cognition and views*, refers to thoughts, points of view, attention patterns, evaluations, stories, and so on. Next is *action and interaction*, which include individuals' behaviors (actions) and interpersonal relationships (interactions). The final class is *neurobiological*, autonomic responses and arousal and sensory experiences. Sensory experiences comprise the visual, auditory, tactile (kinesthetic), gustatory, and olfactory (V/A/T/G/O) realms. Table 6.2 provides a visual illustration of the "Classes of Problems."

Each of the classes represents a broad category within which clients will describe issues with functioning. Most often, client problem descriptions will cross into more than one class as illustrated in Figure 6.1. For example, a client will say, "I keep thinking I'm going to fail. And because of that I don't even try." In this case it can be said that the client's concern falls into two domains: (a) cognition and views, and (b) action and interaction. Further discussion may reveal the problem spanning even more classes.

Models are frameworks that posit explanations for the nature of problems and different ways of intervening with clients to facilitate change in one or

TABLE 6.2

CLASSES OF PROBLEMS

Experiential	Cognition and Views	Action and Interaction	Neurobiological
■ Affect responses ■ Feelings ■ Sense of self ■ Bodily sensations ■ Automatic fantasies and thoughts	■ Thoughts and cognition ■ Points of view ■ Attentional patterns ■ Beliefs, assumptions, interpretations, explanations, evaluations ■ Identity stories	■ Action patterns ■ Interactional patterns ■ Language patterns ■ Nonverbal patterns ■ Time patterns ■ Spatial patterns	■ Autonomic responses and arousal and sensory experiences (V/A/T/G/O) Visual Auditory Tactile (kinesthetic) Gustatory Olfactory

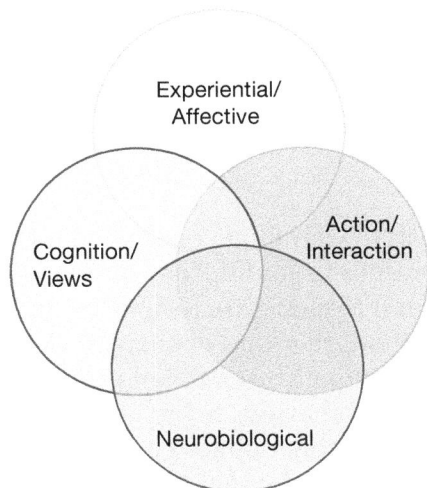

FIGURE 6.1 Classes of Problems.

more of the classes. For example, experientially focused therapists emphasize the expression of emotion. Cognitively oriented therapists focus on changing thinking. Behaviorists target changes in behavior and action. Likewise, systemic family therapists work to change interactions between people. More commonly, however, theories target multiple classes. For example, cognitive behavioral therapies (CBT) often involve the use of behavioral strategies with the ultimate goal of changing thinking. Table 6.3 provides a visual outline of the "Classes of Intervention," which correspond with the "Classes of Problems."

TABLE 6.3

CLASSES OF INTERVENTION

Experiential	Cognition and Views	Action and Interaction	Neurobiological
■ Give messages of acceptance, validation, and acknowledgment. ■ Encourage emotional expression. ■ Use inclusive language to expand acceptance of self.	■ Identify and challenge views that suggest impossibility, blame, invalidation, nonaccountability, or determinism. ■ Develop or increase awareness, insight, or mindfulness. ■ Change thoughts, cognitions, and perceptions. ■ Shift, alter, change, or offer new possibilities for attention.	■ Identify and alter or change problematic action patterns associated with the problem. ■ Identify and alter or change problematic interactional patterns associated with the problem. ■ Identify and utilize solution patterns. ■ Introduce new methods of adjusting and coping.	■ Alter, shift, or change autonomic responses and arousal and sensory experiences (V/A/K/G/O) Visual Auditory Tactile (kinesthetic) Gustatory Olfactory

Psychotherapy models typically target one or two primary forms of change but may incorporate interventions from different classes. For example, the primary goal of cognitive therapies is to change one's underlying thinking. Therapy is not considered successful without this kind of change. However, both emotive and behavioral methods are commonly used to help clients recognize the influence of thinking on emotions and behaviors. So, while a goal of cognitive therapies is not for clients to express emotion, doing so can stimulate change in cognition. Table 6.4 offers a list of some of the major models of psychotherapy and COI that may be active in the service of change.

The therapist's aim is to elucidate information that will help to determine which class or classes are most likely to facilitate change. Prochaska et al. (1992) offer guidance regarding the choice of therapies, "Action-oriented therapies may be quite effective with individuals who are in the preparation or action stages. These same programs may be ineffective or detrimental, however, with individuals in precontemplation or contemplation stages" (p. 1106). Following this advice, with clients who do not see a problem or are not ready to engage in behavior to change their situations, a focus on cognition and views may prove a better fit. On the other hand, when clients identify with a particular problem and express willingness to make changes, therapies that focus on action and

TABLE 6.4

MAJOR MODELS OF PSYCHOTHERAPY AND CLASSES OF INTERVENTION

Model	Experiential	Cognition and Views	Action and Interaction	Neurobiology
Acceptance and Commitment Therapy (ACT)	✓	✓	✓	
Adlerian Therapy (Individual Psychology)		✓	✓	
Behavior Therapies			✓	
Cognitive (CT) and Cognitive Behavioral Therapies (CBT)	✓	✓	✓	
Dialectical Behavior Therapy (DBT)	✓	✓	✓	✓
Existential Therapy	✓	✓		
Eye Movement Desensitization and Reprocessing (EMDR)	✓	✓		✓
Gestalt Therapy	✓	✓		
Hypnosis	✓	✓		✓
Jungian Analysis	✓	✓		
Motivational Interviewing (MI)		✓	✓	
Narrative Therapy		✓		
Person-Centered Therapy	✓	✓	✓	
Psychoanalysis and Psychodynamic Therapies	✓	✓		
Rational-Emotive Behavior Therapy	✓	✓	✓	
Reality Therapy		✓	✓	
Solution-Focused Brief Therapy (SFBT)		✓	✓	
Strategic and Structural Family Therapies			✓	

interaction can be added as options. The 8-KCMS offers other factors of consideration for decisions of models.

Course Corrections

Even the most collaborative therapists will face decisions that can affect the selection of therapy approaches and fit with clients. These decisions result from a relative sea of information that leaves it up to therapists to determine what to let pass or respond to at a later time. Some situations will necessitate use of higher degrees of structure or more directive action. Threats of harm to self or others as well as issues regarding clients' cognitive, developmental, emotional, and physical capacities must be responded to accordingly. To a lesser extent, therapists will choose paths that may not always be in sync with clients; for example, when therapists, either subtly or more directly, challenge clients' perspectives, test ideas or hypotheses, or attempt to engage clients who are less verbal or conversational. Therapists might also deliberately shift conversations to keep therapy focused.

Directive action, particularly in the form of methods, can negatively affect the therapeutic alliance and, in some cases, the overall course of therapy. Even the most skilled clinicians periodically veer off course from time to time. To counter risks that can negatively impact the alliance, we exercise sound judgment, use intuition, and engage in supervision when making critical decisions. In addition, we are cognizant that maps provide only conceptual frameworks; they do not represent the territory. To ensure that they are on track from their points of view and help to minimize risks associated with course deviations, therapists invite and encourage client participation and use feedback as a way to monitor clients' perceptions. All attempts to promote change should also involve feedback. We want to know: What were the results? What was the client's experience in the situation in which the intervention was used? And finally, don't be afraid to fail. As discussed in Chapter 4, an "error-centric" culture is instructive because it provides us opportunities to learn firsthand from clients about what is not working and take corrective action.

A final thought can be found in creativity. Picasso once said that all children are born artists; the problem is to remain an artist as we grow up. Some therapists prefer formulaic interventions for their ease of use. The idea is that by following a series of steps a predictable outcome will occur. But the evidence does not support this approach. Instead, what is needed is creativity combined with routine and ongoing client feedback. It is creativity derived from knowledge of the client, experience, and curiosity that improves the likelihood of success.

In this chapter, we explored ways of selecting and matching interventions to increase the factor of fit between clients and models. Doing so increases the likelihood of successful outcome. We also learned about four classes of problems and interventions, within which models of psychotherapy are aligned. In the next chapter, we explore ways of monitoring and responding to client progress and the benefit of therapy, from subsequent sessions through transition.

REFERENCES

Ackerman, S. J., Benjamin, L. S., Beutler, L. E., Gelso, C. J., Goldfried, M. R., Hill, C., . . . Rainer, J. (2001). Empirically supported therapy relationships: Conclusions and recommendations of the Division 29 Task Force. *Psychotherapy, 38*(4), 495–497. doi:10.1037/0033-3204.38.4.495

Bachelor, A., & Horvath, A. (1999). The therapeutic relationship. In M. A. Hubble, B. L. Duncan, & S. D. Miller (Eds.), *The heart and soul of change: What works in therapy* (pp. 133–178). Washington, DC: American Psychological Association.

Baldwin, S. A., Wampold, B. E., & Imel, Z. E. (2007). Untangling the alliance-outcome correlation: Exploring the relative importance of therapist and patient variability in the alliance. *Journal of Consulting and Clinical Psychology, 75*(6), 842–852. doi:10.1037/0022-006X.75.6.842

Barkham, M., Hardy, G., & Mellor-Clark, G. (Eds.). (2010). *Developing and delivering practice-based evidence*. Chichester, UK: Wiley.

Bertolino, B. (2010). *Strengths-based engagement and practice: Creating effective helping relationships*. Boston, MA: Allyn & Bacon.

Bertolino, B. (2014). *Thriving on the front lines: Strengths-based youth care work*. New York, NY: Routledge.

Bertolino, B., Bargmann, S., & Miller, S. D. (2013). Manual 1: What works in therapy: A primer. In B. Bertolino & S. D. Miller (Eds.), *The ICCE manuals of feedback informed treatment*. Chicago, IL: International Center for Clinical Excellence.

Beutler, L. E. (1989). Differential treatment selection: The role of diagnosis in psychotherapy. *Psychotherapy, 26*, 271–281. doi:10.1037/h0085436

Beutler, L. E., & Harwood, T. M. (2000). *Prescriptive psychotherapy: A practical guide to systematic treatment selection*. New York, NY: Oxford University Press.

Beutler, L. E., Harwood, T. M., Kimpara, S., Verdirame, D., & Blau, K. (2010). Coping style. *Journal of Clinical Psychology in Session, 67*(2), 176–183. doi:10.1002/jclp.20752

Burlingame, G. M., & Beecher, M. E. (2008). New directions and resources in group therapy: Introduction to the issue. *Journal of Clinical Psychology, 64*, 1197–1205. doi:10.1002/jclp.20534

Duncan, B. L., Hubble, M. A., & Miller, S. D. (1997). *Psychotherapy with "impossible" cases: The efficient treatment of therapy veterans*. New York, NY: W. W. Norton.

Duncan, B. L., Miller, S. D., & Sparks, J. A. (2004). *The heroic client: A revolutionary way to improve effectiveness through client directed, outcome-informed therapy*. San Francisco, CA: Jossey-Bass.

Duncan, B. L., Miller, S. D., Wampold, B. E., & Hubble, M. A. (Eds.). (2010). *The heart and soul of change: Delivering what works in therapy* (2nd ed.). Washington, DC: American Psychological Association.

Fisch, R., Weakland, J. H., & Segal, L. (1982). *The tactics of change: Doing therapy briefly*. San Francisco, CA: Jossey-Bass.

Frank, J. D., & Frank, J. B. (1991). *Persuasion and healing: A comparative study of psychotherapy* (3rd ed.). Baltimore, MD: Johns Hopkins University Press.

Held, B. S. (1991). The process/content distinction in psychotherapy revisited. *Psychotherapy, 28*(2), 207–217.

Held, B. S. (1995). *Back to reality: A critique of postmodern theory in psychotherapy*. New York, NY: W. W. Norton

Horvath, A. O., & Bedi, R. P. (2002). The alliance. In J. C. Norcross (Ed.), *Psychotherapy relationships that work: Therapist contributions and responsiveness to patient needs* (pp. 37–69). New York, NY: Oxford University Press.

Lambert, M. J. (2010). *Prevention of treatment failure: The use of measuring, monitoring, and feedback in clinical practice*. Washington, DC: American Psychological Association.

Lazarus, A. A. (1992). Multimodal therapy: Technical eclecticism with minimal integration. In J. C. Norcross & M. R. Goldfried (Eds.), *Handbook of psychotherapy integration* (pp. 231–263). New York, NY: Basic Books.

Madsen, W. C. (2007). *Collaborative therapy with multi-stressed families* (2nd ed.). New York, NY: Guilford Press.

Maslow, A. H. (1966). *The psychology of science*. New York, NY: Joanna Cotler Books.

McAuliffe, G., & Eriksen, K. (2000). *Preparing counselors and therapists: Creating constructivist and developmental programs*. Virginia Beach, VA: Donning.

Miller, S. D., Duncan, B. L., & Hubble, M. A. (1997). *Escape from Babel: Toward a unifying language for psychotherapy practice*. New York, NY: W. W. Norton.

Miller, W. R., & Rollnick, S. (2013). *Motivational interviewing: Helping people to change* (3rd ed.). New York, NY: Guilford Press.

Orlinsky, D. E., Grawe, K., & Parks, B. K. (1994). Process and outcome in psychotherapy—noch einmal. In A. E. Bergin & S. L. Garfield (Eds.), *Handbook of psychotherapy and behavior change* (4th ed., pp. 270–378). New York, NY: Wiley.

Orlinsky, D. E., Rønnestad, M. H., & Willutzki, U. (2004). Fifty years of process-outcome research: Continuity and change. In M. J. Lambert (Ed.), *Bergin and Garfield's handbook of psychotherapy and behavior change* (5th ed., pp. 307–390). Hoboken, NJ: Wiley.

Prochaska, J. O., & DiClemente, C. C. (2005). The transtheoretical approach. In J. C. Norcross & M. R. Goldfried (Eds.), *Handbook of psychotherapy integration* (2nd ed., pp. 147–171). New York, NY: Oxford University Press.

Prochaska, J. O., DiClemente, C. C., & Norcross, J. C. (1992). In search of how people change: Applications to addictive behaviors. *American Psychologist, 47*(9), 1102–1114. doi:10.1037/0003-066X.47.9.1102

Prochaska, J. O., & Norcross, J. C. (2013). *Systems of psychotherapy: A transtheoretical analysis* (8th ed.). New York, NY: Cengage.

Seligman, L., & Reichenberg, L. W. (2017). *Selecting effective treatments: A comprehensive, systematic guide to treating mental disorders* (5th ed.). Hoboken, NJ: Wiley.

Tohn, S. L., & Oshlag, J. A. (1996). Solution-focused therapy with mandated clients: Cooperating with the uncooperative. In S. D. Miller, M. A. Hubble, & B. L. Duncan (Eds.), *Handbook of solution-focused brief therapy* (pp. 152–183). San Francisco, CA: Jossey-Bass.

United Nations. (1948). Universal Declaration of Human Rights. Retrieved from http://www.un.org/en/universal-declaration-human-rights

van der Kolk, B. (2014). *The body keeps the score: Brain, mind, and body in the healing of trauma*. New York, NY: Viking.

CHAPTER 7

Client Progress and the Benefits of Therapy

The primary purpose of this chapter is to monitor the progress of clients in therapy and determine next steps. We are reminded that effective therapy begins with a commitment to routine outcome monitoring (ROM). As discussed in Chapter 1, the absence of ROM therapists leads to three inherent risks: failure to identify client deterioration, overprediction of client improvement, and therapist self-assessment bias. Interestingly, while a large percentage of therapists consistently express interest in regular reports of their clients' progress in therapy (Bickman, 2000; Hatfield & Ogles, 2004), few actually use ROM in their day-to-day work (Gilbody, House, & Sheldon, 2002; Hatfield & Ogles, 2004; Zimmerman & McGlinchey, 2008). A further concern arises in review of clinicians who actually use ROM. Studies indicate that the impact of feedback varies significantly between therapists. While some therapists achieve better results, others see little or no improvement in their outcomes (de Jong, van Sluis, Nugter, Heiser, & Spinhoven, 2012; Sapyta, Riemer, & Bickman, 2005). As it turns out, outcome is largely dependent on *who* uses the feedback. In this chapter, we will explore how feedback-informed treatment (FIT) provides a means for responding to information gleaned from both outcome and alliance measurement, which in this case is the Outcome Rating Scale (ORS) and Session Rating Scale (SRS), respectively.

This chapter will also include a discussion of how to respond to client improvement, lack of progress, and deterioration. In addition, ways of transitioning clients from therapy will be examined.

THE PROGRESSION OF THERAPY IN FUTURE SESSIONS

We begin each subsequent session by administering the ORS (or CORS). Clients are asked to complete the ORS, either on paper or electronically (see Chapter 4), by rating how things have been in their lives since the last session (or over the past week). ORS scores provide a starting point for each session, providing entryways to conversation to determine both the focus of the session and next steps. The SONAR SFC, introduced in Chapter 4 and included in the Appendix can serve as a guide here. In subsequent sessions, therapists skip the "S" part of the SONAR SFC and begin with "O," which is outcome measurement.

Once an ORS has been completed, the therapist or computer-based system plots the results. Although additional sessions will mean we have two or more ORS data points on a graph, the results only reveal so much about a client and his or her progress. Thus, the therapist reviews the results with the client, creating space for the client to convey the idiosyncratic meaning of their scores. The therapist also explores how the client's perceptions relate to the course of therapy including any preestablished goals. As part of the conversation, the therapist continues to acknowledge, validate, employ action-talk, and use language in ways offered in Chapters 4 and 5 to introduce possibilities into client statements that may appear closed-down.

Despite being given instructions, clients will occasionally complete the ORS based on situational events. For example, a client may have a good week overall but have something happen just prior to the session that influences how the ORS is scored. For this reason, therapists inquire about circumstances around scores—factors that may be of influence on clients' ratings. Our aim is to understand what clients are currently feeling and thinking while maintaining focus on the purpose of therapy. We strive for early change, as research makes it clear that the process of change begins early in therapy (Baldwin, Berkeljon, Atkins, Olsen, & Nielsen, 2009; Howard, Kopte, Krause, & Orlinksy, 1986; Kopta, Howard, Lowry, & Beutler, 1994) and the longer therapy goes without improvement the greater the risk of negative outcome and dropout (Duncan, Miller, Wampold, & Hubble, 2010; Howard, Moras, Brill, Martinovich, & Lutz, 1996). However, with a few exceptions (i.e., so-called "epiphanies" or life-changing experiences), lasting change for most clients will be more incremental or gradual. As such, we collaborate with clients to gain clarity about any changes they report, which will be discussed next.

The Reliable Change Index and Clinical Significance

As the therapist reviews with the client the results of his or her most recent ORS and develops an understanding of the meaning of scores, it is important to determine whether the client is progressing from a statistical standpoint. To this end, effective monitoring of client progress involves the use of statistical indices. There are various ways to determine how therapy is progressing, each with benefits and drawbacks. Here we discuss two common indicators.

Client ratings on the ORS or other form of outcomes measurement are part of ongoing discussions with clients. For increases on an outcome measure to be considered reliable, the difference between two scores must meet or exceed a statistical index known as the *reliable change index* (RCI). The RCI is a measure used to assess the magnitude of change necessary to be considered statistically reliable rather than due to chance, maturation (the passage of time), or measurement (statistical) error. It is an average based on the reliability or consistency of an instrument. The RCI for the ORS (and CORS) is 5, meaning that a 5-point increase between two scores is considered a reliable change. Scores that increase by 4 points or less may still indicate progress but cannot be reliably attributed to therapy. The RCI can prove useful in separating successful and unsuccessful cases; however, it can also result in overestimates or underestimates of the amount of change depending on the level of severity (Duncan, Miller, & Sparks, 2004).

A second statistic, *clinical significance* (CS), or clinically significant change, refers to reliable improvement (i.e., 5 points or more on the ORS) that is beyond a trivial amount of "day-to-day" fluctuation and also corresponds to a change in clinical status—movement from a clinical (i.e., distressed) range to a nonclinical (non-distressed, functional) range. Distinctions between clinical and nonclinical ranges are commonly referred to as clinical cutoffs (see Chapter 4). As an example, the clinical cutoff on the ORS for clients ages 20 and over is 25. Therefore, a client who has achieved clinically significant change would, at the end of therapy, have reported an improvement of at least 5 points from his or her first and last session ORS scores *and* have a final ORS score of above 25.

Both the RCI and CS can be useful statistics in determining the client's response to therapy. In the final chapter, we will consider other statistical enumerations for evaluating therapeutic effectiveness. Next, we explore two main categories of client response to therapy: (a) unimprovement or deterioration and (b) improvement. Each form of response includes suggestions for how to use feedback to increase the benefit of services.

CATEGORY 1: UNIMPROVEMENT OR DETERIORATION

Earlier in the book, the story of Cincinnati Children's Hospital (CCH) and its efforts to improve in the treatment of persons diagnosed with cystic fibrosis (CF) was shared. A critical aspect of CCH's approach to achieving better outcomes was its attention to very specific aspects of CF that are correlated with life expectancy. In other words, CCH focused on the 20% of information that matters most in CF treatment. In psychotherapy, we use client feedback to hone in on aspects of clients' lives and situations to increase the fit of therapeutic interventions and monitor the effects of those interventions to increase the likelihood of successful outcomes. This degree of responsiveness is especially critical given the evidence that therapists routinely fail to identify client deterioration. Next, we discuss clients who are not progressing adequately in therapy. These clients typically fall into the unimproved or deteriorated category. Although deterioration is a form of unimprovement, it very often translates to higher client risk. For this reason, deterioration will be discussed separately.

Before we proceed, there is one further reminder about the alliance and client feedback. Sometimes clients will find it difficult to give negative feedback. Duncan and Miller (2008) remarked,

> Sometimes it takes a bit more work to create the conditions that allow clients to be forthright with us, to develop a culture of feedback in the room. The power disparity

combined with any socioeconomic, ethnic, or racial differences make it difficult to tell authority figures that they are on the wrong track. Think about the last time you told your doctor that he or she was not performing well. Clients, however, will let us know subtly on alliance measures far before they will confront us directly. (p. 65)

If clients express apprehension, we acknowledge their reluctance, extend respect for their positions, and invite them to conversations where we can better understand their experiences in therapy. In addition, Chapter 4 provides a series of suggestions to engage clients and increase comfort with the measures should that be an issue. Our hope is to learn from clients what is working, what is not, and how we can partner to achieve the futures they desire.

Unimprovement

When a client's *current* (most recent) ORS increases or decreases but remains within 4 points of his or her initial ORS/CORS score, the client is said to be "unimproved." By comparison, "deterioration" is when a client's most recent ORS score decreases by 5 or more points as compared to the initial ORS. By unimproved we mean that a client is not statistically better or worse as a result of therapy. Recall that between 30% and 50% of clients do not improve from therapy (Lambert, 2010).

It is not uncommon for client scores to vary within a range of a few points, but as we know, the longer clients remain in therapy without measurable progress the greater the likelihood of dropout or negative outcome (Duncan et al., 2010). Figure 7.1 provides a graphical illustration of unimprovement or no progress. In the example, an adult client has an initial ORS score of 20.1, a second session score of 22.4, and a third session score of 20.8. The variance in scores remains small—with no sharp increases or decreases. When the first session ORS score is compared with the most recent session score the change is +0.7, which is an increase, but not a significant one.

If the same client were to have a third session score of 24.2, which would represent a 4.1 point numerical increase from session one (and an overall improvement),

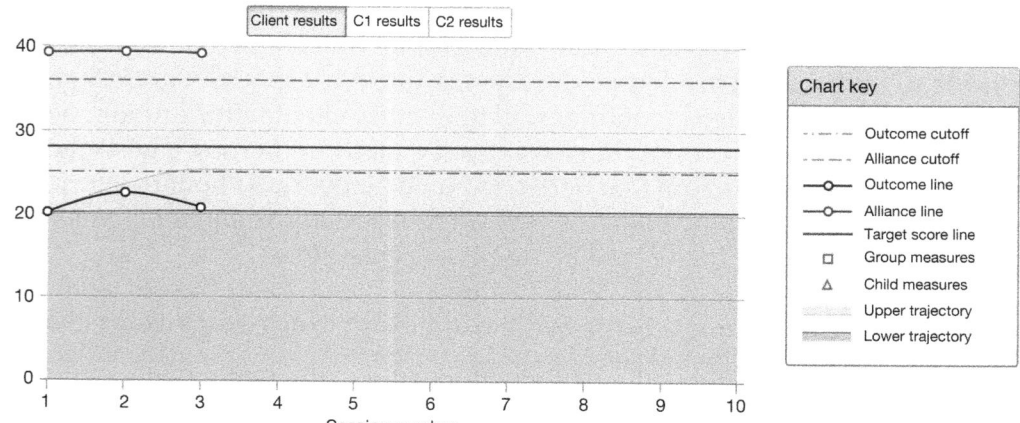

FIGURE 7.1 No improvement.

it still would not be statistically *reliable* or *clinically significant* based on the properties of the ORS. To be considered a reliable change the third session score would need to be 5 points or greater. Then, to be clinically significant, the score would also need to exceed 25, which is the clinical cutoff for ages 20 and over on the ORS.

A second example of "no improvement" can be found with Figure 7.2. In this illustration is an adolescent client with an opening score of 20.3 and a Session 8 score of 22.7. Review of the data reveals that the client improved between Sessions 1 and 3, before experiencing a regression in scores between Sessions 3 and 5. The client then demonstrated a slight improvement leading up to a drop from 27.9 to 22.7 at the most recent session. In fact, at both Sessions 3 and 6, the client's change was both *reliable* and *clinically significant* with improvement of 5 or more points and scores above the clinical cutoff, which is 28 on the ORS for ages 13 to 19. Later in the chapter, ideas for identifying and building on between-session change will be discussed. Here we refer to the current status of the client, which is unimproved. Although the client dropped 5.2 points between Sessions 7 and 8, she is not considered "deteriorated" because the difference between the first and most recent session is +2.5. Of further interest in Figure 7.2 are the SRS scores, which suggest potential problems with the client–therapist alliance. The issue of alliance ruptures will be discussed shortly.

In each session, the therapist checks with the client to see how verbal reports match the rating on the ORS. If a client's verbalizations conflict with ORS scores (i.e., verbalizations are higher or lower than that reported on the measures), the therapist investigates the possible incongruity. For example, a therapist might say, "From what you've said, it sounds like things have gotten worse for you over the past week. But your ORS score is very similar to the last session. Can you tell me about that?" Or, "From what you've described things have been pretty much the same as the last time we met, but your ORS has gone up. What can you tell me about that?" Oftentimes differences between what a client says and actual ORS scores are small and may be statistically insignificant. At the same time, small variations can be building blocks for exploring exceptions and can be meaningful.

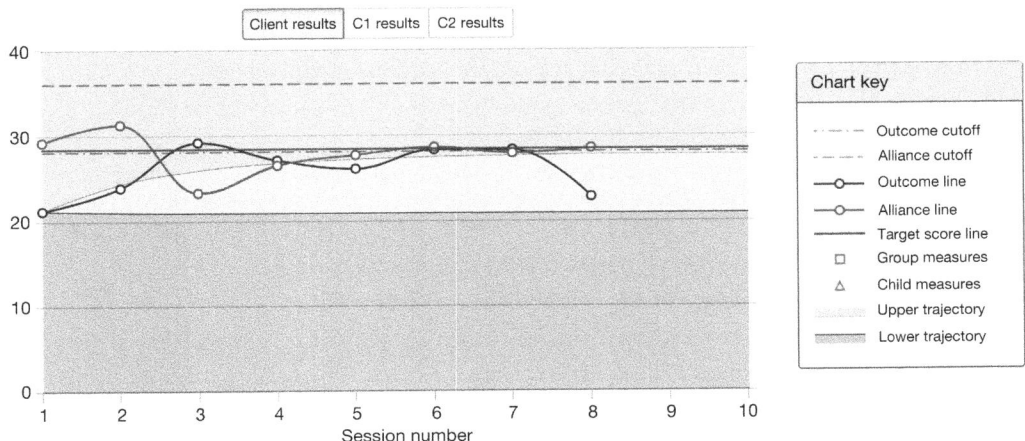

FIGURE 7.2 No improvement.

It is noteworthy that some electronic outcomes management systems (OMS) provide signal alerts and/or feedback messages for both outcomes and alliance measurement. For example, Youth In Need (YIN), Inc.'s cloud-based OMS, Imagine, offers both. Figure 7.3 is an example of an ORS message for a client in the unimproved/unchanged range on the ORS. Further examples will be provided later in this chapter.

Deterioration

Studies indicate that 5% to 10% of adults and between 12% and 20% of adolescents deteriorate while in therapy (Hansen, Lambert, & Forman, 2002; Lambert, 2013; Warren et al., 2010). As with clients who are in the unimproved range, our aim is to increase our effectiveness with such clients so they may experience a greater benefit of services. The more attuned we are to client progress through ROM, the better prepared we can be to respond, session by session.

Again, when there is a decrease of 5 or more points between initial and most recent sessions, it can be said that there is "deterioration." Clients whose outcome scores trend downward will typically say things such as, "My life is going downhill," "I feel like I'm at the bottom," or "It's worse than before." Because clients will have ups and downs, these kinds of reports are to be expected. And

---

Feedback Message

Your client's scores indicate that he/she is in the **moderate risk/unchanged range**.

Actions to Consider:

1. Review the results, and in particular, discuss the subscales to determine if all or some are lower than others.
2. Determine if there has been a change in score from the initial session that is greater than or equal to +5 or -5. Discuss both improving and deteriorating scores with the client.
3. Have an open and transparent discussion with the client about the lack of progress or deterioration.
4. Consider further risk assessment. A change in scores of -5 or more can indicate deterioration, even if the client is not in the high-risk/deteriorated range.
5. If client scores have remained unchanged—in between +5/-5—for two or more sessions, revisit the goals and /or approach.
6. If client scores have remained unchanged for two or more sessions or have dropped by -5 or more since the initial session, consider other service and support options (e.g., another service provider, different dose or intensity, alternative treatment approach, etc.)
7. Talk with the client about what has kept things from getting worse.
8. Review alliance scores to identify and address any problems.
9. Talk with a supervisor or invite a colleague or supervisor to join the session with the client.

ORS, outcome rating scale.

FIGURE 7.3 ORS feedback message for client in "moderate risk/unchanged" (unimproved) range.

yet, what accompanies deterioration is frustration and loss of hope, which are precursors to dropout and negative outcome, two of the most significant threats.

Figure 7.4 offers an example of an adult client who gradually fell into the deteriorated range. Following scores of 23.1, 22.5, and 20.7, which indicated a subtle decrease, the client's score dropped to 17.4 in Session 4. The difference between Session 1 and Session 4 scores is −5.7 points. Over the course of four sessions the client moved from the unimprovement to deterioration range.

In contrast, Figure 7.5 shows an example of marked deterioration of an adolescent client. In this case, the client had ORS scores of 11.1, 29.2, 18.6, and 5.4. There are several crucial elements of this particular example. First, the client's opening ORS score was very low. In some programs, certain scores may trigger more deliberate action on the part of therapists. For example, at my agency, YIN, any client score of 15 or below leads to further risk assessment. A second crucial element of the client example is the dramatic changes in scores. Most often, sharp increases and decreases are in response to situations. Therapists make sure to ask clients about events or changes to their lives that may account for sweeping changes in scores. It is imperative that therapists respond to changes in scores, particularly those that fall into the deterioration range as those clients are at high risk of dropping out of therapy. Later in this chapter we will explore different patterns of scores from clients and how to respond accordingly.

How therapists respond to situations involving unimprovement and deterioration can be the difference between a client staying engaged long enough to reap the benefit of services and dropping out. If clients drop out we may not have another chance to help them and perhaps, they may shy away from seeking assistance in the future, believing that it won't do any good. Figure 7.6 is an example of feedback produced by YIN's OMS, Imagine, for a client whose ORS scores indicate deterioration. When faced with deterioration, therapists respond in a swift and deliberate manner. In the next section, we examine four variations of client outcome patterns and strategies of response for therapists.

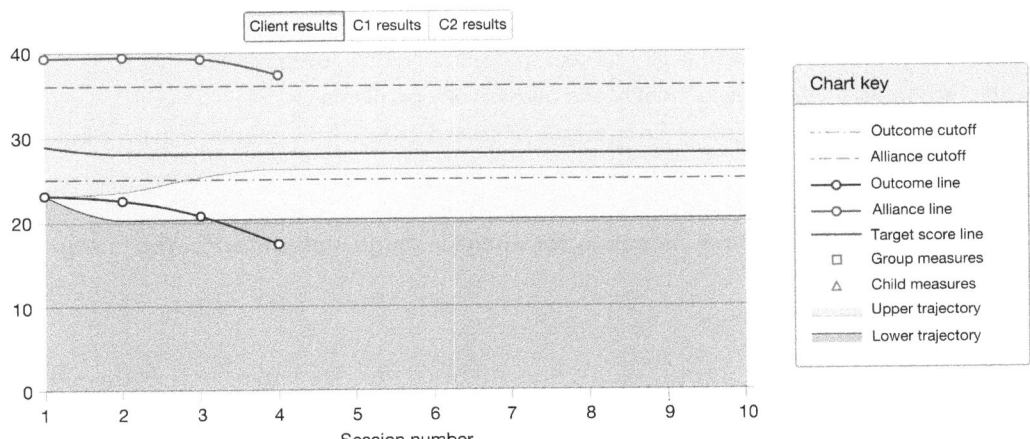

FIGURE 7.4 Deterioration.

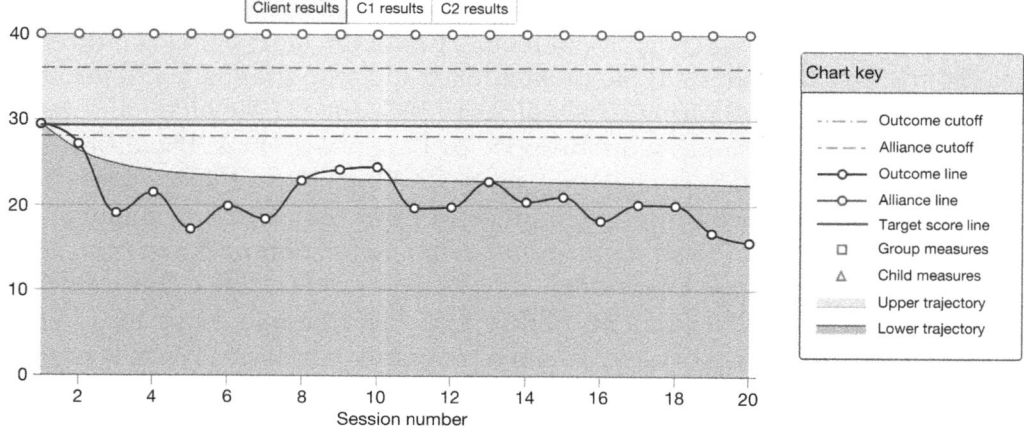

FIGURE 7.5 Deterioration.

Feedback Message

Your client's outcome scores indicate that he/she is in the **high-risk/deteriorated** range.

Actions to Consider:

1. Review the results, and in particular, discuss the subscales to determine if all or some are lower than others.
2. A change in scores of -5 or more from one session to the next indicates deterioration within the high-risk range. Risk assessment is necessary.
3. Determine if there has been a change in score from the initial session that is greater than or equal to +5. Discuss improving scores with the client even if he/she remains in the high-risk range.
4. Have an open and transparent discussion with the client about deterioration.
5. If client scores have remained unchanged—in between +5/-5—for two or more sessions, revisit the goals and/or approach.
6. If client scores have remained unchanged for two or more session or have dropped by -5 or more since the initial session, consider other service and support options (e.g., another service provider, different dose or intensity, alternative treatment approach, etc.)
7. Talk with the client about what has kept things from getting even worse.
8. Review alliance scores to identify and address any problems.
9. Talk with a supervisor or invite a colleague or supervisor to join the session with the client.

ORS, outcome rating scale.

FIGURE 7.6 ORS feedback message for client in "high-risk/deteriorated" range.

Client Outcome Patterns

Of the ways that clients report change on an outcome measure such as the ORS, four distinct patterns emerge most frequently. These patterns are bleeding, dipping, seesawing or fluctuating, and plateauing (Maeschalck, Bargmann, & Miller, & Bertolino, 2013). The first two patterns are associated with clients who fall into the unimproved and deterioration ranges. The second two patterns can involve scores that are in any of the three ranges: unimproved, deterioration, or improvement (which will be discussed shortly). For instance, depending on the slope of the scores, seesawing or fluctuating patterns can occur with clients who may be moving back and forth between improvement and unimprovement or deterioration. A pattern of plateauing scores can also occur within each of the categories of response. Let's briefly examine each pattern.

Bleeding

A frequently occurring pattern in client ORS scores is when the level of distress increases. Clients report feeling incrementally worse, which is reflected in a gradual downturn in scores over the course of a few sessions. Often, though not always, gradual deterioration in scores follows an early and often pronounced improvement in ORS scores early in the treatment process. In such cases, the therapist explores with the client possible reasons for the steady decline and what to do to "stop the bleeding" and help clients maintain gains between visits. Figure 7.4 provides an example of bleeding.

Dipping

Sometimes referred to as "ditching," *dipping* refers to a dramatic drop in ORS scores. Often, dipping will follow an increase in scores, suggesting a rapid onset of distress. Typically, significant drops in scores are attributable to external circumstances outside of the client's and/or therapist's control. In many cases downturns resolve quickly with clients returning to prior levels of functioning within a session or two. In these instances, therapists continue with treatment as usual rather than making the downturn a topic of treatment. However, as discussed previously, sharp drops in scores can also indicate high risk for clients. Therapists always exercise caution by inquiring about the meanings of scores and responding appropriately. This can mean using further risk assessment and

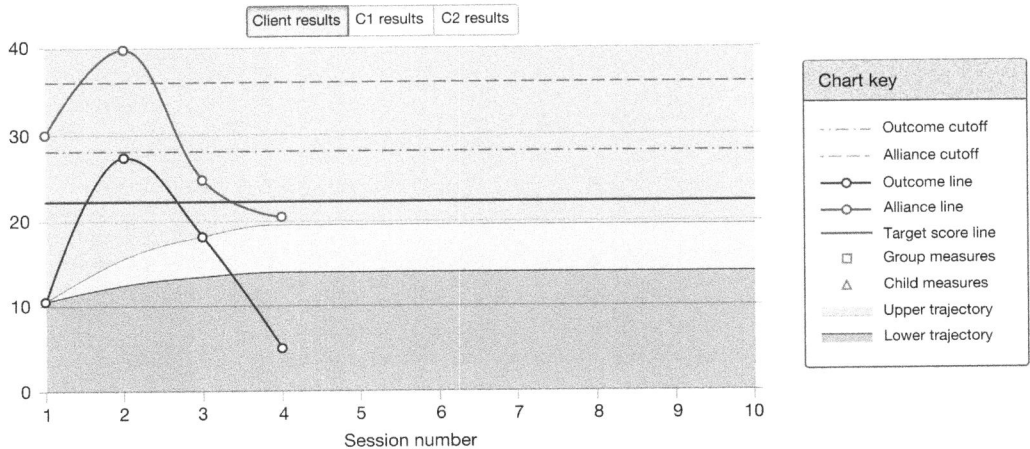

FIGURE 7.7 Dipping.

adjusting the treatment in dosage form, intensity, or referral to a more structured treatment condition. Figure 7.7 provides an illustration of dipping.

Seesawing or Fluctuating

Scores that seesaw involve wide fluctuations in scores from visit to visit. Also referred to as "cycling," these scores represent rapid increases and decreases in client distress levels. Seesawing movements are often attributable to clients scoring based on how they are feeling at the time of measurement completion or an event or situation that occurred just prior to the session. Other reasons for seesawing scores include normal variation in nonclinical levels of functioning (typical of everyday life for a particular client), an expression of a life with large, dramatic, sudden changes in functioning (i.e., chronic illness in which a client does well for a stretch then suffers more during others), and ineffective treatment. If client scores represent a client's sense of instability, the treatment approach can be modified to better fit the client and his or her situation.

Each of the circumstances carries some risk of clients feeling disempowered over time and/or dropping out of services. For example, with clients who start above the clinical cutoff, or who have met or exceeded the benchmark of predicted change, some variation in ORS scores is typical and reflects normal day-to-day (or week-to-week) variation in functioning. Therapists may best serve clients by increasing the length of time between sessions. Doing so minimizes the possibility of needlessly extending services, thereby reducing the risk of discouragement and/or dropout. The supervisor can also encourage the clinician to shift the focus of services to aftercare planning. Figures 7.8 and 7.9 provide different examples of seesawing.

Lack of movement, especially with clients who are in the unimproved or deteriorated range, can tempt therapists to attribute the overall lack of progress to external, extratherapeutic factors or to the client (e.g., "resistance" to treatment). To guard against this, therapists address the failure of the current service

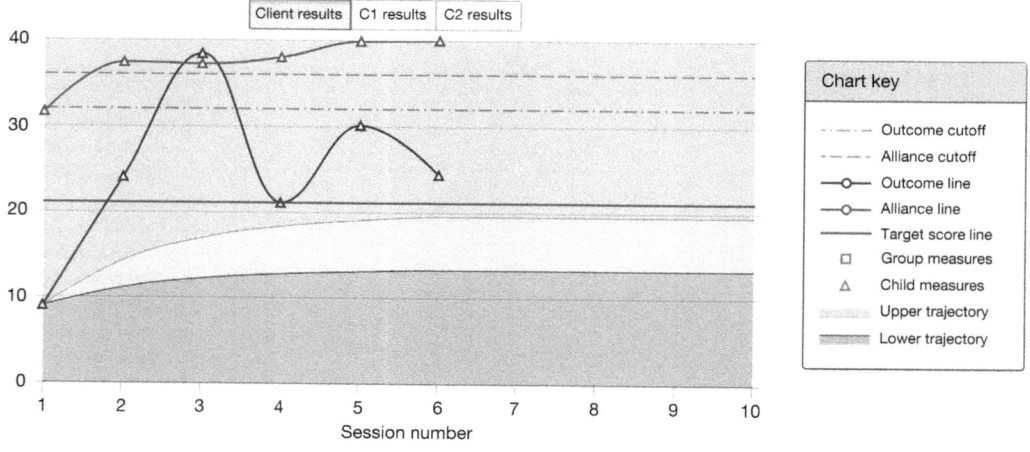

FIGURE 7.8 Seesawing.

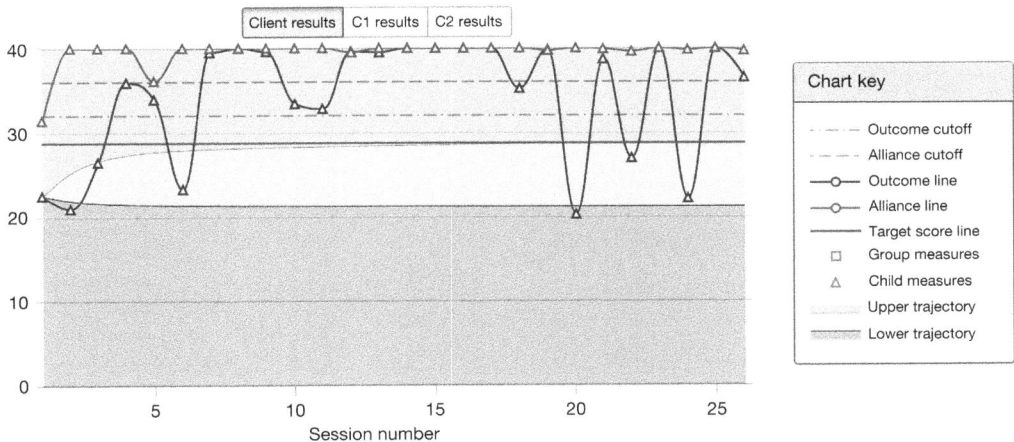

FIGURE 7.9 Seesawing.

to bring about a more stable pattern of change including: (a) having an open and transparent discussion with the client about the fluctuations; (b) identifying and addressing any problems in the alliance; (c) inviting a colleague or supervisor to join the session with the client; and (d) considering other service and support options (e.g., another service provider, different dose or intensity, alternative treatment approach, etc.; Maeschalck et al., 2013).

Plateauing

A final client outcome pattern is when scores plateau. As discussed, plateauing can occur with any of the categories of client response, but is most common when clients have experienced improved functioning. In these cases, therapists work with clients to maintain changes made by exploring strategies for managing setbacks and extending change forward. The dosage form of sessions is often titrated down, with clients coming to therapy less frequently as they transition from services (i.e., therapy is terminated). Because there is a maximum benefit to most forms of therapeutic intervention, when clients plateau in the unimproved or deteriorated ranges, therapists are active in determining next steps including changing the goals and/or approach in therapy, bringing in another therapist to consult in a session, or referral. For reasons already discussed throughout this book, therapists cannot afford to be complacent about the lack of client progress. Instead, conversations with clients about progress and determining how to proceed are recommended. Figures 7.10 and 7.11 offer two different examples of how client scores can plateau at different levels of functioning and distress.

RESPONSES TO UNIMPROVEMENT AND DETERIORATION

We now explore in more detail strategies for responding to client unimprovement or deterioration with consideration given to the four client outcome patterns

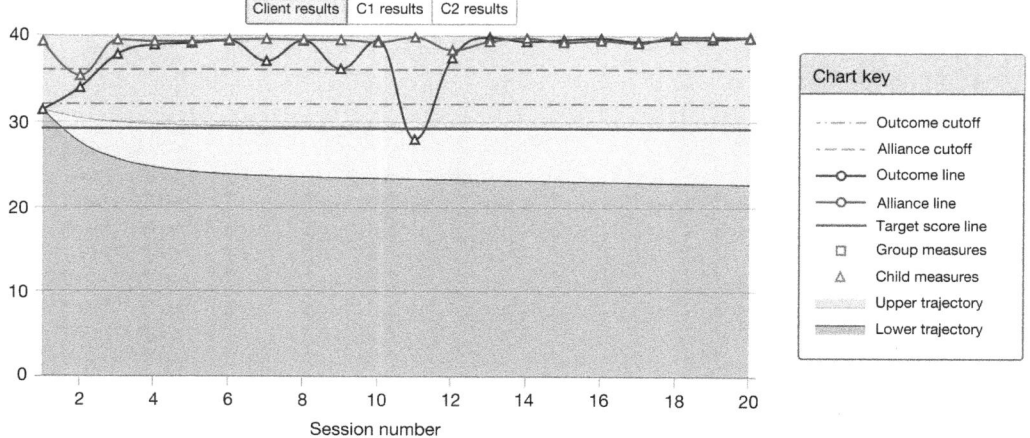

FIGURE 7.10 Plateauing.

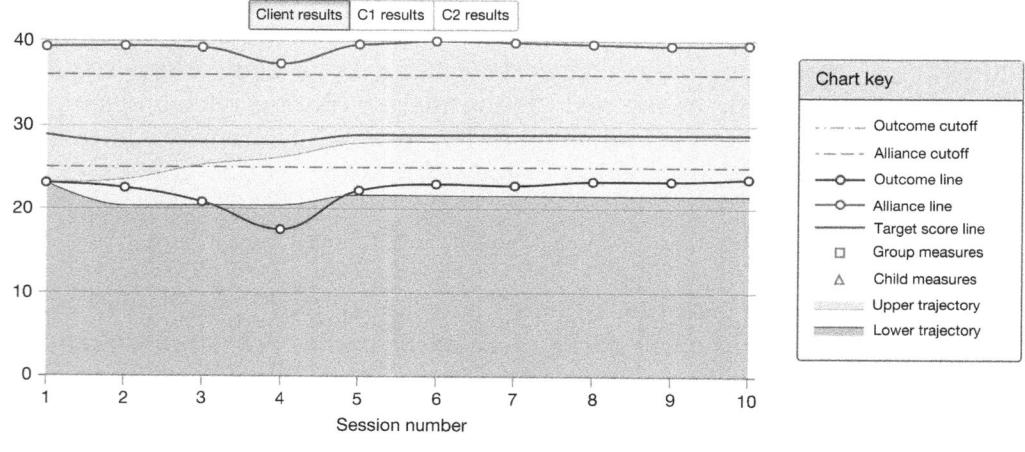

FIGURE 7.11 Plateauing.

described in the previous section. There are three core areas of focus to assist therapists in helping clients who are not progressing. These areas are the following:

1. Reexamine the focus of therapy (three variations of client responses)
2. Activate client strengths
3. Attend to the alliance

Reexamine the Focus of Therapy: Two Forms of Response

When clients are not progressing adequately or deteriorating, we want to connect their ORS scores with their verbalizations of their lives and situations. For example, using Figure 7.11, the therapist might say, "According to your scores, things seem to have been much the same for the past few sessions. How do you see it?" It's not often that clients' verbal reports greatly conflict with their outcome scores. Our aim is to learn the details, which exist in clients' perspectives. As we have learned, out of distress and/or frustration, clients occasionally generalize an event or situation as indicative of how they are doing overall. By listening carefully to clients' stories, we can learn more about what is working, what is not, and ideas for next steps. Equally important is feedback about the direction of therapy and whether goals need to be revisited and perhaps revised. When clients are not progressing, there are two forms of response, each of which will be discussed next.

Reports of new concerns or problems

There are times that completely new concerns or problems will arise that do not appear connected to previously established problem descriptions and goals. Depending on what has transpired between sessions, clients may delve into the details of specific conversations or move between several topics. There are many reasons clients delve into new territory. For example, it can indicate clients' preferred ways of communicating, provide them relief through the sharing of experiences, or be a means of "updating" therapists. Regardless of the rationale, therapists create space for clients to start where they feel most comfortable. Clinicians take care to ensure that clients feel heard and understood.

Through acknowledgment, clients will often shift back to the concerns that led them to seek therapy in the first place. Without prompting, simply by feeling heard and understood, they reorient to their initial complaints and pick up where they left off in previous sessions. In other instances, clients' new concerns represent a theme or are connected to and consistent with previous ones. With further exploration, therapists can explore with clients any possible relationships that may exist between current concerns and those raised at different times.

It is not always clear to therapists whether these new concerns are more significant than previous ones. The most direct path is for therapists to talk with clients to determine the weight of the newly raised concerns. This can be done by summarizing previous concerns and goals along with the current concerns and then asking clients which ones take precedence. Here are some ways to engage clients in these types of conversations followed by a case example.

- Would you say that the concerns you've been talking about today take precedence over the ones we discussed last week?
- In our last session, you mentioned that (problem) was really concerning you and was something that you wanted to focus our attention on. Based on the concerns you've mentioned today, do you think our time might be best spent on what we discussed last week or this week?
- If it's all right with you, I'd just like to make sure we're talking about what you want to talk about. I can see that you've got a few concerns. Would you rather spend this time talking about the concerns you're having now or the ones we discussed last week?

Case Example 7.1: Clarifying New Concerns or Problems

During his initial therapy session, Jalen, a 43-year-old male, expressed concern about being "overwhelmed" with his responsibilities at work. He stated that he wanted to be able to manage his work better and be more efficient. At the start of the second session, Jalen related that he was having trouble with his marital relationship. He described how he felt that his wife didn't value his opinion of things and therefore didn't involve him in important decisions. The therapist acknowledged this new concern and then followed, "Jalen, it sounds like this is really weighing on you. And last week you described some things that were also weighing on you. So, I'd just like to check in with you to make sure we are focusing on what you feel like is most important at this time, knowing that we can change things at any time. Does it make more sense to you to spend this time talking about feeling undervalued and left out of important decisions in your marriage, or do you think it's more important to talk about being able to manage your work better and be more efficient, as we discussed last week?" Jalen replied, "I'm frustrated with what's happened with my wife. But for now, I think we better stick with work stuff. Because work is affecting my marriage. I keep bringing it home with me." The therapist summarized, "That sounds like a good decision. We'll start with work and then move into your relationship with your wife. And if we need to revise things as we move forward, we'll do that."

As in the case example, acknowledging new concerns may be enough for some clients to return to previously established goals. Alternatively, the same client might respond, "I'm really not as worried about work as I am about my relationship with my wife. I think we should talk about my marriage." Another possibility is for the client to say, "I want to work on them both." With the latter two client responses, the therapist would acknowledge a modification in goals. The first would involve a shift to focusing on the client's concerns about his marriage. Although this could change again in future sessions, it is important to accommodate client preferences on an ongoing basis. The second example would entail expanding previous goals by adding the client's interest in focusing on his marital conflict. When there have been additions or changes in concerns resulting in multiple goals, it is a good idea for therapists to go a step further and ask, "Which of these concerns would you like to focus our attention on now/first?" In lieu of potential danger to self or others, clients choose the directions of therapy, including their conversational and relational preferences, which can and do periodically shift (Bertolino, 2010).

When client concerns and/or goals change, it can be helpful to inquire about any changes that have transpired with previous goals. Doing so identifies positive change that may have occurred that might otherwise be overlooked. Identifying progress can reinforce the concept that change is always happening, which can in turn serve as a source of encouragement and empowerment for future change. When clients are able to identify and connect with what they did to bring about change, they may be able to transfer those understandings into the present and future. See Case Example 7.2.

Case Example 7.2: Identifying Progress Along With Goal Revision

Curtis, a 14-year-old male, had been sneaking out at night and staying out until the early morning. In the first session, Curtis' father stated that the sneaking out was the primary issue. The father's concern for Curtis was evident through a score of 17.6 on the ORS. Curtis rated himself at a 36.7 on the ORS, stating that things were "fine" in the initial session. Two weeks later at the next session, the father completed a new ORS which had a score of 18.4—a negligible increase. Curtis' ORS was 37.1, also similar to his score two weeks prior.

At the second session, the father stated that Curtis had skipped school during the past week. After acknowledging his new concern and learning more about it, the father was asked if he was more concerned with Curtis' staying out late or skipping school. The father responded that missing school was the bigger of the two concerns. The father was then asked, "Before we talk about this further, could you give a brief update on what's happened with the situation of Curtis' sneaking out at night?" The father paused for a moment, then replied, "Well, he didn't sneak out this past week, so that's better." The therapist followed, "Really? Were you surprised?" "A little," the father replied.

Before delving into the new concern of school, Curtis was asked questions aimed at evoking exceptions and strengths to build from. These included, "What did you do differently?" and "What was different about last week that you made the decision to remain at home instead of sneaking out?" And the father was asked, "What was it like for you to know that your son was safely inside last week at night before curfew rather than running around?" and "What did you do when you realized that Curtis had stayed home each night instead of sneaking out ?"

In the previous case example, the primary rater's score, in this case the father (because he had the ability to begin and end therapy), remained unchanged. However, a change had occurred with his son, which was important to follow-up on. Although therapy goals can change from session to session, therapists seek opportunities to identify indicators of change to build momentum in the direction of newly identified concerns. Therapists take care not to minimize clients' current concerns or move in directions in which clients are not interested; at the same time, brief reorientations toward previous goals can stimulate stagnant systems and create hope. By identifying positive changes, however small, therapists can help clients to notice that change is always happening and the influence they have over their concerns and problems. This can serve as a catalyst for future change.

Reports that are ambiguous or vague

A second form of subsequent session response with clients who are unimproved or deteriorating is ambiguous or vague reports. When clients are asked about the meaning of ORS scores in which there is either no change or a drop, they will sometimes respond in ways that provide therapists with little direction. For example, a therapist might ask, "The last three sessions your scores have been gradually trending downward. Not a lot, just a little at a time. Your first session score was 23.8 and here in the fourth session your score is 20.6. What have things been like for you over the past week?" To this, clients may respond, "I'm not sure" or "I don't know." There are other instances when clients will remain vague in their replies, but articulate that they are not progressing or getting worse. They will say, "It's the same as last time," "There's nothing new," "It's continuing to go downhill," or "It's worse than ever." It's not until we engage clients in conversations about their scores that we more fully understand what is happening in their lives. Further, it is the therapist's job to use action-talk to gain clear descriptions from clients.

In some cases, a slightly more detailed summarization of ORS scores and client verbalizations may prompt a client to elaborate further. The therapist might say, "I noticed that your score on the ORS is in the higher range, suggesting that you're doing fairly well for someone who is in therapy. Yet you've stated that you're really stuck and haven't felt good. Can you help me to better understand what seems to be out of sync for you?" Another possibility is to say, "In looking at your outcome scores, it makes sense that you are feeling uncertain about where things stand. You've got some concerns, but it has been difficult to pinpoint exactly what they are. What ideas do you have about how we might proceed from here?" Some measures, such as the ORS, also have subscales that can be useful in clarifying ambiguity. After a review of the subscales, the therapist might say, "I noticed that your close and social relationships seem to be satisfactory to you compared to how you feel about yourself. Does it seem that way to you, or am I misunderstanding how you see things for yourself?"

Continuing therapy without clarity has risks. Ambiguity can contribute to frustration for clients and therapists alike and result in misguided attempts at more formal intervention. In addition, clients who score in the nonclinical range tend to have fewer beneficial outcomes because the severity of their problems is relatively low. And as we know, change is predictable, and if therapists do not respond to an absence of subjective change in the first few sessions, the risk of dropout negative outcome is significantly increased. As we try to better understand clients' experiences, we avoid being drawn into stories of impossibility (see Chapter 5). We assume that there have been times when things have gone differently and therefore work with clients to identify and amplify any positive change, however small, that may have occurred. We acknowledge the difficulties that clients face, yet do so in ways that keep open the possibilities for positive change. We can also reorient clients to previous goals through active listening. Doing so reminds clients of specific concerns and allows therapists to search for minute changes. To do this, the therapist can say, "The last time we met you mentioned that you were feeling/experiencing/thinking (description). You commented that you had (symptoms, negative reactions, thoughts). Please tell me a little bit about what has happened since our last session." The following questions can also be useful:

- How have things been in relation to the last time we met?
- What's been different since our last meeting?
- What's your sense about how things are going now as compared to last time?
- The last time we met, you mentioned that on a scale of 1 to 10, things were at a 5. Where would you say things are today?

If these general questions do not provide clarification, therapists can focus on small movements that are typically easier for clients to notice. The questions that follow can help with this:

- What have you noticed about your situation that's been just a little surprising, in a good way?
- How did you get that to happen just a little bit?
- What has been minimally better that could have otherwise gone unnoticed?
- What's something small that indicates to you that maybe things will turn the corner?
- What does noticing do for you?
- What else have you noticed?

Similar to new or changing concerns, therapists are sure to acknowledge and simultaneously search for *counterevidence*, times when things have been different with regard to presenting concerns. We acknowledge and search for possibilities in ways that are not invalidating or suggest that clients should just move past or ignore their struggles. We attend to struggles as hurdles, not barriers. Change is possible even with situations that appear outwardly closed-down.

Activate Client Strengths

A second response to situations of unimprovement or deterioration is to refocus therapy on clients, who, according to research, are the most significant contributor to outcome. As detailed in the second principle of a strengths-based perspective, we search for exceptions to problems, previous solutions, and active clients' strengths and resources, including systems of support. Therapists invite clients into conversations to identify what has or has not worked to any degree and how clients may have used their capabilities to counter deterioration. The following questions can assist with this process:

- How have you managed to keep things the same?
- What specifically seems worse?
- How so?
- How has that affected you?
- What is one thing that you've noticed about your concern that tells you things haven't gotten out of hand?
- What prevented things from deteriorating further?
- What else has helped things from even getting worse?
- How has that made a difference for you/with this situation?
- How did you do that?
- Who specifically did what?
- How did that help?
- How might you get that to happen in the future?
- What kind of help from others, if any, do you need to ensure that that happens?
- What else might help in the future?
- What is the smallest thing that you could do that might make even more of a difference with your situation?
- How could we get that to happen a little now?
- What could others do?
- What is a step that you can take after leaving here today that might help things to get back on track (or keep them from slipping again)?
- What do you need to set that in motion?
- What might help you to hold steady once you set that in motion?
- What will you think to do the next time you feel yourself slipping?
- What specifically will you do?
- What could you do on a more regular basis to keep things from slipping?

Asking about what has kept things from getting worse may surprise clients who are used to talking almost exclusively about problems. The questions offered help orient clients to whatever aspects of themselves, others, or their situations, however small, have worked to any degree. The preventive mechanisms can help build hope for clients who feel or think that nothing is going right. Our purpose is to identify small movements that clients may not have noticed. From session to session, it may seem to clients that their situations are unchanged, and that it is not possible. Problems are contextual and have variations regarding where and when they occur, their intensity, their duration, and so on. Through effective listening and questioning, we can learn about the worst of client situations and then gradually identify shades of intensity with problems. For example, a therapist might say to a client, "From what you've described, things have been worse. I'm sorry to hear that things have been sliding downward. I'm also curious about what has kept things from completely bottoming out. How have you done that?" Case Example 7.3 illustrates a way of using this strategy.

Case Example 7.3: A Shade Better

Client: Nothing's better. I still feel pretty bad. I think I'll always be depressed.

Therapist: You've been feeling bad and have gotten the idea that you'll always be depressed.

Client: Yeah. . . . nothing's worked for me—it's bringing me down.

Therapist: Nothing's worked so far. . . . I can see why that would bring you down.

Client: I just want to feel better.

Therapist: I want you to feel better too. Tell me about the recent time that you still felt depressed, just a little less so—like you had your head just barely above water.

Client: There hasn't been a time. I'm always depressed.

Therapist: It would be helpful if you could tell me a little more about that so that I am sure to understand how difficult it has been for you. Let's start with last week. Even though they were all depressing, which day was the worst—the most depressing day?

Client: Saturday.

Therapist: What was Saturday like?

Client: I couldn't get out of bed until real late. . . . the phone rang, I don't know how many times. . . . but I didn't answer it. I also didn't eat until that night . . . . it was a wasted day.

Therapist: I see. Not the kind of day that you want to repeat too often.

Client: Definitely not.

Therapist: Okay, then tell me about Friday or Sunday because even though you were depressed on those days, they didn't measure up to Saturday, which was the worst. What was different during those other days?

Client: Well, on Sunday I slept too long too.

Therapist: I see. How was Sunday different than Saturday?

Client: Well, I did eventually get up at one o'clock in the afternoon. Saturday I didn't get up until seven in the evening.

Therapist: How did you manage to get yourself up earlier on Sunday than you did on Saturday?

Client: I just knew that I had to function at least a little on Sunday so that I could get to work on Monday.

By starting with the worst a problem or situation has been, there is only one direction to go. Once variations in context have been identified, therapists can work to amplify and expand those exceptions. It is not just clients' perspectives that interfere with change. Throughout therapy, therapists remain aware of how their perceptions affect the way that therapy proceeds, including closing down possible avenues for change. When progress stagnates or things deteriorate, it is essential that therapists not lose sight of their personal philosophies. Therapists who maintain clear perspectives are less vulnerable to negativity and less likely to label clients as resistant, oppositional, unwilling to change, or "up-code" clients with more stigmatizing labels. It is not uncommon when therapy is not progressing for therapists to fall prey to ideas such as "clients have to get worse" or "bottom out" before they get better. In worst cases, clients are left to deteriorate without concerted efforts to respond to unimprovement or deterioration. Failure to respond by adjusting the goals or approach or making appropriate referral and allowing clients to fall into a downward spiral without intervention poses threats to their health and well-being and raises serious ethical and legal concerns.

It is imperative that we respond to the absence of change or deterioration in a timely manner. The risk of negative outcome with clients who do not show improvement in the first few sessions increases without adequate response. Fluctuations are to be expected over time. Some clients will have greater highs and lows than others or have patterns that will repeat. Later in this chapter we will focus on ways to build on improvement; however, it remains very important that deterioration on outcome measures be considered along with professional expertise with an eye on reducing risk. Deterioration is cause for further risk assessment and, if necessary, action, including intensifying or modifying services.

Attend to the Alliance

A third response to client unimprovement or deterioration relates to a point explored throughout this book—the role of client engagement. Recall Principle 2 of a strengths-based perspective: *The therapeutic alliance makes substantial and consistent contributions to outcome* (see Chapter 2). The alliance is the best process predictor of outcome and FIT provides a mechanism for instantaneous feedback about clients' experiences of client–therapist interactions.

Check-Ins

There are two main ways of attending the alliance. One is through periodic checks-in with clients during each session. We say, "I'd like to pause for a moment to check in with you." The therapist can then ask a general question or focus in on a specific aspect of the alliance. A general question might be, "How is our conversation so far for you?" A specific question could be, "Have we been focusing on what is most important to you or do we need to change what we are talking about?" The point is to elicit feedback to keep therapists attuned to clients' experiences in therapy. Information from check-ins is essential in making real-time adjustments, modifications, or referrals to better meet clients' needs and provide a better fit. Examples of questions used to check-in with clients include:

- In terms of our work together so far, what has been helpful or unhelpful? In what way(s)?
- Are there other things that you feel/think we should be discussing instead?
- Is there anything I should have asked that I haven't asked?
- What, if anything, has been overlooked?
- How satisfied are you with how things are going so far on a scale from 1 to 10, 1 meaning you are completely unsatisfied, and 10 meaning you are completely satisfied?
- What changes, if any, should be made at this point?
- What, if anything, should I be doing differently?
- Is the way we've approached your concern/situation fitting with the way you expect change to occur?
- Is there a way to approach your situation that we haven't yet considered?
- What, if anything, has been missing from our sessions?

Responding to SRS Feedback

A second and more formal way of attending to the alliance is through a measure such as the SRS (or CSRS or GSRS), which is described in Chapter 4 with corresponding examples in the Appendix. To recap, the SRS is administered at the end of sessions to learn clients' perceptions of the therapeutic alliance. The clinical cutoff for the SRS is 36, meaning that any overall score of 36 or below or any single subscale score of 8 is a signal for therapists to respond. To better understand the idea of responding to potential problems with the alliance, let's refer back to the client graphs illustrated in Figures 7.2 and 7.7. In both cases, client SRS scores (represented by the top line in each graph) reveal concerns that require action on the part of the therapist. In Figure 7.2, SRS scores begin relatively low, dip, and then flatten at around 28.3. As discussed, our aim is to create an error-centric culture of feedback. That is, we strive to receive negative feedback, which is instructive. In Figure 7.7, the SRS begins at 32.1, again below the cutoff, before rising to 39.7 at Session 2, then dropping substantially at Session 3 and further at Session 4. In each case, the task of the therapist is the same—elicit and respond to client feedback.

To take the pressure off clients, the therapist strives to frame feedback as an "opportunity" to make changes or adjustments. This may involve reorienting clients to the purpose of the measure by saying, "By giving me feedback you're helping me to better help you. You won't hurt my feelings or make me feel bad. You'll actually be helping me to do a better job." Client feedback is not about the therapist himself/herself but instead about the quality of the alliance. Figure 7.12 is an example of feedback produced by YIN's OMS, Imagine, for a client whose SRS scores indicate a possible problem with or rupture in the alliance.

There are different reasons for SRS scores to begin low or fall as therapy progresses. Two common reasons for lower SRS scores from the outset can be found with clients who are mandated to therapy or have little or no trust in mental health professionals. However, there is a growing body of evidence indicating that

---

Feedback Message

Your client's SRS score is at or below the cutoff and indicates possible concerns with the alliance.

Actions to consider:
1. Review the subscales and summarize the results to the client. Invite here-and-now feedback about what is working and what can be improved on.
2. Invite the client to assert any negative feelings about the therapeutic relationship.
3. Accept responsibility for your part in alliance ruptures and in making adjustments.
4. Engage in conversations about the client's expectations and preferences.
5. Discuss the match between the therapist's style and client's preferred ways to relate.
6. Spend more time learning about the client's experience in therapy.
7. Readdress the goals and means or tasks to accomplish those goals.
8. Normalize the client's responses by letting him or her know that talking about concerns, facing challenges, taking action, and/or therapy in general can be difficult.
9. Provide rationale for techniques and methods.
10. Attend to subtle clues from nonverbal behaviors (e.g., patterns such as one-word answers) that may indicate a problem with the alliance.
11. Offer more positive feedback and encouragement (except when the client communicates either verbally or nonverbally that this is not a good match).
12. Talk with a supervisor.

SRS, session rating scale.

FIGURE 7.12 SRS feedback message for alliance score below the clinical cutoff.

client–therapist relationships with early "fits and starts"—that strengthen and improve over time—yield better outcomes compared to those that start and stay good or deteriorate over the course of therapy (Anker, Duncan, & Sparks, 2009; Anker, Owen, Duncan, & Sparks, 2010; Owen, Miller, Seidel, & Chow, 2016).

People often need to get to know and trust each other, which provides insight into why some clients may rate the alliance lower at the start of therapy. In contrast, lower alliance scores as therapy progresses significantly raise the risk of dropout and negative outcome. This is because clients are directly informing therapists that something is not working for them. As such, timely response by the therapist is critical. Because the meaning of client scores is relative, therapists who develop a routine of eliciting feedback are increasing the opportunities to identify and respond to problems in the alliance. In seeking feedback, it is also accepted that there will be times when no further information will be gleaned. The task of the therapist is to elicit feedback about what can be done to strengthen the relationship.

Dependence

There are occasions when alliance scores will indicate dependence. For example, some clients will find their therapists very supportive and rate them as such. There will be little variance in SRS scores, which will remain high, but there will be no improvement in outcomes. Let's revisit Figure 7.11, which illustrates the high SRS, no improvement ORS phenomenon. Often these clients say things such as, "I look forward to seeing you each week. You are the only one who understands me" or "I am so glad I have a therapist like you. You are a great listener." The combination of high SRS, low ORS scores often indicates dependence. In many cases, clients will continue in therapy indefinitely. The therapist's task in such situations is to acknowledge the client's view while addressing the issue of no improvement. The therapist asks, "I here you say that you look forward to seeing me each week. I am glad to hear that. I am also trying to understand how coming to see me is helping you. Your ORS scores indicate that things are much the same. Can you help me to learn more about how therapy is helpful to you?" To this question, the client may respond, "I feel better after seeing you." Accordingly, the therapist would follow, "What has feeling better after our sessions led you to do differently in your life?" The point is to connect therapy to some identifiable and measurable change in life functioning. If the client cannot identify improvement, dependence may be the result.

We are not trying to push clients out of therapy. Instead, our mission is to provide services that facilitate growth, development, well-being, and functioning (see Principle 5 of a strengths-based perspective outlined in Chapter 2). A distinction between psychotherapy and supportive services is that psychotherapy is not only supportive, it focuses on some agreed-upon, goals and improved outcome. Unless there is a mutual agreement that the only purpose of psychotherapy is to provide support, in which case that agreement should be documented, the therapist has a responsibility to ensure that the client is benefitting in a measurable way. Failure to do so by therapists raises serious ethical issues around keeping clients in therapy without sufficient evidence that continuation is beneficial *and* outside of clients' awareness that between 30% and 50% of clients do not improve in therapy, and on average 5% to 10% deteriorate (Hansen et al., 2002; Lambert, 2010, 2013).

Using Subscales

An additional step therapists can take to hone in on potential alliance issues that may be contributing to unimprovement or deterioration is to review subscales. The SRS has four subscales: Relationship, Goals and Topics, Approach and Method, and Overall (see Appendix). Figure 7.13 shows Session 2 subscales of 9.9, 9.7, 9.6, and 9.7 for a total of 38.90. In the next session, illustrated in Figure 7.14, the subscales are 9.2, 7.4, 9.6, and 9.2 for a total score of 35.40.

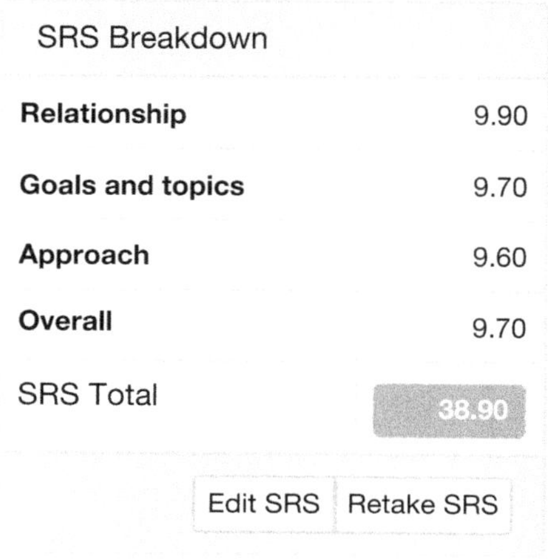

SRS Breakdown	
Relationship	9.90
Goals and topics	9.70
Approach	9.60
Overall	9.70
SRS Total	38.90

Edit SRS | Retake SRS

SRS, session rating scale.

FIGURE 7.13 SRS subscales—Session 2.

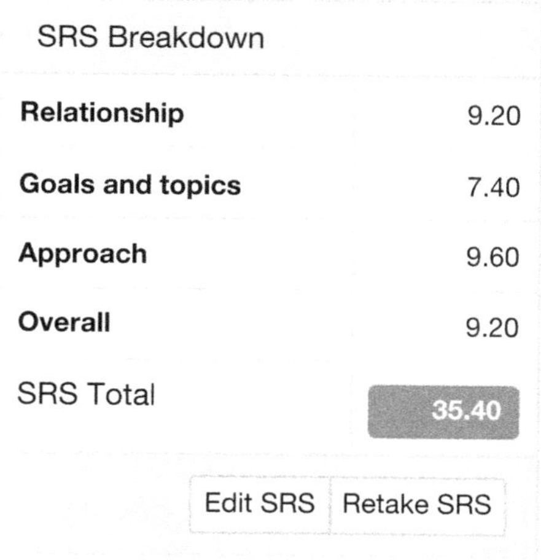

SRS Breakdown	
Relationship	9.20
Goals and topics	7.40
Approach	9.60
Overall	9.20
SRS Total	35.40

Edit SRS | Retake SRS

SRS, session rating scale.

FIGURE 7.14 SRS subscales—Session 3.

Not only is the score below the clinical cutoff of 36, it represents a total score drop of 3.50 from the previous session *and*, in particular, a notable decrease in the second subscale, "Goals and Topics." In addition to requesting feedback about the overall session, the therapist would inquire about the subscale drop. To do this, the therapist would summarize the SRS and simultaneously focus on the SRS, "It seems that you felt listened to and heard and that the approach in the session was okay with you. But something was off in terms of what we focused on in the session. Does that seem right or am I missing something?" The therapist's aim is to generate conversation to learn what he or she can do differently. Failure to respond to feedback is not merely a missed opportunity, it can contribute to dropout.

Responding to Ruptures

Because ruptures in the alliance can happen at any point and often without therapists knowing it, there is no room for shyness when it comes to attending to the alliance. Unmet clients' expectations and preferences are crucial aspects of therapy, and ruptures in the alliance can contribute to frustration and demoralization if not resolved (Safran, Muran, Samstag, & Stevens, 2002). When ruptures are a concern, therapists can do the following:

- Discuss the here-and-now relationship with the client.
- Ask for feedback about the therapeutic relationship.
- Create space and allow the client to assert any negative feelings about the therapeutic relationship.
- Engage in conversations about the client's expectations and preferences.
- Discuss the match between the therapist's style and client's preferred ways to relate.
- Spend more time learning about the client's experience in therapy.
- Readdress the agreement established about goals and tasks to accomplish those goals.
- Reassess the client's readiness to change.
- Accept responsibility for his or her part in alliance ruptures.
- Normalize the client's responses by letting him or her know that talking about concerns, facing challenges, taking action, and/or therapy in general can be difficult.
- Provide rationale for techniques and methods.
- Attend closely to subtle clues (e.g., nonverbal behaviors, patterns such as one-word answers) that may indicate a problem with the alliance.

- Offer more positive feedback and encouragement (except when the client communicates either verbally or nonverbally that this is not a good match).
- Engage in further supervision and/or training.

Unimprovement and deterioration with clients is something that happens to all therapists. The good news is that we can improve on rates of dropout and treatment failure by not simply eliciting, but actively responding to and learning from client feedback. Anderson, Ogles, Patterson, Lambert, and Vermeersch (2009) found that 97% of the variance in therapists' outcomes was due to their ability to form alliances with clients. Similarly, Baldwin, Wampold, and Imel (2007) detailed the value of therapists learning new ways to connect with a diverse range of clients—in particular, clients with whom they typically have had difficulty connecting with. A pathway to improving our connectedness with clients is by monitoring the alliance.

Lack of progress and deterioration are signals to therapists to respond as opposed to react. Accordingly, the strategies discussed throughout this book place clients at the center of decision-making processes. We work with clients, not on clients. The success of therapy is contingent on strong working alliances, which is especially critical when things are not going well. In cases of unimprovement and deterioration, our aim is to partner with clients to improve the fit and effect of therapy.

The three variations of response described in this section also apply to clients who are making progress. In fact, clients who begin therapy above the clinical cutoff—in the non-distressed range and typically the precontemplation or contemplation stages—are often more generalized and less descriptive of their situations. They report fewer symptoms and lower levels of distress—which can make it challenging to pinpoint their concerns—what they would like to have different in their lives. In cases where clients are progressing but there appear to be some impediments to therapy, the same ideas in this section apply. We still aim to gain further clarity about concerns, rework goals as necessary, and determine other changes that may be needed to support clients to achieve their goals. As discussed, for those who use electronic OMS, alerts and feedback messages are often provided to offer further guidance for clinicians.

Arguably, it matters little whether or not clients *need* therapy if they do not *benefit* from it (Bertolino, 2014). Because we are monitoring progress from the outset of services, we are better able to distinguish clients in an unimproved or deteriorated range from those who are improved. In the next section we will focus on how to identify and build on client improvement, which is the main focus of psychotherapy.

CATEGORY 2: IMPROVEMENT

The second category of response in subsequent sessions is improvement. From a standpoint of reliable change, when a client's current ORS increases by less than 5 points of his or her initial score, it can be said that there is "no improvement." To be clear, an increase in ORS scores from one session to the next is to be explored by the therapist to determine the veracity of the change. We want to learn what was different for the client that could serve as a building block for larger, more substantial changes in the future. We simply cannot attribute a change of less than 5 points on the ORS to the work done in therapy. Rather, the change is likely to be an artifact of maturation, measurement error, or chance.

In contrast, a client who achieves a change that is 5 points or greater on his or her most recent ORS as compared to the initial session score is said to be making reliable change. If that same client's most recent ORS score also places the client above the clinical cutoff for the ORS, which is 25 for most adult clients, then the client is also said to have achieved change that is clinically significant (CS). To further recap, CS change results when both the criteria for reliable improvement and exceeding the clinical cutoff are met, indicating a change in clinical status.

Figures 7.15 and 7.16 provide different examples of client improvement. While the illustrations differ, a starting point with each is to have a conversation with the client to determine the meaning of the scores. The therapist might ask, "Looking at the graph, what do you see happening?" Or, the therapist may choose to lead with a statement and follow with a question, "In looking at your graph, it appears that your scores have increased. Increasing scores can indicate that people are doing better, but that's not always the case. How do the results of your ORS scores match up with how you see things in your life?" Scores reveal little information-wise until therapists engage clients in conversations about their meaning. For the purposes of discussion, let's assume that with Figures 7.15 and 7.16, the clients had been talked with about their scores.

Figure 7.15, for example, is of an 8-year-old, whose primary caregiver, his grandmother, has reported gradual improvement of her grandson over the course of six sessions. Review of the graph in Figure 7.15 reveals some seesawing of

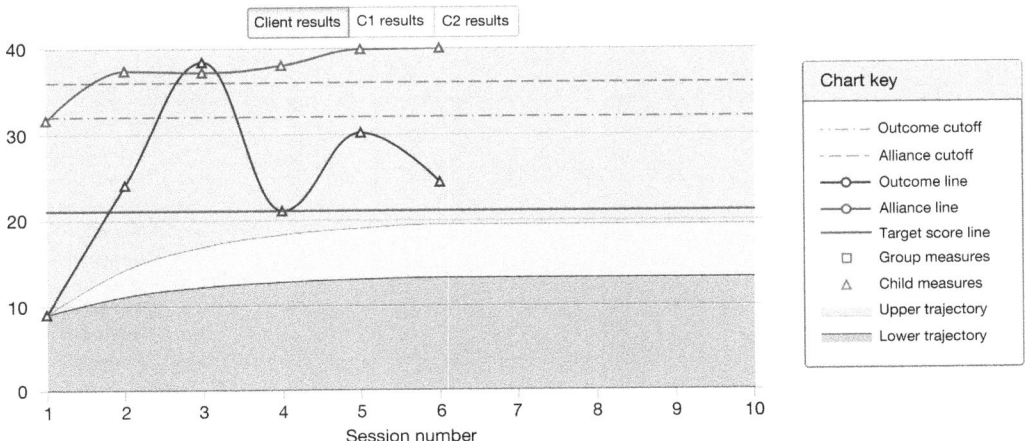

FIGURE 7.15 Improvement.

scores. For example, the child's opening ORS score (as rated by his grandmother, who attended each session) was 9.8. The next few session scores were 23.8, 38.5, 21.0, 29.2, and 23.7. The child had achieved reliable change by virtue of his current session score being 13.9 points higher than his first session score. However, in order to achieve clinically significant change, the child's most recent ORS would have to exceed 32. That may be possible by the end of therapy since it did already happen once, during Session 3, when the grandmother rated her grandson's functioning at 38.5. In this case, it would be a good idea to discuss the seesawing scores to help the grandmother with ways to respond to any significant behavior that she views as disruptive and/or distressing.

In contrast, Figure 7.16 is of an 18-year-old female with an opening ORS score of 19.8. The young woman reported a sharp increase at Session 2 with a score of 33.1. In many cases, when there is a steep slope of change, that change is situational and does not maintain. However, in this case the client maintained her progress as evidenced by her Session 3 to 5 scores of 32.4, 35.2, and 37.1. In the two cases described, the therapist works with the clients to identify what specifically had changed and other indicators of improvement related to the problem(s) that led to therapy. What follows is a series of questions to assist in identifying change:

- What have you noticed that has changed with your concern/problem/self/situation?
- What specifically seems to be going better?
- Who first noticed that things had changed?
- Who else noticed the change?
- When did you first notice that things had changed?
- What did you notice happening?

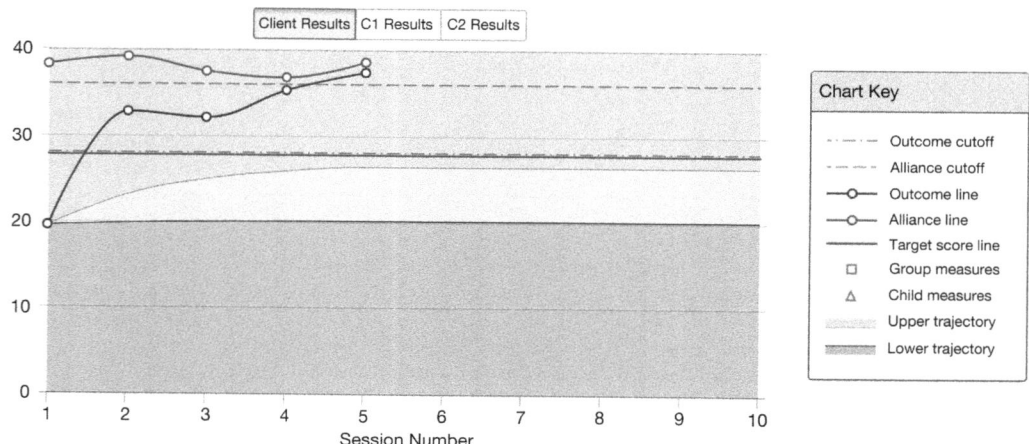

FIGURE 7.16 Improvement.

The therapist then inquires as to *how* the change occurred and *what* factors may have contributed to it. As discussed in Chapter 4, 4WH questions can be useful in learning about the role clients and supportive others have in change processes. Therapists also explore any differences that the current change may have had in relation to the goals of therapy. The following questions are used to learn more about the details of client change:

- How did the change happen?
- What do you think might have influenced that positive change (family, supportive others, etc.)?
- What worked for you to bring about this change?
- What specifically did you do?
- How did you get yourself to do that?
- How was what you did different than before?
- Where did you get the idea to do things that way?
- What role, if any, did others play in helping to move things forward?
- How specifically did others support and/or help you?

Information gathered from the previous questions helps therapists to understand the role clients have in changing their situations and lives, how interventions are working, and about next steps in therapy. Because 4WH questions are largely exploratory and generative (see Chapter 4), they provide opportunities for clients to notice positive changes and the influences that contributed to changes, thereby leading to the construction of new meaning. As with any form of questioning, in this case about improvement, clients may respond with ambiguity (e.g., "I just did it"; "I wanted things to be different"). In these instances, therapists continue to use action-talk to translate vague descriptions into clear, observable behaviors. Should clients struggle with questions such as the previous ones, it may be an indication that the questions are too large or too general. A modification is to focus on questions to draw on smaller changes. A therapist might say, "How did you get that change to happen just a little?" or "What did you do a little differently than in past situations?" We need only identify tiny moments or small ripples, such as when a pebble splashes into a pond. Little changes can then be developed into bigger, more profound ones.

As clients improve, a key question emerges: To what do clients attribute their improvements? In other words, do clients see themselves as initiators and contributors to their improvement or do they see external factors such as other people, medication, and so on, as the reasons for their improvement. As it turns out, how clients view their improvement influences whether positive change will be fleeting or lasting. In the section, we address the topic of influences on client change and strategies to "anchor" change going forward.

Attribution of Change

Therapists facilitate positive change through client engagement, eliciting and activating client strengths, focusing on client capacities to change, creating hope and expectation, and utilizing strategies that fit with and benefit clients. Similarly, in each client situation, there will be factors outside of the client's control that are the result of others' actions, happenstance, factors such as medication, and other external entities that are influential to clients' progress. But as we know, all change is self-change. Clients are what makes therapy work. Approximately 87% of the variance in outcome is due to clients and factors associated with clients' lives (Wampold, 2001). Therefore, what clients attribute their improvement to is critically important when it comes to lasting change. The more clients view factors or forces outside of themselves and their control as the primary reasons for their improvement, the greater the likelihood that their change will fade, sometimes sharply. This is in part because personal accountability dissipates once external factors have been removed or diminish as causal agents of change.

"Blame" the Client for Change

It is the task of therapists to enhance the effects of change by helping clients to view change and its maintenance as a consequence of their own efforts (Duncan, Miller, & Sparks, 2004). We engage in efforts to attribute the major part of the change to clients' actions and who they are as people. In a sense, therapists "blame" clients for changing for the better. To do this, therapists ask questions to assist in assigning change to clients:

- How is it that you have been able to face so many challenges and not lose sight of _____?
- Who are you such that you've been able to _____?
- What does the fact that you've been able to face up to _____ say about you?
- What kind of person are you that you've been able to overcome _____?
- Where did the wherewithal come from to _____?

We enhance the effects of change by helping clients to see change and its maintenance as a consequence of their own efforts and their character. In a sense, therapists positively "blame" clients for changing for the better. In doing so, we are careful to acknowledge and not dismiss the contributions of external influences that serve as catalysts for change. Instead, we convey the idea that even though external factors may be triggers in producing change, it is clients themselves who are in charge of their lives. The following questions can assist in both identifying the contributions of external factors and promoting accountability and self-efficacy:

- You mentioned that _____ seems to be helping. How are you working with _____ to better your life?
- In your mind, what has _____ allowed you to do that you might not have otherwise done?
- You said that _____ (i.e., partner, family member, caregiver, friend, other form of support, etc.) has always been there for you. How has _____'s involvement helped you with what you've been going through? How did you use _____'s support as a stepping-stone to take steps toward your future?
- You mentioned that _____ (e.g., medication, therapy) is helping. How are you working with _____ (e.g., medication, therapy) to better your life?
- What percentage of the change you've experienced is a result of _____, and what percentage do you think is the result of your own doing?
- As a result of feeling better from _____, what are you then able to do?

Even the most experienced therapists encounter clients who are unable to identify what has brought about or contributed to positive change. Some clients, particularly adolescents, often respond to therapists' questions with "I don't know." These kinds of replies do not mean that clients are purposely withholding information or are resistant; they may not have given much thought to it, do not know, or perhaps are not interested. Rather than pushing clients to come up with answers or labeling them "resistant" or "noncompliant," we consider clients' responses only as communication; and such communication calls for therapists to do something different.

Speculate About Change

A different approach would be to *speculate* about how the change might have come about. Speculation involves combining conjecture or curiosity with guesswork about how change might have come about (Bertolino, 2003). For example, a therapist might have a client speculate or guess by asking, "If you had to guess, and there were no wrong answers, what would you say made a difference for you?" or "If (e.g., a close friend, your partner, mother, boss) were here, what would he/she say has contributed to things changing?" If this does not reveal anything, therapists can do their own speculating, "What do you think about the idea that you might have had a role in your situation improving?" These questions assist with using speculation:

- I'm wondering if perhaps part of the reason things are going better for you is that you are becoming (e.g., more in tune with what you want, more responsible, more mature, wiser, growing up). Perhaps you are becoming the type of person you want to be and learning new ways of managing your life. What do you think about this idea?

- Is it possible that the change you've experienced might be related to your (action)?

- What do you think about the idea that the change you've experienced might be related to your (e.g., wanting to lead a different life, being ready for the next stage of your life)?

- What do you think about the idea that the change you've experienced might be an indication that you're taking back control of your life?

- How might the change you've experienced be a sign of a new, preferred direction for you?

When we attribute speculations to client qualities and actions they are less likely to be rejected. Most clients will not say, "No, I'm becoming less responsible." Even if speculations are off target, because they highlight competencies, clients will at least consider them. Case Example 7.4 provides an example of how speculation can be used.

Case Example 7.4: Speculating About Change

A woman came to therapy stating that she was "depressed." Discussion of her concern revealed that she had suffered a series of events including the loss of her job. After making gains and then experiencing periodic setbacks, she accepted a new job that paid less but had the potential to be more fulfilling. At first the woman appeared to remain mired in self-defeat; then, over the course of a couple weeks, her depression seemed to lift. This was evidenced by a change in her demeanor, voice, and posture. As the next few weeks passed, the woman's physical appearance changed as she took more of an interest in her self-care. After two months, the woman was back in charge of her life. Her therapist asked , "How did you get your life back from the throws of depression?" She replied, "That's a good question. I've actually thought about that but I'm still not sure." The therapist asked, "I've been wondering if something inside you, that's been dormant for a while, came to life. Perhaps you realized that it was time to reclaim your life and use the wherewithal that's kept you afloat over the years." In tears and seeming to connect with the therapist's words, the woman followed, "I think you know me better than I know myself."

Attribution and speculation not only draw attention to the roles clients have in creating positive change, they also support evolving new stories of growth, resiliency, and hope that run counter to the problem-saturated ones. New stories serve as an "anchor" for change, meaning that clients are better able to connect with their internal experiences, including feelings and sensory perceptions (Bertolino, 1999). By moving to an experiential level, the change may be more profound. To further assist clients in connecting with internal experiences, therapists ask questions such as:

- When you were able to (action), what did that feel like?
- How did you experience that change inside?
- How was that feeling similar or different than before?
- What does it feel like to know that others may also benefit from the changes you've made?

Sharing Credit for Change

When working with couples and families, the "client" is actually multiple persons. Likewise, both problems and solutions involve two or more people. In these cases, it can be helpful to share the credit for change. As a parallel to attribution, sharing the credit involves focusing on relationships and acknowledging each person's contribution to improving overall situations. Sharing the credit serves several purposes. First, as you have learned, the quality of each person's participation in therapy is an important factor in outcome. When involved persons are left out of therapeutic processes, they can appear as noncompliant, resistant, and unmotivated. By recognizing the contributions of each person involved in therapy, we are extending change to those who are important to the stability of a family and/or relationships. For example, sharing change can be especially important with couples so that each partner feels he or she contributed to the improvement of the relationship.

Sharing the credit can also act as a countermeasure in situations where positive change has occurred but is being negated in some way. This is most often evidenced by a member of a couple or caregiver who makes statements such as, "It will never last"; "He's done that before"; or "You haven't seen the real _____ (name of other client) yet." These comments sometimes originate from people who do not feel as if they have made a valued or positive contribution to the improvement of a situation. To better understand this idea, let's consider what a caregiver, such as a parent, might experience when change happens quickly in therapy. A parent gives her all to raise her son. Because her son gets into trouble she begins to feel her efforts were to no avail. So, the mother attends family therapy with her son and things begin to improve. Although the intent of family therapy was to improve the family situation, the change actually leads the mother to blame herself. She thinks, "I'm a bad parent," "I obviously don't know what I'm doing," and "I failed. I should have been able to fix this." It is not uncommon for clients to feel or think that they should have been able to resolve their problems without seeing a relative "stranger," a therapist who prior to therapy knew nothing about the family or couple.

Experiences of invalidation and feelings of failure can, at times, undermine progress. The irony is that although family members are sometimes considered the cause of problems, they do not always get credit for their contributions when things go better. By identifying the contributions of everyone who may be involved, therapists counter negative statements that can minimize change and prove invalidating. There are several possibilities for sharing the credit for change. One way is to give others involved with services credit by saying:

- I wonder how you were able to instill the value of _____ (specific value) in _____ (name).
- Like you, _____ (name) seems to hold the value of _____ (specific value). I can't help thinking that he/she learned it from you.
- It seems to me that (name) has learned the value of _____ (specific value) from you.

Another possibility is to evoke from those involved something that they feel contributed to the change process:

- How do you think your _____ (relationship, parenting, etc.) has contributed to (name)'s ability to (action)?
- In what ways do you think you have been able to help _____ (name of other client) to stand up to adversity?
- In what ways do you think you were of assistance in helping _____ (name of other client) to stand up to _____ (problem) and get back on track?

A third way is to ask one client what contributions another client, typically another family member, in therapy has made to his or her life and then to share the answers with others who are involved:

- What did you learn from _____ (name of other client) about how to overcome _____ (problem)?
- Who taught you the value of _____ (specific value)?
- From whom did you learn about _____ (action, thing)?

The previous questions do not create conflict in attributing change to the qualities and actions of individuals but offers "both/and" as opposed to "either/or." Therapists both attribute the major portion of significant change to those individuals who have made behavioral changes and share the credit with those who are either directly involved in therapy or who have provided care and support. For example, it can be effective to acknowledge supportive others such as teachers, coaches, employers, community members, and the like, who have lent their support to clients. By sharing credit for change, we can neutralize feelings of negativity and in turn help those involved to experience a new sense of togetherness or spirit of family.

Amplifying Change

As clients improve, we continue to explore how a change in one area can lead to one or more in another. Therapists scan for ways in which positive change may produce a ripple effect, like a snowball traveling downhill, expanding as it gains speed and momentum, or a domino starting a chain reaction of knocking over others. The questions that follow can assist with searching for additional changes:

- What else have you noticed that has changed?
- What else is different?
- How has (have) that (those) difference(s) been helpful to you?
- What difference has the change made with school/work/home/friends/etc.?
- Who else has noticed these other changes?
- Who else has benefited from these changes?

Although we have collaborated with clients on goals identified from the outset of services, it is not uncommon for secondary gains to be made. In this context, secondary gains refer to additional benefits of change. For example, using the ORS, a primary goal may have been for a client to develop more fulfilling social relationships, which corresponds with the third subscale which is the "social" domain. As a result of improving social relationships, the client may also experience an improved sense of self, perhaps having more energy, which aligns with the "individual" domain. Or, the same client may experience an increase in satisfaction with intimate relationships—the second subscale of the ORS. The idea is for therapists to scan for additional changes that may not have been the original focus of services.

REVISITING GOALS AND OUTCOMES: THE MEANING OF PROGRESS

A cornerstone of any evidence-based approach is a focus on improved outcomes. As clients progress in therapy, conversations include discussion of the meaning of improvement, which then informs next steps. There are different ways to gauge both progress and its meaning. In this book, we have focused on two different forms of corroborating improvement: goals and outcomes. To restate, goals are clearly delineated, observable changes described through action-talk. Outcomes refer to clients' interpretations of the benefit of services. We have used the ORS, an evidence-based index for measuring clients' overall functioning and well-being. The psychometrics of the ORS are discussed in Chapter 4 and are described in greater detail elsewhere (see Seidel & Miller, 2013; Schuckard & Miller, 2016). The ORS subscales—individual, interpersonal, and social functioning—also provide specific areas of focus related to client functioning.

In some instances, as is the case with families or external stakeholders, there may be entities that have the ability to end services. In these cases, therapists work with such persons to ensure there is clarity as to when the goals and/or outcomes of therapy have been achieved. For this reason, it is a good practice in couples, families, and when there are external stakeholders to have each person complete an ORS that corresponds with the primary client's ORS. This way ORS scores can be compared, discussed, and used as guidance for sessions to ensure everyone is working together toward the same end.

Let's refer back to the ORS graphs illustrated in Figures 7.15 and 7.16. In Figure 7.15, an 8-year-old was brought to therapy by his grandmother. The grandmother was the primary rater of her grandson's functioning, which she rated as relatively low at the first session, resulting in a score of 9.8 on the ORS. Subsequent sessions revealed improvement with a seesaw pattern of scores. The grandmother saw the variance in scores (i.e., seesawing) as indications of her grandson "adjusting to the new situation," which involved the grandmother becoming the primary custodian. At Session 6 the ORS scores had improved by 13.9 points, which is a substantial change. The grandmother was satisfied with her grandson's improvement, stating, "He's a different boy. He now goes to school on his own and is trying. He didn't do that before." Not only was the young man improving outcome-wise, he had also achieved the goal of attending school at least 85% of the time. With these changes, a decision was made to titrate down the dosage form by seeing the family every other week instead of weekly.

Figure 7.16 is the case of an 18-year-old female who after reporting a 13.3 point increase between the first and second sessions continued to progress. At Session 5, her score was 37.1. The client stated that therapy had helped her to "get a new perspective on things." She and her therapist agreed that therapy was no longer needed.

In contrast, Figure 7.17 involves a 17-year-old who began therapy in the non-distressed range with a first session ORS score of 34.0. Because the risk of

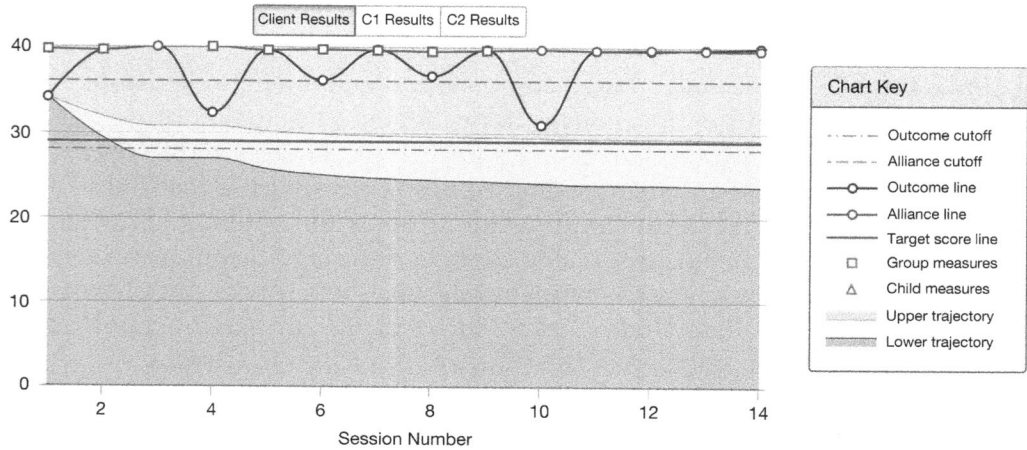

FIGURE 7.17 Improvement.

dropout is high when clients begin therapy with reports of little or no distress, therapists determine whose idea it was for the client to attend therapy and, if possible, seek feedback from a collateral rater—a person who has the ability to begin and end services. Therapists also seek to find what clients might be motivated to work on. Doing so also helps to clarify clients' readiness for change. In this case, the client was admitted to a transitional living program due to conflict at home. The client sought independence from her mother and an interest in moving toward living on her own when she turned 18. Upon admission she stated, "I just need a place to live." Aside from conflict with her mother, the client revealed little distress in other aspects of her life. She simply wanted a place to "get things done" such as completing her General Educational Development (GED) certificate, attend community college to study art, and be self-sufficient.

Over the next 13 sessions, the client's ORS scores indicated some seesawing, which were the result of life challenges. She made adjustments to meet her challenges and after less than 4 months and just after turning 18, she was transitioned into a scattered site apartment arranged by the agency. Because the client met her goals and remained in the non-distressed range, she was moved to a less restrictive environment in which her goals were modified to meet the next stretch in her life.

In conversations to understand the meaning of change, we address both goals and outcomes. A central question is: How does the change that has occurred relate to the goals and outcome established at the start of therapy? Further questions include: Have the concerns or problems been resolved? What else needs to happen for services to be considered successful/for goals to be met? To understand how change is situated in relationship to goals, the following questions can be helpful:

- What difference has the change made in your life?
- How are you benefiting from the change you've experienced?
- What will be different in the future as these changes continue to occur?
- In the future, what other changes do you think might occur that might not have otherwise come about?
- Who else might benefit from these changes? How?
- In the future, what will indicate to you that these changes are continuing to happen?
- How does the change that's happened relate to the goals that we set?

Throughout this book, the role of both goals and outcomes has been discussed. And yet, not all clinicians will track both. Let's review some concerns with evaluating progress exclusively on the basis of one or the other, beginning with goals.

Monitoring Goals Versus Outcomes

A primary concern is that clients can meet goals without necessarily having improved outcome. For example, a client may report that he is meeting goals such as getting to work on time, completing his tasks and projects on schedule, and that his boss is pleased with his performance. However, if the same client does not report improvement on an outcome measure, further exploration is necessary. This is because the same client may remain depressed or anxious or continue to have trouble in close relationships, and so on. If goals have been met but outcome scores have not improved, a therapist might approach and say, "You've accomplished the goals you set out to achieve when you began therapy. And yet, you've expressed some _____ (concern, worry, etc.—summarize what has been indicated in the outcome measure) in terms of how you see your life at this time. Does that seem right to you?" Clients who meet goals without measurable improvement in functioning and well-being are at risk of relapse.

Monitoring Outcomes Versus Goals

The same can also occur when outcomes improve without goals being met. Because real-time data provide snapshots of recent times, therapists are cognizant that single scores can be reflective of one-time events or what is most on clients' minds. Large changes in scores are likely to reflect situational changes (e.g., positive events or crises) that may not give an accurate depiction of clients' lives as a whole. Therapists best serve clients by comparing and contrasting scores over several sessions. Whether improvement or deterioration, gradual change and flattening of scores (i.e., very small changes over a span of multiple sessions) are likely to provide a more reliable picture of client functioning.

An important point arises when working with couples and families. When the "client" is a couple or family, improvement is based on multiple ORS scores. For example, for a couple to achieve a reliable change, both partners would have to report a change of 5 points or more between the first and last sessions. Clinically significant change would be achieved when each partner in the couple reached a reliable change *and* finished with scores above the clinical cutoff. In the largest clinical trial with couples ($N = 410$), clients were randomly assigned to one of two arms: (a) treatment as usual (TAU), routine marital therapy without feedback; or (b) routine marital therapy with feedback. Couples in the feedback condition demonstrated significantly greater improvement than those in the TAU condition. At posttreatment, the former achieved nearly four times the rate of clinically significant change, and maintained a large advantage on the primary measure at six-month follow-up while attaining a 50% lower rate of separation or divorce (Anker et al., 2009).

Since both goals and outcomes can produce anomalies, using multiple sources of data while sticking to the 80/20 rule (i.e., focus on information that is most meaningful and essential to decision making) is a best practice. The duo of goals and outcomes provides a consistent way of evaluating improvement. At the same time, research makes it clear that if a choice has to be made in terms of what kind of data best indicate improvement, an outcomes focus is far more reliable.

TRANSITION FROM THERAPY

Because therapy takes place in different settings and populations, transition or termination will vary based on factors such as the current type of service, program, and improvement achieved. Options can include: decreasing service dosage or type of service, establishing new goals (particularly if clients choose to remain in therapy after goals have been met and outcomes have improved), residential or long-term services such as foster care, and/or transition from services, also known as termination. An example of adjusting the service dosage would be by lengthening the time between meetings, which can help with managing challenges that occur over the life span. Another way to transition clients is through "well-being check-ups," which involve clients returning periodically for sessions (Bertolino, 2010). Checkups can assist clients with more severe or chronic concerns to stay on track and maintain their progress.

As in Figure 7.17, new goals and/or transition to less structured settings that provide more independence may be called for in some contexts—particularly in long-term care programs. In setting new goals, therapists keep in mind that there is a threshold of benefit to therapy and most mental health and health service. More is not always better. Figures 7.9 and 7.10 provide examples of clients who have had 20 or more sessions and are in the improved range. In such cases, when client scores have plateaued and the benefit of therapy appears to have been reached, serious consideration needs to be given as to what is best for clients. The longer clients remain in therapy in a state of stasis (unimproved or improved), the greater the risk they will deteriorate. Consider that physicians do not continue to treat patients for problems that have been resolved and when patients are functioning in an acceptable range. Treatment is concluded, with or without follow-up, with the understanding that patients may return if there is a reoccurrence of the same problem, if they should experience a new one, or if they would like a checkup.

Apprehension to Transition

It is not uncommon for clients to express apprehension about transitions from therapy. These concerns are often perpetuated by difficulties clients may have experienced with getting appointments, authorization for payment, and so on. Long waitlists, limited access to services, and affordability are but a few of the challenges clients face. For others, concerns with transitions will be more related to the prospect of having a setback, which will be discussed shortly. Part of the job of clinicians is to work with clients during therapy to manage future challenges and ensure they have support in their social systems to be successful.

In doing so, it can also be helpful for therapists to practice an "open door" approach (Bertolino, 2010). Such an approach does not mean clients can show up anytime and expect to be seen. Instead, the message parallels the general practitioner (GP) model employed by physicians. The idea is that clients are encouraged to make contact when they first have concerns, instead of allowing those problems to exacerbate. Our aim is to reduce barriers to reentry and provide a timely response to clients when there is a need. This approach can reduce suffering from problems worsening, the intensity and length of services, and the cost of therapy or more intensive behavioral health or health services. A message throughout this book has been the importance of accountability in demonstrating the efficacy and benefit of therapy while exercising stewardship resources.

Building on Progress for the Future

To help clients transition from therapy we engage in conversations about potential setbacks and hurdles. These kinds of conversations are preventive because they involve the use of strengths and resources as a buffer to challenges that may arise as clients continue with their lives. Next, we explore ways to build on the progress made in therapy to prepare for and cope with potential future challenges.

Hurdles and Setbacks as Opportunities

The stages of change (SOC) model (see Chapter 6) teaches us that client progress is seldom linear. Clients will make progress, then face a new challenge, and in some cases have a minor setback before getting back on track. Said differently, they will move from the action to maintenance stage, back to the action, then forward to maintenance again. As a preventive measure, therapists can talk with clients about possible future hurdles or perceived barriers. We ask, "Is there anything that might come up between now and the next time we meet that might threaten the changes you've made?" or "Can you think of anything that might come up over the next (few weeks/months) that could present a challenge for you in staying on track?" If a client responds in the affirmative, we then explore, in detail, what those challenges might be and how the client will meet them. The following questions help to identify and address perceived hurdles or barriers:

- What have you learned about your ability to stand up to _____?
- What might indicate to you that the problem was attempting to resurface?
- What might be the first sign?
- What will you do differently in the future if you face the same or a similar problem?

- How can what you've learned help you in solving future problems?
- If you feel yourself slipping, what's one thing that can stop that slipping and get you back heading in the direction you prefer?
- What's one thing that can bring a slippage under control or to an end?

Another strategy is to develop and role-play scenarios that will require clients to use what they have learned, including any new skills. As an example, a therapist might say, "If you were to encounter a new concern such as _____ and it caught you off guard, how might you use what you've learned to keep it from overwhelming you?" Another possibility would be, "If in a few weeks or months you were to have a little setback, what would you do differently than in the past?" The following is an illustration of how a client coped with a potential hurdle to his progress.

Case Example 7.5: He Wasn't Going to Get to Me

A 16-year-old boy was in services for fighting at school. During his last session, he was asked if he could think of anything that might throw him off track. When he said he couldn't, he was asked specifically how he might handle things in the future if someone were to start something with him. He immediately said, "That already happened. A kid threatened to pop my bike tire. I stood there and told him to go ahead. I told him I wasn't going to fight him. The kid walked away." I wasn't going to let him get to me.

It's neither possible nor is it necessary to address the infinite range of situations that could derail a client. Instead, we scan for critical situations, discuss them, and explore ways that clients can utilize their strengths more deliberately in the future. Effective therapy prepares clients for coping with life beyond the concerns that led to services. By asking questions that orient clients toward future change and progress, clients often become more resilient to everyday problems. It is as if their psychological and relational immune systems are less likely to be compromised because they are focusing on health, well-being, and the future. To invite clients into conversations to explore how change can be extended into the future, therapists ask:

- How can you put your new understandings to work in the future?
- What have you been doing that you will continue to do once therapy has ended and in the future?
- How will you continue to solidify and build on the changes that you've made?
- What will you be doing differently that you might not have otherwise been able to do?

- After you leave here, what will you do to keep things going in the direction you prefer?
- What else will you do?

A vision of the future can affect how clients act in the present and how they view the past. Instead of focusing on how they may have been held captive by past events, clients focus on where they are going and the kind of futures they want for themselves. As such, when setbacks do occur, we respond to them as part of life. Setbacks may be a source of frustration, and yet, they are to be expected as opportunities for further learning. Lapses or setbacks infrequently result in substantial loss of gains and full-blown returns to old patterns. Therapists can prepare clients for potential hurdles to their progress by openly discussing those areas of risk that accompany growth. We are not suggesting that there will be setbacks, only that setbacks do happen and are a part of life. They do not need to knock clients off track. By taking stock of progress made to date and having a realistic view of the future, clients can be prepared to face and effectively cope with the challenges that may come their way.

One way to prepare clients for the future is by employing their "muscles of resilience," strategies that they have used in the past to minimize the impact of setbacks and get back on track (Bertolino, 2003). Therapists assist clients in activating their muscles of resilience by using questions offered early in this chapter to learn how clients kept problems from getting worse. For example, a therapist might ask, "When you felt yourself slipping, what did you do to keep things from getting worse?" Central to exploring this kind of resiliency is to help clients to identify *what* they did and *how* they did it as opposed to explaining *why* they did what they did. The following questions can further assist with the identification of small differences that demonstrate how clients managed those setbacks to any degree:

- Given what you've been through, how did you manage to (continue to go to school or work, make it to this appointment, etc.)?
- When you hit that rough spot, what kept things from going downhill any further?
- How did you manage to bring things to a halt?
- What did you do?
- What helped you to bring it to an end?
- Who else helped you?
- How were those persons helpful to you?
- How might they be helpful to you in the future?
- What signs were present that things were beginning to slip?

- What can you do differently in the future if things begin to slip?
- What have you learned about this setback?
- What will you do differently in the future as a result of this knowledge?
- What do you suppose _____ (name of person) would say that you will do differently as a result of this knowledge?
- What do you suppose will be different as a result of doing things differently?
- What might be some signs that you were getting back on track?
- How will you know when you're out of the woods with this setback?

Setbacks are opportunities to understand how clients adjust to their everyday experiences, and put to use what they have learned to both keep things from getting worse and get back on track. Although we don't wish for setbacks, they can provide valuable insight into how clients keep moving forward in lieu of life circumstances. Acknowledgment that setbacks are part of life often adds perspective which can neutralize disappointment that clients may express. Even when setbacks are more serious, in nearly every situation, at least some gains have been retained. And in most cases, setbacks are more akin to a brief rain shower than a hurricane. In contrast, when single setbacks become patterns (i.e., two or more instances), therapists are more explicit in the search for triggers or precursors to those setbacks. Detailed information can help to determine what methods are most applicable in preventing future setbacks.

A final consideration with setbacks relates to outcome measurement. By monitoring outcome scores, patterns sometimes become evident, bringing forth some predictive value. The example that follows illustrates this point:

Case Example 7.6: "I Never Noticed"

A 43-year-old woman had seesaw scores on her ORS, a pattern that unfolded over the course of 10 sessions of therapy. The client would make progress only to have a setback shortly thereafter. After one particularly rough stretch, her therapist asked the client if she noticed anything about her ORS scores over the time they had met together. The client said, "Wow. I never noticed how up and down they were. All those low scores are times my boyfriend has been off work and we hung out more. It's stressful. He says mean stuff to me and makes me nervous." The therapist followed, "Does that mean the higher scores were around times when he was working more and you spent more time apart?" The young woman confirmed this observation and said, "It's so tense around him. The rest of my life is going much better now but I don't know what to do when it comes to him." The therapist asked the client if she wanted to work on a plan to address her relationship. The woman replied, "No. I really just want to get away from him. He only brings me down and I'm sick of it." The pair then proceeded to develop a plan for how the woman would separate from the boyfriend, which included a safety plan given her fear of him.

Outcome scores can also be helpful with clients who attend therapy sporadically (i.e., their periodical attendance is mixed with cancellations and "no shows") and then call-in crisis. Exploration of their scores often reveals distinct patterns that may be helpful in predicting more challenging or stressful times and an increased risk of setbacks. Services become more preventive when possible "trouble zones" are identified and plans are created by which clients use their strengths and resources to stay on track.

A critical determinant between those who learn from their experiences and those who do not is *mindset*. The concept of mindset has been discussed at different junctures of this book. Here mindset relates to how clients perceive the "hand" they have been dealt and their subjective experiences rather than the events themselves. Clients will experience ups and downs, transitions, and movement through different phases of life. What is most important is the meanings that clients attribute to their experiences. We invite clients into conversations where they can explore the relevance of change as they move through the various phases of life.

In this chapter, we have explored the topic of subsequent sessions. From unimprovement and deterioration to improvement and transition from therapy, a myriad of ideas, processes, and strategies has been offered. As we know, therapy unfolds moment by moment, interaction by interaction, and session by session. The better therapists stay attuned to clients' experiences of therapy, particularly as those experiences relate to fit and effect, and respond to client feedback, the greater the likelihood of successful outcomes.

In the final chapter, our journey comes full circle, as we examine ways for therapists to improve their overall effectiveness. As detailed in the opening chapter, some therapists consistently achieve better outcomes than others. So far you have learned core principles, practices, and strategies for improving performance. But improvement over the course of one's career requires even more calculated, concerted effort, which we'll learn about in the final pages of this book.

REFERENCES

Anderson, T., Ogles, B. M., Patterson, C. L., Lambert, M. J., & Vermeersch, D. A. (2009). Therapist effects: Facilitative interpersonal skills as a predictor of therapist effects. *Journal of Clinical Psychology, 65*(7), 755–768. doi:10.1002/jclp.20583

Anker, M. G., Duncan, B. L., & Sparks, J. A. (2009). Using client feedback to improve couple therapy outcomes: A randomized clinical trial in a naturalistic setting. *Journal of Consulting and Clinical Psychology, 77*(4), 693–704. doi:10.1037/a0016062

Anker, M. G., Owen, J., Duncan, B. L., & Sparks, J. A. (2010). The alliance in couple therapy: Partner influence, early change, and alliance patterns in a naturalistic sample. *Journal of Consulting and Clinical Psychology, 78*(5), 635–645. doi:10.1037/a0020051

Baldwin, S. A., Berkeljon, A., Atkins, D. C., Olsen, J. A., & Nielsen, S. L. (2009). Rates of change in naturalistic psychotherapy: Contrasting dose-effect and good-enough level models of change. *Journal of Consulting and Clinical Psychology, 77*, 203–211. doi:10.1037/a0015235

Baldwin, S. A., Wampold, B. E., & Imel, Z. E. (2007). Untangling the alliance-outcome correlation: Exploring the relative importance of therapist and patient variability in the alliance. *Journal of Consulting and Clinical Psychology, 75*(6), 842–852. doi:10.1037/0022-006X.75.6.842

Bertolino, B. (1999). *Therapy with troubled teenagers: Rewriting young lives in progress.* New York: Wiley.

Bertolino, B. (2003). *Change-oriented psychotherapy with adolescents and young adults: The next generation of respectful and effective therapeutic processes and practices.* New York. NY: W. W. Norton.

Bertolino, B. (2010). *Strengths-based engagement and practice: Creating effective helping relationships.* Boston, MA: Allyn & Bacon.

Bertolino, B. (2014). *Thriving on the front lines: Strengths-based youth care work.* New York, NY: Routledge.

Bickman, L. (2000). Summing up program theory. *New Directions for Evaluation, 87*, 103–112. doi: 10.1002/ev.1186

de Jong, K., van Sluis, P., Nugter, M. A., Heiser, W. J., & Spinhoven, P. (2012). Understanding the differential impact of outcome monitoring: Therapists variables that moderate feedback effects in a randomized clinical trial. *Psychotherapy Research, 22*, 464–474. doi:10.1080/10503307.2012.673023

Duncan, B. L., & Miller, S. D. (2008). When I'm good, I'm very good, but when I'm bad I'm better: A new mantra for psychotherapists. *Psychotherapy in Australia, 15*(1), 62–70.

Duncan, B. L., Miller, S. D., & Sparks, J. A. (2004). *The heroic client: A revolutionary way to improve effectiveness through client directed, outcome-informed therapy.* San Francisco, CA: Jossey-Bass.

Duncan, B. L., Miller, S. D., Wampold, B. E., & Hubble, M.A. (Eds.). (2010). *The heart and soul of change: Delivering what works in therapy* (2nd ed.). Washington, DC: American Psychological Association.

Gilbody, S., House, A., & Sheldon, T. (2002). Psychiatrists in the UK do not use outcome measures: National survey. *The British Journal of Psychiatry, 180*, 101–103. doi: 10.1192/bjp.180.2.101

Hansen, N., Lambert, M. J., & Forman, E. M. (2002). The psychotherapy dose-response effect and its implication for treatment delivery services. *Clinical Psychology: Science and Practice, 9*(3), 329–343. doi:10.1093/clipsy.9.3.329

Hatfield, D. R., & Ogles, B. M. (2004). The use of outcome measures by psychologists in clinical practice. *Professional Psychology: Research and Practice, 35*, 485–491. doi:10.1037/0735-7028.35.5.485

Howard, K. I., Kopte, S. M., Krause, M. S., & Orlinsky, D. E. (1986). The dose-effect relationship in psychotherapy. *American Psychologist, 41*(2), 159–164.

Howard, K. I., Moras, K., Brill, P. L., Martinovich, Z., & Lutz, W. (1996). Evaluation of psychotherapy: Efficacy, effectiveness, and patient progress. *American Psychologist, 51*(10), 1059–1064. doi:10.1037/0003-066X.51.10.1059

Kopta, S. M., Howard. K. I., Lowry, J. L., & Beutler, L. E. (1994). Patterns of symptomatic recovery in psychotherapy. *Journal of Consulting and Clinical Psychology, 62*(5), 1009–1016. doi:10.1037/0022-006X.62.5.1009

Lambert, M. J. (2010). *Prevention of treatment failure: The use of measuring, monitoring, and feedback in clinical practice.* Washington, DC: American Psychological Association.

Lambert, M. J. (2013). The efficacy and effectiveness of psychotherapy. In M. J. Lambert (Ed.), *Bergin and Garfield's handbook of psychotherapy and behavior change* (6th ed., pp. 169–218). Hoboken, NJ: Wiley.

Maeschalck, C., Bargmann, S., Miller, S. D., & Bertolino, B. (2013). Manual 3: Feedback-informed supervision. In B. Bertolino & S. D. Miller (Eds.), *The ICCE manuals of feedback informed treatment.* Chicago, IL: International Center for Clinical Excellence.

Owen, J., Miller, S. D., Seidel, J., & Chow, D. (2016). The working alliance in treatment of military adolescents. *Journal of Consulting and Clinical Psychology, 84*(3), 200–210. doi:10.1037/ccp0000035

Safran, J. D., Muran, J. C., Samstag, L. W., & Stevens, C. (2002). Repairing alliance ruptures. In J. C. Norcross (Ed.), *Psychotherapy relationships that work: Therapist contributions and responsiveness to patients* (pp. 235–254). New York, NY: Oxford University Press.

Sapyta, J., Riemer, M., & Bickman, L. (2005). Feedback to clinicians: Theory, research, and practice. *Journal of Clinical Psychology, 61*(2), 145–153. doi:10.1002/jclp.20107

Schuckard, E., & Miller, S. D. (2016). Psychometrics of the ORS and SRS: Results from RCTs and meta-analyses of routine outcome monitoring and feedback. Retrieved from http://scottdmiller.com/wp-content/uploads/2016/09/Measures-and-Feedback-2016.pdf

Seidel, J., & Miller, S. D. (2013). Manual 4: Documenting change: A primer on measurement, analysis, and reporting. In B. Bertolino & S. D. Miller (Eds.), *The ICCE manuals of feedback informed treatment*. Chicago, IL: International Center for Clinical Excellence.

Wampold, B. E. (2001). *The great psychotherapy debate: Models, methods, and findings.* Mahwah, NJ: Lawrence Erlbaum.

Warren, J. S., Nelson, P. L., Mondragon, S. A., Baldwin, S. A., & Burlingame, G. A. (2010). Youth psychotherapy change trajectories and outcomes in usual care: Community mental health versus managed care settings. *Journal of Consulting and Clinical Psychology, 78*(2), 144–155.

Zimmerman, M., & McGlinchey, J. B. (2008). Why don't psychiatrists use scales to measure outcome when treating depressed patients? *The Journal of Clinical Psychiatry, 69*, 1916–1919. doi:10.4088/JCP.v69n1209

CHAPTER 8

Professional Development and Clinical Excellence

In this final chapter, our focus is squarely on increasing the benefit of psychotherapy by improving clinician effectiveness. By design, this chapter is meant to be concise, and a starting point for those committed to achieving clinical excellence. As such, we will explore ways of improving their clinical performance through supervision, training, and individual practice strategies. It is hopeful that these ideas will inspire clinicians to engage in lifelong learning.

UNDERSTANDING THERAPIST EFFECTIVENESS

At no time in the history of psychotherapy has there been more well-designed studies on therapist effectiveness and efforts to improve its practice than in the present. In accordance, a wealth of materials and resources has become available, offering guidance for those who desire to take their performance to its next level. Despite studies questioning the veracity of supervision and training as it relates to therapist performance and outcomes (see Chapter 1), it is clear that clinicians want to continue to develop their skills and effectiveness. Orlinsky and Rønnestad (2005), together with members of the Society for Psychotherapy Research, conducted a large-scale, 20-year study involving 11,000 multinational clinicians in which the researchers confirmed the deeply held desire of clinicians to improve (Orlinsky & Rønnestad, 2005; Rønnestad & Orlinsky, 2005). Similar results were found by Jennings and Skovholt (2016) in their study of clinicians from seven cultures.

Building on therapists' drive to develop professionally, this chapter examines practical ideas and strategies to assist with improvement over the course of one's career. As we do so, we consider a question that is asked in virtually every discipline: Are successful people born that way? In psychotherapy, it is reasonable to consider that some therapists are more gifted and talented than the rest. Following this discussion, we'll tackle the issue of therapist effectiveness. In other words, how do we reliably measure effectiveness? Thirdly, the topic of how therapists improve is addressed. In doing so, various strategies will be provided as well as suggestions of strategies for professional development.

THE ROAD TO EXCELLENCE: NATURAL AND TALENTED?

We've all heard those interested in becoming helping professionals say, "I've been told I'm a good listener" and "My friends say I'm the one to go to when they have problems." Is it possible that the most effective therapists are born with a set of innate abilities? After all, the word *talent* has become synonymous with expert performance. We say, "Elizabeth is a talented gymnast" and "Alex has an aptitude for chess." By now you've probably become at least a little suspicious of the idea that talent is the main cog behind success. How, then, do some therapists consistently achieve better outcomes than others? A hint can be found through the study of an array of disciplines.

In a review of historical figures, it may seem that most simply "came out of nowhere" by way of their extraordinary abilities and accomplishments. Consider that Wolfgang Amadeus Mozart wrote his first composition at the age of 5 and then his first symphony by the age of 8. In all, Mozart wrote over 600 pieces of music, including 41 symphonies during his short life of 35 years. Pablo Picasso made over 20,000 paintings in his lifetime and created a new type of art called "cubism," comprised of different overlapping shapes. Hockey player Wayne Gretzky holds 61 National Hockey League (NHL) records including most all-time goals, assists, and points. Many of his records are considered unbreakable. The Beatles, disbanding in 1970 after just 7 years together, remain the top selling musical group of all time with estimates of having sold over 1 million disks and tapes worldwide. Then we have Bill Gates, whose accomplishments are part of our everyday lives. These are just a few of the remarkable achievements of people considered by many as gifted and, perhaps, even deserving of the moniker *genius*.

It's hard to look at the lives of successful persons and not think, "They're naturals." But to view such persons—and countless others not listed here—in a way that suggests they were born with exceptional abilities and skills would be to overlook the very heart of what led to their success. Mozart, for example, had a father who taught music and practiced more by the age of 7 than most who were twice his age. But that is a side of the story not often raised in discussions of Mozart's accomplishments. Mozart was prolific, but there is little to support the idea that he was born that way. Although a very different field, similar things are often said about clinicians who consistently outperform the rest. We find ourselves saying, "She has such a gift for working with others. I'll never be that good." It seems we have created a story that equates raw talent with success.

It is reasonable to consider that Mozart had some innate talent. Similarly, it is difficult to explain how Srinivasa Ramanujan, who grew up in India with little formal education and resources, would in his very short life (he died at the age of 32) make substantial contributions to mathematical analysis, number theory, infinite series, and continued fractions, including solutions to mathematical problems considered to be unsolvable (Kanigel, 1991). It seems that some do have a knack for certain disciplines or fields. The story begins to break down, however, when we study the paths to achievement persons have taken, regardless of the field.

As it turns out, there is a wealth of evidence to suggest that the concept of talent has been greatly exaggerated. In the first chapter, researcher K. Anders Ericsson, who is widely considered the "expert on expertise," was mentioned for his study of musicians, physicians, chess players, mathematicians, and athletes, to name a few. In their research of persons who had achieved excellence in their respective disciplines, Ericsson and colleagues found a distinct lack of evidence to support the concept of "naturals" (Ericsson, Charness, Feltovich, & Hoffman, 2006). Still, if talent does not explain how excellence is achieved, what does? While research continues to evolve, it does provide insight into performance improvement, which, as it turns out, has little to do with natural born ability.

It seems that success has more to do with factors that are within our grasp. Let's now learn about three precursors for performance improvement and achieving excellence: grit and determination, learning from failures, and practice. Collectively these factors create an "improvement-driven mindset."

1. Grit and Determination

Former president of Apple Computer, John Sculley, often tells the story of how Steve Jobs convinced him to leave PepsiCo. to work for the future computer giant. Sculley described a meeting with Jobs, "He looked up at me and just stared at me with the stare that only Steve Jobs has and he said, 'Do you want to sell sugar water for the rest of your life or do you want to come with me and change the world?' and I just gulped because I knew I would wonder for the rest of my life what I would have missed." Mythologist Joseph Campbell famously encouraged others to pursue their passions or "follow their bliss":

> If you do follow your bliss, you put yourself on a kind of track that has been there all the while waiting for you, and the life you ought to be living is the one you are living. . . . If you follow your bliss, doors will open for you that wouldn't have opened for anyone else. (Campbell & Moyers, 1988, p. 120)

If you have chosen to become a clinician, there is a passion within to do your best to improve the lives and well-being of others. There is no competition when it comes to following your passion, just a desire to do your absolute best. As such, there will be times when it will be challenging to muster up the energy and drive to continuously work at improvement. Poet David Whyte (2011) has spoken of the importance of staying the course and facing challenges head on:

> If you are sincere about your vocation you will get to thresholds where you will not know how to proceed . . . and where you will forget yourself . . . and where you will start to imprison yourself with the very endeavor that was first a doorway

to freedom. And if you don't become disappointed in yourself you're not trying. There is actually no path a human can take with sincerity, with real courage that doesn't lead to heartbreak. It's astonishing how human beings spend an enormous amount of their energy and time turning away from that possibility.

Success requires commitment, patience, and passion. Still, *passion* is a tricky and potentially ambiguous word. Passion refers to grit, and grit refers to "perseverance and passion for long-term goals" (Duckworth, Peterson, Matthews, & Kelly, 2007, p. 1087). When it comes to performance improvement, focused determination to reach a reasonable, long-term goal is necessary. This is because meaningful skill acquisition is hard work that requires persistence and continuous effort despite delayed gratification (Ericsson, 2006). Without focused determination and a drive to improve, it is very difficult to maintain the energy long enough to see the benefits of efforts. Rousmaniere, Goodyear, Miller, and Wampold (2017a) observed, "It is our impression that most clinicians remain intellectually curious throughout their professional lives, but that once they attain basic competence the curiosity is manifest in more diffuse then focused ways" (p. 13). And while therapists' degrees of motivation will vary, it is important to set the compass in the direction that is reachable. Our aim is not to achieve *supershrink* status. It is to improve over the course of our careers. A starting point, then, is simply having the passion and drive to improve—to achieve excellence—and not give up when hurdles appear. Should your inspiration wane, consider revisiting your personal philosophy (see Chapter 1)

2. Learning From Failures

At several junctures in this book, the concept of an error-centric culture has been discussed. Error-centric refers to learning from situations that are either failing or have already failed. The idea of learning from failures is closely associated with grit. This is because failure, when not viewed through the lens of growth, can lead to, well, a sense of *being a failure*. For example, when Abraham Lincoln turned to politics, he was defeated in his first try for the legislature, again defeated in his first attempt to be nominated for Congress, defeated in his application to be commissioner of the General Land Office, defeated in the senatorial election of 1854, defeated in his efforts for the vice-presidency in 1856, and defeated in the senatorial election of 1858. The effects of his defeats were substantial. Lincoln wrote to his friend, John T. Stuart, "I am now the most miserable man living. If what I feel were equally distributed to the whole human family, there would not be one cheerful face on the earth" (Basler, 1953, pp. 229–230). Fortunately, Lincoln did not view his defeats as failures of character, but of performance, and therefore something that can be improved upon. Later, Lincoln recounted to his best friend, Joshua Speed, that he had an "irrepressible desire" to accomplish something while he lived (Shenk, 2005).

Let's further explore the idea of failure as *actionable*. Consider that both Einstein and Thomas Edison had far more failures than successes. In fact, Edison made 1,000 unsuccessful attempts at inventing the light bulb. When a reporter asked, "How did it feel to fail 1,000 times?" Edison replied, "I didn't fail 1,000 times. The light bulb was an invention with 1,000 steps." Bill Gates spent hours and hours building computers and developing software that did not see the light of day. Accomplished authors E. E. Cummings, J. K. Rowling, James Joyce, and Dr. Seuss were rejected over and over for manuscripts that would become classics. And Peter Vegso, publisher of the *Chicken Soup for the Soul* series, once told me that Jack Canfield's first book for the series was rejected by over 260 publishers before being published and becoming a best seller. If you're a sports fan, you might relate to Michael Jordan, who failed to make his high school basketball team. The Hall of Famer with six NBA championships remarked, "I've missed more than 9,000 shots in my career. I've lost almost 300 games. Twenty-six times I've been trusted to take the game winning shot . . . and missed. I've failed over and over and over again in my life. That is why I succeed" (Goldman & Papson, 1999, p. 49). Even Sigmund Freud was booed from the podium when he first presented his ideas to the scientific community of Europe. He returned to his office and kept on writing.

An error-centric culture is not one in which therapists purposely try to fail. Instead, it refers to acceptance of failure as part of learning. Railton (2016a) remarked, "Memory must be active and constructive, not passive or fixed—it must metabolize information into forms that are efficient and effective for the forward guidance of thought and action" (p. 15). We do want to recognize good performance—what we do well—so that we repeat skills that are uniquely tied to successful outcomes. But it is our failures that prove more instructive when it comes to performance improvement. Rather than focusing energy on the skills already mastered, time and energy are on areas less developed. As a way to become familiar with the concept of learning from failures, both new and experienced clinicians can ask of themselves, "When was the last time I failed and how did I overcome it?"

In the context of psychotherapy, "failures" refer to opportunities to learn from clients who are unimproved or deteriorated in a non-blaming atmosphere. In this way development occurs when small errors in the application of knowledge and skills are identified, thereby allowing for remedial action. Both the Outcome Rating Scale (ORS) and the Session Rating Scale (SRS) provide therapists with opportunities to learn. This is because ORS scores represent client's views of he subjective impact of therapy. ORS scores also provide therapists with feedback as to whether clients are unimproved (and moderate risk) or deteriorated (high risk). Figure 8.1 is an example of clients who are in the unimproved (moderate risk) range. Figure 8.2 is an example of clients in the deteriorated (high risk) range. Sorting cases by the ORS is one way to identify failing cases. Similarly, the SRS is a mechanism to elicit negative feedback. With alliance feedback, the therapist can respond to possible ruptures to reduce dropout and negative outcome. The client's rating of the alliance is second only to the client's rating of distress at the start of therapy as the best predictor of outcome (Martin, Garske, & Davis, 2000; Norcross, 2011). In most electronic systems, sorting can also be done by SRS scores.

Only by decreasing these "deficits" can performances rise above average (Ericsson et al., 2006). Through an error-centric focus and developing and

Clients

Client Name	Client ID	DOB	First Session Date	Program	Recent Session	Outcome Rating	Session Rating	Risk Rating	Target
	20389		8/24/2015		8/24/2015	ORS: 26.3	40	7	29.26
	24066		9/11/2014		9/18/2014	ORS: 26.1	39.8	6	29.15
	25654		3/20/2014		10/1/2014	ORS: 26	36	6	29.15
	28619		6/10/2015		6/14/2015	ORS: 26	39.2	6	29.29
	26401		8/18/2015		8/18/2015	ORS: 26	34.4	8	29.24
	25086		8/19/2015		8/25/2015	ORS: 26	39.8	7	29.27
	24153		8/24/2015		8/24/2015	ORS: 26	40	6	29.24
	25323		8/25/2015		8/25/2015	ORS: 26	14.4	6	29.24
	27264		8/25/2015		8/15/2015	ORS: 26	39.9	6	29.24
	32471		7/8/2016		7/15/2016	ORS: 26	39.5	6	28.99

FIGURE 8.1 List of clients in the unimproved (moderate risk) range.

Clients

Client Name	Client ID	DOB	First Session Date	Program	Recent Session	Outcome Rating	Session Rating	Risk Rating	Target
	25032		1/9/2014		1/21/2015	ORS: 11.5	16.1	6	24.12
	27447		11/21/2014		1/16/2015	ORS: 11.4	34	7	27.13
	25275		8/20/2015		8/25/2015	ORS: 11.1	35.5	3	21.55
			8/25/2015		8/26/2015	ORS: 11	28.4	3	25.27
	25521		7/23/2015		8/5/2015	ORS: 10.8	39.6	3	25.2
	15252		8/18/2015		8/18/2015	ORS: 10.7	37.5	6	22.33
	21371		8/20/2015		8/24/2015	ORS: 10.6	31	5	23.76
	15650		8/26/2015		8/26/2015	ORS: 10.6	31.9	5	22.25
	28701		6/23/2015		8/18/2015	ORS: 10.5	24.9	8	22.18
	28934		8/21/2015		8/25/2015	ORS: 10.5	40	3	27.71

FIGURE 8.2 List of clients in the deteriorated (high risk) range.

implementing "deliberate practice" (DP) strategies—which will be discussed later in this chapter—we can improve areas of weak performance. The idea of focusing on deficits may appear counter to a strengths-based perspective, but is not. Rather, attention is placed on the perseverance and commitment of learners to build further skills and capacities to better themselves and, in the case of therapists, the lives of others.

Given that grit and failure are inextricably connected, therapists are encouraged to continuously revisit their areas of development and their motivation to continue the path toward excellence. Orlinsky and Rønnestad (2015) observed,

> Presumably a certain portion of therapists at each career level may fail to master the challenges that confront them, perhaps because of a lack of aptitude and preparation or a lack of adequate support and supervision, with the result being either stagnation or deterioration. Those who struggle or fail to meet career-specific developmental challenges may be more likely to discontinue their work as therapists. (p. 1135)

As with any discipline, excellence as a psychotherapist comes at a cost. And yet, vitality and enthusiasm to do good therapeutic work serve as excellent catalysts for professional development. In the next section, we will add a third element to an improvement-driven mindset, practice.

3. Practice

It would stand to reason that the longer therapists practice, the better outcomes they would achieve. On the contrary, studies have shown that psychotherapy is a field in which clinicians' proficiency does not automatically increase with experience (Goldberg et al., 2016; Owen, Wampold, Rousmaniere, Kopta, & Miller, 2016; Tracey, Wampold, Goodyear, & Lichtenberg, 2015; Tracey, Wampold, Lichtenberg, & Goodyear, 2014). In fact, in a longitudinal study, Goldberg et al. (2016) found that on average clinicians' performance decreased as they gained experience. However, this apparent contradiction between effectiveness and experience may not be as puzzling as it seems. Let's explore this issue from several different points of view, each of which returns to the theme of practice.

Gathering and Responding to Feedback

Lack of therapist improvement has been a central theme of this book—specifically, therapists' failure to (a) track the outcomes of their clients in reliable and valid ways and (b) respond effectively to client feedback to client unimprovement and deterioration. The value of monitoring both the outcome of therapy and the strength of the alliance is well established and a starting point for all therapists. This leaves us with the second part of the equation, responding to client feedback.

An example of the impact of reviewing client outcomes is A Collaborative Outcomes Resource Network (ACORN, 2013), a project in which researchers reviewed therapists' outcomes over a period of 12 months. In the project, researchers found that the amount of time therapists spent reviewing outcome data was directly correlated with their effectiveness. Three groups emerged from the study. The first included therapists who either did not review their outcome data or reviewed their data less than 50 times over the 12 months. The second group was of therapists who reviewed their outcome data between 50 and 200 times during the year. The third and final group was of therapists who reviewed their data more than 200 times during the year.

The differences in outcomes between the groups were substantial. Therapists in the first group had effect sizes (ES) that either remained unimproved or deteriorated. Meanwhile, therapists in the second group showed solid improvement in their ES. But it was the third group that made the most significant gains, which were more than double those made by the second group. The ACORN (2013) study draws attention to continuous monitoring of client outcomes accompanied by timely responses to client lack of progress. But as we know, the impact of feedback can vary significantly depending on who uses the feedback (Schuckard, Miller, & Hubble, 2017). As such, feedback alone is not sufficient to improve outcomes.

As we have learned, a first-order response is to commit to routine outcome monitoring (ROM). Second is to learn to use feedback, particularly with cases of unimprovement and deterioration. Doing so provides solid countermeasures to the three risks to therapist effectiveness and outcomes detailed in Chapter 1: overprediction of client improvement, failure to identify client deterioration, and self-assessment bias. Building on grit and determination, therapists use ROM while simultaneously honing their skills to improve effectiveness through practice. Practice is critical to learning how to nuance the introduction of ROM and the specific measures chosen, and to respond to various outcome patterns, and potential problems with the alliance. Each of these areas is discussed in detail in previous chapters.

Practice Perfect: Mastering the Basics

Whether in private or public settings, it is clear that some therapists consistently achieve better outcomes than others (Wampold & Brown, 2005). Outcome variations may result in part with differences in skills of therapists. Although time and experience are not predictors of therapist effectiveness, it is also clear that effective therapists have a high degree of mastery when it comes to the basics of psychotherapy. In their study of 1,102 therapists 60 years of age and older, Orlinsky and Rønnestad (2015) found that "these hardy 'surviving' therapists typically had succeeded in mastering the developmental tasks of previous phases of professional development" (p. 1128). A good starting point, then, would be to ensure therapists are competent with core relational skills related to empathy, positive regard, and genuineness. A second level would be for therapists to achieve the kind of relational responsiveness and flexibility demonstrated in the facilitative interpersonal skills (FIS) approach (Anderson, Ogles, Patterson, Lambert, & Vermeersch, 2009). The FIS approach assists therapists with learning skills to manage interpersonally challenging encounters with clients, thereby strengthening the alliance. Wampold (2017) makes it clear that therapists give particular emphasis to enhancing the strength and quality of their therapeutic alliances, their levels of empathic responding, and their ability to deliver a cogent rationale for treatment that will match clients' expectations for change.

Let's further reflect on the idea of mastering fundamental skills by momentarily stepping outside of the world of psychotherapy. Consider that the average age of Nobel Laureates the year they were awarded the Nobel Prize between 1901 and 2016 is 59. The most frequent age bracket for winning a Nobel Prize is 60 to 64. In physics, for example, a researcher may take 40 or 50 years to reach a point in which he or she "knows enough" to create something truly world-changing. In other disciplines, psychotherapy notwithstanding, it takes years to develop and master basic skills before becoming adept and competent with advanced ones.

This again brings us back to Mozart. In addition to access to an accomplished instructor in his father (which will be discussed later in this chapter), a very young Mozart practiced and rehearsed many hours each day. And although they began to hone their individual crafts at different ages, Picasso, Gretzky, the Beatles, Gates, and Ramanujan all practiced intensively to acquire the various abilities that would underscore their success. Whether it's employing the basics of physics, shooting hockey pucks, singing harmonies, solving math problems, or the like, it simply takes a while to get the basics down before making a novel contribution to one's field.

For therapists, ROM provides a starting point for improvement. With feedback in hand, therapists can practice different forms of response to develop their skills in nuancing feedback. For example, through formal and ongoing feedback (i.e., the "N" in the SONAR SFC, Chapter 4), a therapist may learn that for one client, empathy is felt through eye contact, whereas another client experiences empathy through a fist bump. The tailoring of feedback is especially important to increase the fit between the approach and the client.

Advanced Skills

One of my friends and mentors, psychologist Steve Gilligan, a student of Milton Erickson, tells a story about the first Evolution of Psychotherapy Conference in 1985, the first of its kind, following the passing of Dr. Erickson in 1980 (see Chapter 1). Steve said he was struck by the number of people dressed in purple. Erickson had acquired color blindness as a result of two episodes of polio and purple was the only color he could see well. He was so fond of the color, he almost always wore purple clothing. And while many at the conference were just paying homage and respect to a true innovator, Steve commented that it didn't end there. Numerous followers would attempt to emulate Erickson's work including his mannerisms, methods, and so on. Even today, therapists invest in training to learn from experts in the field, hoping to replicate the methods they learn, perhaps unaware that therapeutic models contribute to only about 1% of the variance in outcome.

At the surface, it makes sense. It has been said that the highest form of flattery is imitation. In the case of psychotherapy, once basic skills have been mastered, a focus on replication carries the consequence of losing sight of the uniqueness of the client. The essence of Erickson's brilliance was in his ability to tailor his approach to each patient. In fact, in a review of over 300 of Erickson's patients, O'Hanlon and Hexum (1990) could find no consistency in Erickson's choice of methods. In other words, Milton Erickson was not an "Ericksonian." To be clear, there is nothing wrong with learning creative and clever techniques. What Erickson seemed to understand and stands as an example for all clinicians is that mastering methods involves *knowing what to do* and *when to do it*.

So how do therapists learn advanced skills (i.e., what to do) and when to use them? As with basic skills, advanced skill development begins and ends with practice. Mozart, who may have played and wrote music at a very young age, did not produce his first masterwork (N. 9, K. 271) until the age of 21—which, of course, is still remarkable, but nonetheless relative to his years of practice (Howe, 1999). It took thousands of hours of practice over many years for Mozart to create anything of consequence. To create something novel, he first had to learn the basics, then advance his abilities to become "creative." Today, a scan of YouTube reveals a myriad of very young children who can play, note for note, the works of compositions that were once considered unplayable but by a few. But how many of these so-called prodigies, as adults, create original works? There are, of course, major differences between musicians, mathematicians, athletes, and therapists, to name a few. There is a place for what amounts to flawless replication. For example, professional violinists need to be able to play pieces of music to perfection should they expect to be part of a world-class symphony. Unlike performing a particular classical piece for a symphony performance, in which the purpose is to play it impeccably, no two hockey games are ever the same. Therefore, hockey players may practice a variety of plays that are never used in game conditions. But practice prepares players should situations arise.

An extraordinary example of this can be found in the 1996 NCAA championship hockey game between the University of Michigan Wolverines and Minnesota Golden Gophers. In what is arguably the greatest college hockey goal of all time, from behind the Gophers' net, Wolverine player Mike Legg used a "lacrosse shot" by lifting the puck onto his stick and carrying it around the front of the net before "throwing" the puck into the net, similar to what a lacrosse player would do. According to college teammate, goaltender, and future NHL player Marty Turco, "Mike did that shot all day, every day." But it wasn't until the precise opportunity presented itself that Legg tried the shot.

Putting in the work is part of a process of learning, developing, and performance improvement. Study of high performers in virtually every field reveals similar practices. Therapists can advance their skills by practicing for situations that require creative thinking, nontraditional methods, and allowance of failure.

Real-World Practice

By the time the world had heard the Beatles, they had played hundreds of gigs (which translated to thousands of hours) in clubs throughout Europe. They played the same songs (a mixture of original tunes and covers of other artists) over and over, sometimes multiple times a night in venues with poor acoustics, often unable to hear themselves or their band mates. Central to the group's development was repetition in "real-world" situations. It's one thing to practice in settings where you can stop and start again and there is no added pressure. It's another to practice in the type of climate in which the skill will likely be used. For therapists, there is no substitute for real-world learning. Later in this chapter, ideas for simulating real-world learning in psychotherapy will be offered.

Putting in the Time

The amount of practice time also matters. Ericsson and colleagues have estimated that it takes about 10,000 hours (about 10 years) to achieve the kind of expertise shown by persons including *international chess champions and Olympic athletes* (Ericsson, Krampe, & Tesch-Romer, 1993). In pop culture, writers such as Malcolm Gladwell (2008) in his book, *Outliers: The Story of Success*, have taken the "10,000 hour rule" as a generality in an effort to challenge the notion of talent and unpack the mystery of success (also see Colvin, 2008; Syed, 2010). This has sparked a debate with dissenters arguing that 10,000 hours in and of itself does not make one an expert—which misses the point.

Ericsson and colleagues do not say that all domains of expertise require the same amount of effort. Many domains will require fewer hours (5,000–6,000 in many cases) to achieve what is considered expertise for that specific skill set (Ericsson et al., 1993). Said differently, the number of hours required for mastery varies by field (Ericsson, 2006). And not just any kind of practice counts when it comes to developing ability. Ericsson is fond of saying, "Just because you've been walking for 50 years doesn't mean you're good at it." Thousands of hours of routine work experience does not itself lead to expert performance. Researchers have actually found something quite more challenging: Thousands of hours of *DP* (a topic that will be discussed in detail shortly), on top of hours spent in routine work performance, is usually required for expert performance. The amount of time invested on improving ability is dependent on both what is practiced and, more importantly, how practice occurs. Bruce Lee once said, "I fear not the man who has practiced 10,000 kicks once, but I fear the man who had practiced one kick 10,000 times." Practice dedicated to intensive honing of skills is what seems to matter. Let's now explore how practice can improve performance specific to therapy.

Each of the three aspects previously discussed—grit and determination, learning from failures, and practice—forms an "improvement-driven mindset." This mindset is a precursor to performance improvement and achieving excellence, which will be explored in more detail in the sections that follow, beginning with what researchers have deemed a "cycle of excellence (COE)."

CYCLE OF EXCELLENCE

Miller, Duncan, and Hubble (2007) proposed a model—a COE—to improve the performance of therapists (see Figure 8.3). More recently, this model has been expanded to help therapists in their growth and in achieving clinical excellence (Rousmaniere et al., 2017b). This chapter provides an overview of the basics of the framework with the hope that therapists will explore it in greater detail through a growing body of available literature and resources (see Prescott, Maeschalck, & Miller, 2017; Rousmaniere, 2017; Rousmaniere et al., 2017b).

The COE framework is based on a universal set of processes that both account for the development of expertise as well as a step-by-step process that can be followed to improve their performance within a particular discipline (Ericsson et al., 2006). The COE includes three core components: (a) determining a baseline level of effectiveness, including strengths and skills that need improvement; (b) obtaining systematic, ongoing, formal feedback; and (c) engaging in DP.

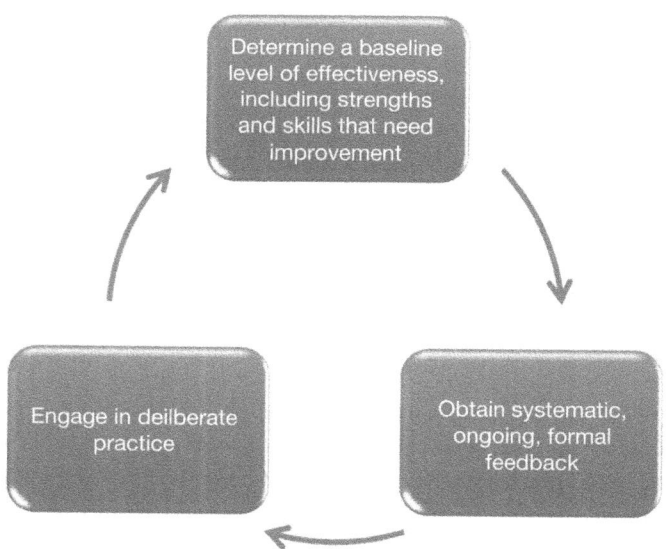

FIGURE 8.3 Cycle of excellence.

Source: From Miller, Hubble, & Duncan, 2007; Rousmaniere, T., Goodyear, R. K., Miller, S. D., & Wampold, B. E. (Eds.). (2017b). *The cycle of excellence: Using deliberate practice to improve supervision and training.* Washington, DC: American Psychological Association.)

Determining a Baseline Level of Effectiveness

In fields such as sports, music, medicine, and now behavioral health, top performers are able to accurately assess their knowledge, skills, and effectiveness. Top performers are also consistently comparing their current performance to their own personal best, the performance of others, and existing standards or baselines (Ericsson et al., 2006). The purpose of establishing a baseline level of effectiveness is to know how well one fares in a given practice domain, including strengths and skills that need improvement. As we have learned, there are numerous outcome measurement systems (OMSs) available to psychotherapists for assessing their baseline (Miller et al., 2013). These systems provide therapists with real-time comparisons of their results (Lambert, 2010; Miller, Duncan, Sorrell, & Brown, 2005). Throughout this book, the partners for change outcome management system (PCOMS) has been used as an example given its reliability, validity, and feasibility. It is important to note that to determine one's baseline a minimum number of completed cases of psychotherapy will be needed. In most cases, between 30 and 60 inactive clients will provide a point of reference. With enough data, supervisors, trainers, and/or peers, depending upon the developmental level of the therapist, can review data to assist with therapist development and for quality assurance.

There exists a variety of ways to determine a baseline level of effectiveness, each with strengths and drawbacks. Although a detailed overview of statistical calculations is beyond the scope of this book, a few options will be discussed here in brief. There are excellent resources available for clinicians to determine the best way to measure their effectiveness (see Lambert, 2010; Rousmaniere et al., 2017a).

Effect Sizes

A commonly used statistical measure is the effective size. ES provides estimates of client progress compared to no treatment controls. Standard ES measures change from point A to point B. An example of an ES is Cohen's D, which is calculated by subtracting the mean of the client's first session scores from the mean of the most recent session scores, then dividing that score by the standard deviation for the measure or pooled group. An ES for no treatment is typically reported to be around .20 and for therapy around .80. Therefore, an ES of .20 is considered small, and indicates client improvement is no better than no treatment at. By comparison, a medium ES is around .50, whereas a large ES is generally considered to be .80 and above. An ES will be lower for active clients than inactive clients in the database because they have not completed therapy or services. The larger the number of clients in the data pool, the more confidence in the ES. In contrast, typically a relative (RES) or corrected effect size (CES) compares client progress to progress of clients in the normative sample who have the same intake score (compares like to like). Again, in most cases a RES or CES of .0 indicates average; .01 is better than average; and −.01 is below average. As with the ES, the larger the number of clients in the data pool, the more confidence in the CES. In their article, "Effect Size Calculations for the Clinician: Methods and Comparability," Seidel, Miller, and Chow (2013) describe various ways to calculate ES for clinicians.

Reliable Change, Significant Change, Predictive Trajectories (Target Scores), and Expected Treatment Response

A second way to create a baseline is to determine the number of clients who complete therapy with a reliable change, which is the difference between the first and most recent session scores. A third form of enumeration is to calculate how many clients complete therapy at the level of clinically significant change, which includes both a reliable change and a final score above the clinical cutoff for a particular measure. Both reliable change and clinically significant change were discussed in detail in chapter 7. A final option is to use client target scores (based on national datasets and predictive algorithms) and expected treatment responses (ETRs), which are typically part of electronic OMSs.

There are two areas to bear in mind when it comes to establishing a baseline rate of effectiveness. First, despite considerable evidence that psychotherapists are not alert to treatment failure and strong evidence that clinical judgments are usually inferior to actuarial methods, therapists' confidence in their clinical judgment alone stands as a barrier to implementation of monitoring and feedback systems (Chow, 2017). Second, efforts to implement an OMS in an agency-type setting should be done with respect to the clientele, staff, and organizational mission. Key components include sufficient planning, involvement of key stakeholders, ongoing support, and patience. The success of implementation is largely based on collaboration. Although the specifics of large-scale implementation of an OMS is outside the scope of this book, numerous resources are available to guide and support organizations and group practices (see Bertolino, 2011, 2017; Bertolino, Axsen, Maeschalck, Miller, & Babbins-Wagner, 2012; Moss & Mousavikizadeh, 2017).

Obtaining Systematic, Ongoing, Formal Feedback

With a baseline rate of effectiveness, therapists move to the second phase of obtaining systematic, ongoing, formal feedback. If you have read this far in this book, you probably do not need to be convinced of its role in outcome data to improve performance, outcomes, and the benefit of therapy to clients. It's likely you also have a passion for improvement. You may already be seeking feedback, or planning to do so in the near future. If this describes you, your role in supporting others may be called upon. This is because for a percentage of therapists, the process of collecting, analyzing, and learning from data will not be an invitation for improving services but instead a mandate to "get on board." In these circumstances, a move to begin tracking and monitoring the effects of therapy will be void of rationale and seen as "another thing we have to do to satisfy administration." Under such conditions, this second step can come slowly. Grit, determination, and patience are keys to success.

There are two sources for obtaining feedback: (a) empirical outcome measures and (b) coaches and teachers. The use of ROM has been detailed throughout this book to monitor the effects of behavioral health interventions and in creating systems of response to improve the benefit of those services. The role of feedback cannot be overstated. In the world of sports, for example, the role of accurate information is critical to performance improvement. Railton (2016b) remarked, "Expert models in competitive sports and games must include accurate *evaluative* information, because successful competitors must make trade-offs involving risks, benefits, and costs" (p. 71). A first step of clinicians involves commitment to using outcome measurement to generate client feedback. Real-time client feedback procedures help to compensate for therapists' limited ability to accurately detect client worsening in psychotherapy. Clients are best served when standardized procedures are used by clinicians to monitor clients' response to psychotherapy and satisfaction with the therapy relationship (Rousmaniere et al., 2017a). Such feedback improves psychotherapy outcomes and assists with identification of client patterns, such as those detailed in Chapter 7. Through identification, therapists can then consider ways of responding effectively to such patterns and reduce the risk of deterioration or dropout.

A critical second step is to recognize that feedback alone does not improve outcomes (Goldberg et al., 2016; Miller, Hubble, Chow, & Seidel, 2013; Tracey et al., 2014). Therapists who receive routine and ongoing feedback from supervisors about individual clients can alter the treatment for those clients, particularly when that feedback relates to specific clinical skills, such as the ability to build a strong therapeutic working alliance (e.g., Hill et al., 2015; Hilsenroth, Kivlighan, & Slavin-Mulford, 2015). However, receiving the feedback does not appear to reliably generalize to other cases or improve the therapists' overall clinical skills (Schuckard et al., 2017).

A second source for obtaining feedback is through coaches and teachers. Without feedback, our attempts to improve are suspect to "confirmation bias," in which we believe what we want to believe. And in some cases, subpar performance is reinforced because there is not enough feedback for a person to accurately reflect on the performance itself (Bertolino, 2014). The Beatles ultimately stopped playing live when they could no longer evolve as a band outside the studio. Onstage sound-monitoring systems were woefully inadequate and the band continued to struggle to hear what they were playing. In most cases the crowd noise surpassed the level of the music. Although the band's performances in live settings had benefits in terms of gaining experience through repetition in a "natural" environment, the Fab Four reached a point when they could not improve further without hearing the nuances of their playing. The studio, on the other hand, provided an opportunity to listen very discreetly, break down each track into smaller segments, reflect on their individual and collective performances, and then work to improve upon them. They also had the likes of George Martin, an expert producer, who provided direct feedback about their efforts. In short, the Beatles had feedback in the studio to improve the quality of their performance.

In psychotherapy, coaches and teachers are most often referred to as supervisors. When it comes to improving clinical performance, the role of the supervisor is to identify the skills that need to be developed and provide suggestions and training experiences specifically designed to enhance the individual's performance (Rousmaniere et al., 2017a). Supervision can be provided by on-site staff or external persons. Hunt (2006) noted that high performers seek out recognized experts to learn from and also have more access to such persons. Whereas connecting with others in the field may have once been very challenging, innovations in technology have made it less so. It's now common to do "live" workshops and supervision in real time, across the world. Research indicates that the idea of learning from peers and experts is highly valued across cultures. In their meta-analysis, Jennings and Skovholt (2016) found that "master therapists" from multiple cultures (i.e., Canada, Czechoslovakia, Japan, Korea, Portugal, Singapore, United States) rated professional development, which included learning from their peers both within and outside of their area of practice, as essential to becoming an effective and proficient clinician.

The idea of interdisciplinary learning experiences appears to be integral in an ever-evolving, diverse world. In his book *The Medici Effect: Breakthrough Insights at the Intersection of Ideas, Concepts, and Cultures*, Frans Johansson (2002) described how varying independent perspectives and disciplines intersect, leading to the resolution of problems—many of which are global. Although individual disciplines and theories within those disciplines maintain their integrity and usefulness as stand-alone approaches (i.e., an approach may provide a good fit for a particular person or situation in which there is a specific, well-defined concern), collectively each viewpoint contributes to an expanded perspective with potentially far greater benefits. Such an idea not only places impetus on the study of disciplines outside of psychology and psychotherapy, it represents a response to an ever-changing world through a more globalized view of psychotherapy. Marsella (1998) remarked, "Psychology can best respond to the emerging global challenges and opportunities by developing a new psychology that is responsive to our emerging global life contexts, conditions, and consequences–a global community psychology" (p. 1284).

A step toward multidisciplinary learning is for clinicians to gain exposure to a wider array of supervisors, mentors, coaches, and teachers who represent different cultures and experiences and provide opportunities to understand the etiology of distress, healing rituals, and change from very different points of view. It appears that top performers not only expand their awareness through exposure to new cultural experiences, but also take action to connect with experts who can provide guidance.

Engaging in Deliberate Practice (Successive Refinement)

Following the first two steps, determination of a baseline and a process for obtaining feedback, we add a third to complete the COE—*DP* (Ericsson, 2006). Ericsson and Lehmann (1996) defined DP as "individualized training activities especially designed to . . . improve specific aspects of an individual's performance through repetitive and successive refinement" (pp. 278–279). DP is focused, systematic, and carried out over extended periods of time. Areas of focus for

DP are identified through review of one's performance to determine potential shortcomings. In the case of psychotherapy, a therapist's baseline performance provides one possible starting point. Once one or more areas of focus have been identified through evaluation of performance, guidance is sought from experts. Next, the therapist sets time aside to reflect on the feedback provided. Following this, a plan of improvement is developed.

Central to DP is a clear focus on practicing specific skills through repetition. This repetition continues until the skills become part of the therapist's routine. Doing so requires sustained concentration and ongoing, corrective feedback from a mentor or supervisor, the purpose of which is to move the therapist outside of his or her comfort zone, which is where learning occurs. DP also requires what Kahneman (2011) describes as System 2 modes of decision making. Whereas System 1 is intuitive—fast and automatic and affective rather than calculating with "little understanding of logic and statistics" (p. 24)—System 2 is conscious and deliberative. It involves conscious thought and is capable of logical and statistical reasoning. However, System 2 also requires substantial effort and is slow.

Truly, DP is hard work, and not generally experienced as enjoyable or immediately rewarding (Coughlan, Williams, McRobert, & Ford, 2014; Ericsson & Pool, 2016). Strenuous, DP creates conditions in which learners, therapists in this case, are able to "seek out challenges that go beyond their current level of reliable achievement—ideally in a safe and optimal learning context that allows immediate feedback and gradual refinement by repetition" (Ericsson, 2009, p. 425).

Deep Domain-Specific Knowledge

What constitutes DP differs across domains of expertise (i.e., musicians practice different than athletes). All forms, however, include the highly focused, repetitious practice of skills focused on improving the parts of performance that are not yet mastered. Over time, DP results in the acquisition of what researchers refer to as "deep domain-specific" knowledge—mental maps that guide planning, analysis, execution, and monitoring of their performance (Ericsson, 2006). Domain-specific knowledge involves knowing "what" to do, "how" to do it, and "when" to do it. For example, a therapist may learn about a specific technique in a book. Then, he or she learns how to execute the technique in practice. Thirdly, the therapist must determine when to use the technique in actual client situations. The application of knowledge and skills is contextual. By engaging in DP, performers are continuously pushing themselves to expand and refine the three types of knowledge with the goal of achieving a higher level of functioning. Because DP is stressful, its success can be increased through a supportive social context involving networks of people, places, and resources.

Deliberate Practice in Psychotherapy

Although in its infancy, DP has been applied to the field of psychotherapy. In the first study on the impact of DP on the development of therapists, Chow et al.

(2015) examined a series of therapist variables to determine their relationship to outcome (i.e., demographics, work practices, participation in professional development activities, beliefs regarding learning and growth as a therapist, and personal appraisals of therapeutic effectiveness). Consistent with earlier studies, neither age, gender, gender match, qualifications, profession, years of experience, time spent conducting therapy, or clinician self-assessment of effectiveness were related to outcome (Anderson et al., 2009; Blatt, Sanislow, Zuroff, & Pilkonis, 1996; Malouff, 2012; Walfish, McAlister, O'Donnell, & Lambert, 2012; Wampold & Brown, 2005).

The findings from the study of Chow et al. (2015) showed a correlation between the time therapists spent on activities intended to improve their ability and their outcomes. The top performers spent 2.5 to 4.5 more hours reflecting on actions, consulting about cases, reading, attending professional development activities, planning, and engaging in other learning activities than average therapists. Researchers also estimated that "the accumulative time spent by the top quartile (most effective therapists) was, on average, about 2.8 times more hours per week engaged in DP activities aimed at improving effectiveness than the rest of the other therapists" (p. 341). However, Chow et al. were unable to identify any one specific activity that reliably led to an increase in outcomes. Although this was an unexpected finding, it is consistent with previous research (Ericsson et al., 1993), and may reveal the importance of targeting very specific areas of knowledge and skill development for each clinician. One interesting finding, which serves as an impetus for future research, is the most effective therapists indicated requiring more effort in reviewing therapy recordings alone than did the rest of the cohort (Chow et al., 2015). This may be because more cognitive processing is needed in the identification and remediation of errors in performance recordings.

STRATEGIES FOR PRACTICE TO IMPROVE THERAPEUTIC EFFECTIVENESS

Research to date has demonstrated the efficacy of DP activities to improve therapist effectiveness. Top performers are dedicated to improving their performance. They are willing to do the necessary work, with the understanding that doing so is mentally challenging and uncomfortable. And although there are various activities that therapists can engage in to increase their individual effectiveness, research has yet to identify any one activity that unequivocally improves performance across the board.

DP involves two kinds of learning: (a) skill refinement: improving the skills you already have; and (b) skill development—extending the reach and range of your skills. The enormous concentration required to undertake these twin tasks limits the amount of time one can spend doing them. Because DP is taxing, sustainability of motivation is at the forefront in the pursuit of expertise. Therefore, organizational support is both a necessary and effective mechanism of accountability (Goodyear, 2015). This is especially true for licensed clinicians who may be less compelled to continue skill development and challenge themselves instead of engaging in ongoing DP.

Making a Plan for Deliberate Practice

It is interesting to note that across a wide range of experts, including athletes, novelists, and musicians, very few appear to be able to engage in more than a few hours of high concentration and DP at a time. In fact, most expert teachers and scientists set aside only a couple of hours a day, typically in the morning, for their most demanding mental activities, such as writing about new ideas. While this may seem like a relatively small investment, it is 2 hours a day more than most executives and managers devote to building their skills, since the majority of their time is consumed by meetings and day-to-day concerns.

DP has to be planned for and factored into daily activities such as meetings, trainings, and "down time," when full attention can be given to practicing. Mornings are often a good time because we have more energy and fewer distractions. To determine a plan we ask: When is the best time to reflect? When am I best focused and for how long? Define the time and place specifically. Be consistent and persistent about the habit (Ericsson et al., 2006).

We now explore two areas of focus with DP: skill refinement and skill development.

Skill Refinement

As therapists gain experience, a degree of emphasis remains on the preservation of already acquired skills. This point echoes back to a quote in Chapter 4 by K. Anders Ericsson (2006), "The enemy of excellence is proficiency" (p. 683). Automaticity is critical when it comes to everyday activities such as walking and talking. However, moving through the same actions without awareness in therapy can lead to a one-size-fits-all approach and increase the likelihood that nuances in client verbal and nonverbal communication may be missed. A way of countering the potential effects of "ineffective" proficiency is by practicing skills at which the therapist is already competent as separate exercises (Rousmaniere & Goodyear, 2017).

One way to approach skills refinement is to break up various strands of an interaction into pieces, which breaks up automaticity. For example, a therapist may practice the opening moments of a session. Another example would be for a therapist to practice getting into a particular role (i.e., individual therapist, couples therapist, case manager). A further possibility might be to think in terms of a treatment model or framework, including practicing questions and/or techniques associated with that model. Doing so can serve as a form of "warm up" in preparation for sessions. This form of exercise can help to put the therapist in the right frame of mind. When engaging in skill refinement activities, therapists should eliminate any potential disruptions to practice (Rousmaniere & Goodyear, 2017).

Skill Development

A second approach to DP is through the use of skill development exercises. Here the approach is to focus on skills that are just beyond the therapist's current level of proficiency (Goodyear & Rousmaniere, 2017). Because skill development requires the acquisition of new proficiencies, the exercises tend to be longer and in some cases, more detailed. Exercises aimed at skill development stretch therapists just beyond the edge of their ability. Let's consider a few options.

Review Video Recordings

As discussed previously, in a study by Chow et al. (2015), top performers considered the review of video recordings cognitively challenging but important to their growth. Review of live performance is used in different disciplines. Ericsson (2003) described its use with surgeons:

> The methodology of using video recordings and their independent assessment seems to offer a potential loop through which weaknesses and potential problems can be identified. These areas requiring improvement could then be addressed through targeted training focused on the relevant technical skills, the perceptual skills necessary . . . the ability to plan . . . and/or the capacity to detect and deal with unexpected deviations or events. (pp. 8–9)

Video Review Strategies

As a supervisory tool, video can be used to help identify particular sequences that contribute to deviations and perhaps unimprovement or deterioration. Because video can be paused, slowed down, rewound, and so forth, it provides opportunities that live supervision does not. In contrast, moments can be identified that facilitate client improvement.

A specific exercise that can be used with video is to have therapists first watch a section of their work without audio. Be sure to choose short passages of 5 minutes or less. Next, only the audio of the section is played with the screen off or unable to be seen. In each case, the therapist pauses after the chosen sequence to reflect. What was seen or heard without the benefit of the audio or video? What was different about the sequence when viewing it as a recording versus doing the session live? Critical to learning is reflection. An additional way to choreograph the exercise is to have a supervisor follow the same process. The supervisor and therapist then compare their notes.

There are many possibilities for using videos. A further variation is to have therapists view a lengthier segment of video—15 to 20 minutes. After each client response, the therapist writes down his or her response, then compares each written response with what he or she actually did in the live session. For poignancy, it can be more efficient to target specific sequences that appear to contribute to a client who is unimproved or deteriorated.

A further option for using video recordings involves a therapist and supervisor identifying a challenging part of a client–therapist exchange on video. Then, the exchange is role-played until the therapist attains mastery of the skills needed to navigate the particular situation. Repetition is key to this form of learning experience.

A final example in this section is to have therapists review sessions of other experts. With the availability of video recordings for rental, purchase, or through streaming systems, there are many avenues for therapists to review sessions of experts in the field of psychotherapy. Review of videos can be especially useful, but should be done with a task in mind. We ask, "What do I want the therapist to focus on?"

Simulation-Based Learning

Studies involving simulation-based learning with military pilots, surgeons, nurses, and musicians, to name a few, indicate that this method of practice provides value in replicating situations that such persons may encounter in real life. Through preestablished or contrived situations that simulate problems, events, conditions, or opportunities, learners are able to practice their responses and gain valuable feedback about their performance (McGaghie, Issenberg, Barsuk, & Wayne, 2014). Ericsson (2004) described a value of using simulators, "Practice in the simulator can be stopped at any time, allowing trainees an immediate chance to correct mistakes and even repeat challenging parts of procedures" (p. S78).

The results are compelling. For example, studies of military pilots trained in a specific emergency situation were more effective in their response when the same situation occurred during an actual flight mission (Ericsson, 2004). Likewise, surgeons who train in rare emergency procedures when mentally ready are better prepared should those situations arise unexpectedly during actual operations. Similarly, nurses are routinely trained using simulators (i.e., simMan, simBaby) that replicate patient vital signs and symptoms. Musicians, in turn, "spend hundreds of hours mastering challenging pieces in their practice room by working on selected difficult passages" (Ericsson, 2004, p. S78).

In psychotherapy, simulations are typically in the form of role-plays or observations of such. The purpose is to place therapists in situations that replicate client situations. This can be especially useful with specific interactions or sequences that are associated with unimprovement or deterioration. Simulations can also be used to create situations or dilemmas that require therapists to change their engagement style, therapy model, or some other aspect of their approach. For example, a supervisor may select a challenging part of therapy to simulate. The supervisor first demonstrates how to use a specific skill in a role-play. Then, the therapist practices using the same skill until it is mastered (Rousmaniere, 2017). Other therapists and students can also be used in such role-plays to vary the characteristics of the clientele and the dynamics of the interactions.

Facilitative Interpersonal Skills

Anderson et al.'s (2009) study involving the use of FIS provides further opportunities for therapist learning. In their study, therapists were assessed with a performance task that measures therapists' interpersonal skills by rating therapist responses to video simulations of challenging client–therapist interactions. The researchers found that therapists' ability to handle interpersonally challenging encounters with clients accounted for the significant portion of variance between therapists. An example would be to use a scaffolding method in which skills such as eye contact, body posture, voice tone, and so on, are demonstrated, then practiced. Next, a new set of skills is taught that build on the previous set. For example, a supervisor or trainer may demonstrate active listening using reflecting, paraphrasing, and summarizing. The supervisee or trainee would then practice the new set of skills. Each set of skills might first be taught with the supervisor role-playing a client who is responsive and easy to talk with. Once the supervisee has achieved a level of comfort and mastery, the degree of difficulty with the client is increased. Again, as the supervisee acquires skill and confidence, the degree of difficulty is sufficiently increased. The process outlined allows for skills to be learned in more easily digestible pieces that are just beyond the supervisee's level of performance.

Another exercise using the FIS method that can be used in group trainings is for supervisors to formulate scenarios that involve the same presenting problem but a different relational style for each client. To do this, first have therapists form dyads to role-play scenarios. In Group 1, the "client" is told to present with the concern of being depressed and to do so with a passive relational style. For Group 2, the same presenting problem is used but the client is asked to use a confrontational relational style. The same setup is used for as many groups as there are in the exercise. The person role-playing the "therapist" should not be told of the "client's" relational style. If observers are used, they are to note how the "therapist" engages the "client," including verbal and nonverbal communication, and any adjustments made to strengthen the alliance. Feedback is given to the therapist in the roleplay with opportunities to repeat the exercise to master necessary skills. Rotations with role-plays are encouraged to train therapists in a variety of different potentially challenging encounters. For those interested in video recording, role-plays can be recorded and used in supervision to assist with skill building.

Ericsson (2004) described that this form of learning can assist athletes in their responses to unplanned situations, "The rapid reactions of athletes are not due to greater speed in their nerve signals, but depend rather on their ability to better anticipate future situations and events by reactions to advanced cues" (p. S74). Therapists who can learn to make course corrections through simulations will be more prepared to respond should such occasions arise in actual client sessions. Although some therapists may view simulation-type exercises as mechanical or as inauthentic, this usually passes after they engage in simulation activities. Once therapists experience the benefits of "thinking on their feet," learning the nuances of applying domain-specific knowledge—"what" to do, "how" to do it, and "when" to do it—they see its value. Therapists will often report that they were able to expand their repertoires of typical responses and interventions during simulations. This kind of growth occurs as therapists move outside of their comfort zones. Therapists who are able to manage their own anxieties will be better able to respond to actual client situations.

Professional Development in Action: Further Ideas

As the study of therapist growth evolves, more will be learned about effective ways of training therapists. In the meantime, four additional exercises are offered to assist with professional development. Each of these will be discussed next.

Behavioral Rehearsal

A specific way of helping therapists to develop skills is through solitary behavioral rehearsal (Rousmaniere, 2017). Here a therapist first reviews a video with his or her supervisor to identify areas of correction. Later, the therapist practices skills to develop those that correspond to areas identified. For example, a therapist might practice using silence, asking open-ended questions, or refocusing a conversation. As with most forms of practice, it can be helpful to have the therapist write about the experience for a few minutes afterward.

Next, to help therapists to think from different theoretical points of view, therapists can be asked to reflect on a client situation and describe at least three ways to intervene, each from a different theoretical approach (Bertolino, 2010). Given the risk of compartmentalizing clients and problems, doing so can train therapists to challenge their own explanations and orientations. Doing so can be especially helpful with cases that are not progressing adequately.

Visual Rehearsal

Athletes, musicians, and public speakers are routinely taught to do reviews of past performances and run-throughs of future ones before they happen. The same process can be useful to clinicians. Chow et al. (2015) stated, "Mentally running through and reflecting on the past sessions in your mind" and "Mentally running through and reflecting on what to do in future sessions" are behaviors related to DP. This form of mental preparation puts the clinician in a growth mindset.

Attunement

Beutler et al. (2004) found that therapists' emotional well-being and cultural attitudes—which are often sources of emotion—are positively correlated with outcome. In situations where therapists seem to struggle with their personal responses and attunement to client encounters or in which their anxiety levels seem to spike, mindfulness-oriented exercises may be used. To do this, therapists are asked to tune into their internal experiences while observing videos of their sessions, those of colleagues, or experts in the field. We ask therapists to note their thoughts, feelings, body sensations, and so on, to become more mindful of such responses and how they may influence therapeutic interactions, decisions made in sessions, and so on. This exercise can be used to identify with session experiences that are both comfortable (i.e., contribute to therapists feeling more secure and aligned with clients, confidence about their abilities, etc.) and uncomfortable, especially those experiences that may lead to avoidance and/or distraction.

Endurance

An additional area of professional development for therapists relates to endurance. Although some therapy sessions seem to move quickly, others can be much more challenging and taxing. Therapists can develop the endurance to remain attuned to client interaction and on task through practice. To do this, the therapist finds a colleague to role-play with and extends the length of the role-play beyond that of a typical session. For example, a therapist who usually does 50-minute sessions would extend the role-play to 60 minutes. In performing the exercise, the therapist attunes to some aspect of the client interaction such as the client's verbal responses, nonverbal responses, or their own experience. Because it is a role-play, the interaction will feel awkward. In addition, the therapist will struggle to keep focus. This is understandable and can help the therapist to recognize things that can throw him or her off track. This exercise can also be done in isolation, with the therapist pretending to have a conversation with a client. This idea is much the same as preparing to do an hour speech in front of a large audience, with minimal or no notes as a guide. This form of activity can also assist therapists with developing procedural memory or "flow," which occurs when a person is very focused on a task that can be pursued without interruption for the purposes of growth (Csikszentmihályi, 1990).

DELIBERATE PRACTICE IN CONTEXT

As discussed, DP involves hard work. It is not as intrinsically enjoyable as the practice of psychotherapy. Even the most committed psychotherapists will need support and encouragement to sustain it. There is also the issue of time. Therapists have clients to see, documentation, meetings, and the infamous job descriptor, "other duties as assigned." The reality is that psychotherapy practice is not something that most organizations account for, whereas professional athletes, for example, are expected to practice through drills, simulations, video review, and so on. The benefits of such efforts are well documented in terms of responses to situations, efficiency, and, most importantly, effectiveness. For example, Railton (2016b) stated:

Elite athletes appear to differ from merely excellent athletes not in the speed of their reflexes, ability to jump, or degree of training of basic motor patterns. The crucial difference appears to be that they possess more detailed and accurate models of complex movements and competitive situations, which allow them to get the drop on their rivals (e.g., placing a tennis shot where it can't be returned, identifying a fast-emerging scoring opportunity before the opponent can spot and close it) and to achieve more efficiency and effectiveness in exploiting the body's resources (just how to take off and twist in a high jump). (p. 71)

Finding time to practice can be difficult. Tony Rousmaniere (2017) has suggested that therapists map the logistics of their DP. Areas of focus include location, scheduling (i.e., days and times of day), timing (i.e., when you are most mentally alert and able to engage in activities), and duration of DP activities. A further suggestion is to keep a DP journal (Chow et al., 2015; Ericsson et al., 1993). Rousmaniere (2017) recommends the following areas of focus for journaling (or notes):

- My response to practice (e.g., did it feel helpful or not?).
- My energy level during practice.
- Any issues in my personal life that may have affected practice.
- Emotional responses or experiential avoidance. (p. 123)

Throughout this book, the focus has been largely on the identification of clients who are unimproved, deteriorating, or improved and perhaps plateauing. A good starting point for DP is to devote 1 hour per week focusing on cases that are unimproved or at risk of deterioration. This process can be made easier when outcomes data are stored in an electronic OMS or sophisticated spreadsheet that can be easily sorted for client severity. Another consideration is to compare groups of inactive clients. For example, a therapist might compare client cases from January to June with July to December. In this way, statistical enumerations such as those discussed earlier can be used to determine therapist improvement over time. In turn, this can influence future directions with DP.

A final yet extremely important point with DP is downtime. Intensive learning is strenuous. It is cognitively taxing and draining. While expert performance does require ritualized planning and commitment, squeezing in a little extra work or lengthening the time invested in performance improvement does not itself provide a payoff when compared to the benefits of downtime. Rest aids with developing insights, recovery, and rejuvenation.

Although difficult, available evidence indicates that deliberate practice is essential to improving therapist outcomes. In a study of over 150 clinicians and 550 clients in an agency setting, Goldberg et al. (2016) found that therapists improved year after year over the course of 7 years. At the core of therapist improvement was a climate in which deliberate practice was valued and incorporated as part of standard operating procedures. Similar results in therapist performance have also been found at my agency, Youth In Need, Inc. (Bertolino, 2017).

FUTURE-FORWARD: SUPERVISION REVISITED

As we know, supervision is widely considered an essential component of successful therapy outcomes (Bernard & Goodyear, 2014); however, evidence concerning its impact on improving client outcomes is mixed at best (Bernard & Goodyear, 2014, Beutler & Howard, 2003; Ladany, 2007; Ladany & Inman, 2012; Rousmaniere, Swift, Babins-Wagner, Whipple, & Berzins, 2014). Watkins (2011) minced no words in his remarks, "We do not seem to be any more able now, as opposed to 30 years ago, to say that supervision leads to better outcomes for clients" (p. 252). Recall that Rousmaniere and colleagues' study of 6,521 clients of 175 trainee therapists supervised by 23 supervisors found that supervision accounted for only .01% of the variance in outcome (Rousmaniere et al., 2014).

Our task may appear monumental but it is not unachievable. Supervision remains a standard in psychotherapy and it is imperative that we explore ways of improving its effectiveness. Throughout this chapter, various ideas have been presented for improving outcomes, some of which relate directly to supervision and training. The purpose of this closing discussion is to continue moving the conversation forward to elevate the usefulness of supervision.

Let's first be mindful that supervisors, similar to therapists, juggle numerous responsibilities and are typically in a position of being evaluated. And even though teaching and evaluation involve different responsibilities for the supervisor, they also share a common thread. Supervisors want their supervisees to have better outcomes and endeavor to help them to improve. By virtue of collecting and monitoring outcome data, therapists (supervisees) are helping their supervisors by pointing to specific areas of growth, as opposed to sitting together and coming up with random professional development goals. Said differently, the roles of supervisors and supervisees may be different but the mission should be the same. Our aim is not to have an office full of supershrinks, which is not statistically possible, but to instead have an office full of persons committed to improving their craft to the benefit of those served by pushing themselves, every day, to improve from their baseline rates of performance.

Purpose of ROM in Supervision

Therefore, for learning to take place, what must be established from the outset is how ROM will be used in supervision. Its purposes are to monitor the benefit of services to clients and serve as a mechanism for improvement of therapist performance. To be clear, utilization rates, hours worked, timely completion of documentation, and the like are examples of actions and responsibilities most therapists understand as part of the job and evaluation of their performance. These tasks have to be identified as responsibilities and separate from therapist outcomes. Organizational cultures that use ROM—for example, as an evaluative tool for personnel—are inevitably contributing to a culture of fear. It is my strong opinion that client outcome data should not be used as a punitive measure to determine whether a therapist should be reprimanded, fired, and so on. Without such an understanding, it is unreasonable that therapists will feel safe, secure, and supported in their efforts to improve their performance.

Clinical supervision has remained largely unchanged for decades. At the same time, there is sufficient evidence that supervision and training can be helpfuin developing basic therapy skills (Hilsenroth et al., 2015; Reese, et al., 2009; Wampold & Imel, 2015). Some of the exercises outlined earlier are designed to help students and newer therapists, in particular, with basic skills. Supervision also provides opportunities to be more data driven in therapy. We are able to bring clients' experiences of therapy into supervision in the form of direct feedback about both the benefit of therapy and satisfaction with the alliance.

Supervisee (Therapist) Performance and Supervision

Goodyear and Rousmaniere (2017) suggest the following three areas for supervisors in terms of determining where to direct attention regarding their supervisees' performance.

Observation of Therapist's Performance

Supervision involves supervisees sharing their descriptions of clients, situations, and other details they find relevant. The inevitability of such a process is that supervisees' accounts will be represented with limitations associated with memory, language, culture, and other influences. In their book, *The Structure of Magic*, Bandler and Grinder (1975) described how people often delete (omit), distort (modify descriptions), or generalize (make general conclusions about) parts of an experience that they remember. To illustrate, if you were asked to sit in a room for 10 minutes, then step outside the room and describe what you saw to another person, you would provide a limited description. You might leave out the fact that there were six tables and only recall having seen four (deletion). You might also remember the walls as white when they were beige (distortion). And you might describe the chairs as all being covered with fabric when 12 of the 20 were fabric and the other eight were fiberglass (generalization). The consequence of deletions, distortions, and generalizations in supervision is that supervisees will describe situations as they experience them, but in effect, may be leaving out key aspects. To create more alignment between supervisees' descriptions and supervisors' interpretations and to neutralize possible artifacts of the supervision process as a whole (time limitations, need to discuss other issues related to performance, supervisees' apprehension about disclosure, etc.), routine observation is recommended.

Outcome Information Obtained From Clients

Gathering information about client progress, especially with clients who are unimproved or at risk of deterioration, is essential to professional development. Simply using ROM provides instantaneous feedback to review and keeps track of client progress.

Information Obtained From Simulations

As discussed earlier, simulations provide a means of evaluating supervisees' processes and practices, which is necessary to determine targets for performance improvement.

With information about supervisee's performance, supervisors and supervisees can collaborate to determine what will indicate the desired performance. In most cases there will be multiple indicators tied to performance improvement. For example, an indicator may be for a therapist to improve on the number of clients who discharge either above the clinical cutoff or in the clinically significant range, or to reduce the number of premature terminations (dropouts) (Callahan et al., 2009). Other indicators of performance improvement are likely to be more qualitative and related to how therapists handle challenging client encounters, the quality of alliances with clients, or perhaps refinement of a current skill, or development of a new one. In such cases, this form of indicator is usually tied to the supervisee's results. As we have learned, a therapist must have first established a baseline rate of effectiveness and compared that baseline to available standards or benchmarks. Standards serve as the basis for the feedback that supervisors and consultants will deliver. Some performance goals inevitably will be informed by the supervisor's own subjective interpretations and theoretical model(s) that form the mental maps from which they work. Although subjectivity cannot be completely removed nor should it be, goals that are more specific to the particular supervisee are to be identified.

The Quality, Timing, and Usefulness of Supervisor Feedback

Standards and benchmarks provide specific targets for improvement, but without quality feedback many therapists are left to learn without proper guidance or in isolation. As such, supervisors provide feedback that is constructive, timely, incremental, and perhaps most importantly, useful (Goodyear & Rousmaniere, 2017). Quality feedback begins with therapist (supervisee) performance data and preparedness on the part of the supervisor. It is the task of the supervisor to be ready and able to provide feedback that is specific and performance related. Lack of preparation on the part of the supervisor can be deflating to the supervisee and, in many cases, a poor use of time.

An example of supervisor preparation is to sort the supervisees' caseloads according to unimprovement and/or deterioration as well as those whose scores have plateaued. Figures 8.1 and 8.2, from earlier in this chapter, provide examples of the first two categories. Figure 8.4 is an example of how plateauing scores can

Clients

Client Name	Client ID	DOB	First Session Date	Program	Recent Session	Outcome Rating	Session Rating	Risk Rating	Target
	23707		8/21/2014		8/6/2015	ORS: 40	40	9	29.25
	24617		8/27/2014		11/19/2014	ORS: 40	40	9	28.5
	21894		9/2/2014		12/15/2014	ORS: 40	40	8	29.25
	25756		9/2/2014		12/15/2014	ORS: 40	40	8	29.25
	26406		9/3/2014		11/5/2014	ORS: 40	33.7	7	29.29
	23152		9/8/2014		12/15/2014	ORS: 40	39	9	29.07
	23066		9/8/2014		12/8/2014	ORS: 40	39.7	9	29.25
	26628		9/18/2014		1/14/2015	ORS: 40	39.9	6	29.2
	26705		9/25/2014		11/18/2014	ORS: 40	40	7	29.22
	23753		8/11/2015		8/11/2015	ORS: 40	40	6	29.25

FIGURE 8.4 Clients who have plateaued with outcome scores.

be sorted in an electronic OMS. Sorting of client scores allows for supervisors to delve deeper into the client record to review graph results, alliance measures, subscores, case notes, and other details that provide context to the specific client situation. Additionally, supervisors can prepare by formulating questions for their supervisees about specific clients.

Time constraints and client caseloads can require both supervisors and supervisees to bring more focus to supervisory conversations from the outset. In most cases, 1 hour of supervision per week is insufficient to adequately discuss more than a few clients in each meeting. This puts the impetus on the process of selecting which clients to review. For this reason, in most instances beginning with clients who fall into the unimproved or deteriorated categories will be a good starting place.

Another possibility is to employ structure to client discussions. For example, at Youth In Need, Inc., there is a 5-minute supervision model, which includes discussion of ORS scores, therapist risk ratings (to identify areas that may indicate risk of harm to self or others and act as hurdles to achieving their preferred futures), and a plan of action (Bertolino, 2017). In each conversation, the client's voice (ORS score) is combined with the therapist's assessment of risk (risk rating; 1–3 = high risk; 4–7 = moderate risk; 8–10 = low risk) and the plan the therapist and client(s) have created. Graphs such as the examples posted in previous chapters are used to identify client patterns of response and any particular issues that may be influencing client progress. Although there are exceptions—for example, with issues related to safety—as a rule, longer discussions about clients do not typically translate to better ideas and better outcomes. Time limits help to keep conversations moving and focused to ensure that as many clients are discussed as needed during a particular supervision session. The same structure is used in client staffings and follows the 80/20 rule described earlier in the book (see Juran & De Feo, 2010).

The issue of what constitutes quality supervisory feedback is certainly worthy of debate. In this case, quality feedback is considered "actionable" and tied to performance improvement (Larson, Patel, Evans, & Saiman, 2013). Hattie and Timperley (2007) describe quality feedback as intended "to reduce discrepancies between current understandings and performance and a goal . . . [and which] must answer three major questions. . . . Where am I going? (What are the goals?), How am I going? (What progress is being made toward the goal?), and Where to next?" (p. 86). Through quality feedback, supervisors can reduce the likelihood of therapists overestimating their levels of performance (Walfish et al., 2012) by targeting specific aspects of a client's situation or actions of a therapist in need of refinement or development.

One of the factors related to usefulness of feedback is timelines. Ideally, supervisees have opportunities to get feedback outside of supervision sessions. Technology advances make it possible for client data to be reviewed quickly and for conversations to occur when needed. However, not all systems are set up to operate in this way. In such cases, a starting point is to address current processes and make revisions needed to meet the needs of service providers and clientele. When possible, supervisors and supervisees should coordinate systems in which client data are readily accessible and the degree of feedback occurs both at the level of number of clients served and on the basis of progress. In other words, larger caseloads require greater oversight. Having such a system does not mean that supervisors must always be available in a moment's notice. Instead, when therapists have access to their data, they are able to self-monitor in between supervision sessions and staffings and contact their supervisors for additional support as needed. A parallel process is that supervisors can do periodic scans of data to potential problems, particularly with clients at risk of dropout and negative outcome. The timeliness of feedback increases when both therapists and their supervisors engage in a mutually agreed-upon process of oversight with an eye on client progress.

An additional consideration in terms of the usefulness of supervision is the degree to which it is specific and descriptive or "actionable," as stated earlier. Feedback that is too general, global, and vague is typically of little use to the supervisee. The greater the ambiguity, the greater the likelihood of misunderstanding. To reduce incidences of confusion or misunderstandings, supervisors can ask supervisees to summarize what occurs in supervision sessions and state how the feedback impacts his or her work. A supervision alliance index such as the Leeds Alliance Supervision Scale (LASS) can also be used to facilitate feedback between the therapist and the supervisor. The LASS, which can be found in the Appendix, is a parallel to the SRS.

Maximizing the Effects of Feedback

The utility of feedback is contingent on the interplay of multiple factors. First, as supervisors, we concentrate on providing simple and precise feedback. When it comes to early learners, the simpler the better. Too much feedback, too continuously can create cognitive overload, increase anxiety, and interfere with learning. As expertise develops, the feedback should also evolve, meaning that persons providing feedback need to have evolved with their own expertise. For advanced learners, feedback that is too fundamental can actually inhibit development. Ideally, therapists will, over time, develop their own cognitive maps that enable self-monitoring of their performance. The ability to discriminate what constitutes a good or expected response is a prerequisite to being able to demonstrate that response.

Next, supervisors have the responsibility to maintain a sense of self-awareness. A good practice is to do a self-check to ensure their comfort level with giving feedback. Check-ins can also help with identification of potential hurdles to giving feedback and the growth of supervisors. An example of a hurdle is the cultural differences between supervisors and supervisees that can contribute to difficulties in providing feedback (Burkard, Knox, Clarke, Phelps, & Inman, 2014; Constantine & Sue, 2007). Although there are consequences to not getting feedback, poor quality feedback can also prove detrimental. Each presents a threat to client improvement and to the development of expertise.

Perhaps the most poignant question when it comes to supervision is also a very simple one: What will you do differently as a result of our supervision? If the supervisee does not have an answer to this question, there is more work to be done. Like therapy, supervision is intended to be remedial. When it is not, a reexamination of the supervision process is necessary.

THE PATH TO EXCELLENCE

The path to clinical excellence is both difficult and rewarding. To get better at anything takes a grinding determination for betterment. Some people simply don't care enough to face the difficulty—this is true in all professions and walks of life. Repetition is dull. It is why so few people become true experts. The good news is that our end goal is not expertise. As we learned in Chapter 1 from surgeon Atul Gawande, our aim is to push beyond average. Jennings and Skovholt (2016) suggest that long-term therapist development is multidimensional, and is akin to a three-legged stool comprised of learning from clients, research, and personal life. These three elements combined form a path toward growth and expertise. And as it turns out, maintaining a sense of professional growth and resiliency serves as a buffer to burnout and stagnation (Orlinsky & Rønnestad, 2013, 2015).

Through my experience as a therapist, supervisor, teacher, and trainer, I have had the good fortune of meeting many who are considered experts both within and outside of psychotherapy. One such expert is a friend and colleague, Colorado psychologist Jason Seidel. Jason offers practical tips for clinicians devoted to performance improvement:

1. Feedback is there for the asking, but not always freely given.
2. At first, feedback can be surprising and intimidating.

3. It's about humility, not humiliation.
4. Not everyone will buy the quality of what you are selling.
5. Actions speak louder than words when you respond to feedback.
6. A focus on service quality keeps "client experience" front and center.
7. Reaching for clinical excellence is both unnecessary and insufficient for financial success and a great reputation.
8. Save your breath, but be a helpful resource.
9. Go wrong or go home.
10. If you collect no evidence, you are basking in reflective glory, not doing "evidence-based practice."
11. Seek out smart and insightful but highly-divergent colleagues.
12. We sink or we swim together.
13. Use extreme caution before considering or even talking about a pay-for-performance plan.
14. Make outcome tracking an easy, automatic, and expected part of daily work.
15. Reduce sources of friction with clear communication.
16. Act like a guinea pig. (Seidel, 2017)

Experts, by and large, are not simply great at what they do; they are devoted to what they do and accepting of failure. The amazing people I have met also do not apply the label of expert to themselves. They are a humble bunch. They are confident but modest. What I have experienced from these friends, colleagues, and mentors is an insatiable curiosity, high motivation, humility and some degree of professional self-doubt, and strong work ethic. And there is one last quality among all—a willingness to connect with others and share knowledge. Each in his or her own way is committed to doing the best for others.

So, while it is up to each of us to make a pledge to improve our performance, we also have the ability to band together, en masse, to improve the outcomes of psychotherapy. We can create what researcher Etienne Wenger deemed, "communities of practice," which are, "Groups of people who share a concern or a passion for something they do, and who interact regularly to learn how to do it better" (Bertolino, 2011, p. 35). Communities of practice have a common interest, work together, and share information and resources. More than a group of friends or network of personal connections, a community of practice represents a "domain of interest"—a profession, a hobby, a field of expertise, an art or craft, even a common concern. Wenger (cited in Bertolino, 2011) writes that such communities:

> Engage in a process of collective learning in a shared domain of human endeavor: a tribe learning to survive, a band of artists seeking new forms of expression,

a group of engineers working on similar problems, a clique of pupils defining their identity in the school. (pp. 35–36)

We heed the call for more concerted efforts to improve the effectiveness of psychotherapy as individuals and as a field, not by invention of more methods and models, but through devotion to improving the benefit of psychotherapy as lifelong learners.

REFERENCES

ACORN, A Collaborative Outcomes Resource Network. (2013). *Measurement + feedback = improve outcomes*. Retrieved from http://www.psychoutcomes.org

Anderson, T., Ogles, B. M., Patterson, C. L., Lambert, M. J., & Vermeersch, D. A. (2009). Therapist effects: Facilitative interpersonal skills as a predictor of therapist effects. *Journal of Clinical Psychology, 65*(7), 755–768. doi:10.1002/jclp.20583

Bandler, R., & Grinder, J. (1975). *The structure of magic: A book about language and therapy*. Palo Alto, CA: Science and Behavior Books.

Basler, R. (Ed.). (1953). *Collected works of Abraham Lincoln* (8 vols.). New Brunswick, NJ: Rutgers University Press.

Bernard, J. M., & Goodyear, R. K. (2014). *Fundamentals of clinical supervision* (5th ed.). Boston, MA: Allyn & Bacon.

Bertolino, B. (2010). *Strengths-based engagement and practice: Creating effective helping relationships*. Boston, MA: Allyn & Bacon.

Bertolino, B. (2011). Building a culture of excellence: Anatomy of a community agency that works. *Psychotherapy Networker, 35*(3), 32–39.

Bertolino, B. (2014). *Thriving on the front lines: Strengths-based youth care work*. New York, NY: Routledge.

Bertolino, B. (2017). Feedback-informed treatment in an agency serving children, youth, and families. In D. S. Prescott, C. L. Maeschalck, & S. D. Miller (Eds.), *Feedback-informed treatment in clinical practice: Reaching for excellence* (pp. 187–209). Washington, DC: American Psychological Association.

Bertolino, B., Axsen, R., Maeschalck, C., Miller, S. D., & Babbins-Wagner, R. (2012). Manual 6: Implementing feedback-informed work in agencies and systems of care. In B. Bertolino & S. D. Miller (Eds.), *The ICCE manuals of feedback informed treatment*. Chicago, IL: International Center for Clinical Excellence.

Beutler, L. E., & Howard, M. (2003). Training in psychotherapy: Why supervision does not work. *Clinical Psychologist, 56*, 12–16.

Beutler, L. E., Malik, M., Alimohamed, S., Harwood, T. M., Talebi, H., Noble, S., & Wong, E. (2004). Therapist variables. In M. J. Lambert, A. E. Bergin, & S. Garfield (Eds.), *Handbook of psychotherapy and behavior change* (pp. 227–306). Hoboken, NJ: Wiley.

Blatt, S. J., Sanislow, C. A., Zuroff, D. C., & Pilkonis, P. A. (1996). Characteristics of effective therapists: Further analyses of data from the National Institute of Mental Health treatment of depression collaborative research program. *Journal of Counseling and Clinical Psychology, 64*, 1276–1284.

Burkard, A. W., Knox, S., Clarke, R. D., Phelps, D. L., & Inman, A. G. (2014). Supervisors' experiences of providing difficult feedback in cross-ethnic/racial supervision. *The Counseling Psychologist, 42*(3), 314–344. doi:10.1177/0011000012461157

Callahan, J. L., Aubuchon-Endsley, N., Borja, S. E., & Swift, J. K. (2009). Pretreatment expectancies and premature termination in a training clinic environment. *Training and Education in Professional Psychology, 3*(2), 111–119. doi:10.1037/a0012901

Campbell, J., & Moyers, B. (1988). *The power of myth*. New York, NY: Doubleday.

Chow, D. L. (2017). The practice and the practical: Pushing your clinical performance to the next level. In D. S. Prescott, C. L. Maeschalck, & S. D. Miller (Eds.), *Feedback-informed treatment in clinical practice: Reaching for excellence* (pp. 323–355). Washington, DC: American Psychological Association.

Chow, D. L., Miller, S. D., Seidel, J. A., Kane, R. T., Thornton, J. A., & Andrews, W. P. (2015). The role of deliberate practice in the development of highly effective psychotherapists. *Psychotherapy, 52*(3), 337–345. doi:10.1037/pst0000015

Colvin, G. (2008). *Talent is overrated: What really separates world-class performers from everybody else.* New York, NY: Portfolio.

Constantine, M. G., & Sue, D. W. (2007). Perceptions of racial microaggressions among Black supervisees in cross-racial dyads. *Journal of Counseling Psychology, 54*(2), 142–153. doi:10.1037/0022-0167.54.2.142

Coughlan, E. K., Williams, A. M., McRobert, A. P., & Ford, P. R. (2014). How experts practice: A novel test of deliberate practice theory. *Journal of Experimental Psychology, Learning, Memory, and Cognition, 40*(2), 449–458. doi:10.1037/a0034302

Csikszentmihályi, M. (1990). *Flow: The psychology of optimal experience.* New York, NY: Harper & Row.

Duckworth, A. L., Peterson, C., Matthews, M. D., & Kelly, D. R. (2007). Grit: Perseverance and passion for long-term goals. *Journal of Personality and Social Psychology, 92*(6), 1087–1101. doi:10.1037/0022-3514.92.6.1087

Ericsson, K. A. (2003). Development of elite performance and deliberate practice: An update from the perspective of the expert performance approach. In J. L. Starks & K. A. Ericsson (Eds.), *Expert performance in sports: Advances in research on sports expertise.* New York, NY: Human Kinetics.

Ericsson, K. A. (2004). Deliberate practice and the acquisition and maintenance of expert performance in medicine and related domains. *Academic Medicine, 79*, S70–S81. doi:10.1097/00001888-200410001-00022

Ericsson, K. A. (2006). The influence of experience and deliberate practice on the development of superior expert performance. In K. A. Ericsson, N. Charness, P. J. Feltovich, & R. R. Hoffman (Eds.), *The Cambridge handbook of expertise and expert performance* (pp. 683–703). Cambridge, UK: Cambridge University Press.

Ericsson, K. A. (Ed.). (2009). *Development of professional expertise: Toward measurement of expert performance and design of optimal learning environments.* New York, NY: Cambridge University Press.

Ericsson, K. A., Charness, N., Feltovich, P. J., & Hoffman, R. R. (Eds.). (2006). *The Cambridge handbook of expertise and expert performance.* New York, NY: Cambridge University Press.

Ericsson, K. A., Krampe, R. T., & Tesch-Romer, C. (1993). The role of deliberate practice in the acquisition of expert performance. *Psychological Review, 100*, 363–406. doi:10.1037/0033-295X.100.3.363

Ericsson, K. A., & Lehmann, A. C. (1996). Expert and exceptional performance: Evidence of maximal adaptation to task constraints. *Annual Review of Psychology, 47*, 273–305. doi:10.1146/annurev.psych.47.1.273

Ericsson, K. A., & Pool, R. (2016). *Peak: Secrets from the new science of expertise.* Boston, MA: Houghton Mifflin Harcourt.

Gladwell, M. (2008). *Outliers: The story of success.* New York, NY: Little, Brown.

Goldberg, S. B., Rousmaniere, T., Hoyt, W. T., Miller, S. D., Babibs-Wagner, R., Berzins, S., Whipple, J. L., & Wampold B. E. (2016). Creating a climate for therapist improvement: A case study of an agency focused on outcomes and deliberate practice. *Psychotherapy, 53*(3), 367–375.

Goldberg, S. B., Rousmaniere, T., Miller, S. D., Whipple, J., Nielsen, S. R., Hoyt, W. T., & Wampold, B. E. (2016). Do psychotherapists improve with time and experience? A longitudinal analysis of outcomes in a clinical setting. *Journal of Counseling Psychology, 63*(1), 1–11. doi:10.1037/cou0000131

Goldman, R., & Papson, S. (1999). *Nike culture: The sign of the swoosh.* Thousand Oaks, CA Sage.

Goodyear, R. (2015). Using accountability mechanisms more intentionally: A framework and its implications for training professional psychologists. *American Psychologist, 70*(8), 736–743. doi:10.1037/a0039828

Goodyear, R., & Rousmaniere, T. (2017). Helping therapists each day become a little more than they were the day before: The expertise-development model of supervision and consultation. In T. Rousmaniere, R. K. Goodyear, S. D. Miller, & B. E. Wampold (Eds.), *The cycle of excellence: Using deliberate practice to improve supervision and training* (pp. 67–95). Washington, DC: American Psychological Association.

Hattie, J., & Timperley, H. (2007). The power of feedback. *Review of Educational Research, 77*(1), 81–112.

Hill, C. E., Baumann, E., Shafran, N., Gupta, S., Morrison, A., Rojas, A. E. P., . . . Gelso, C. J. (2015). Is training effective? A study of counseling psychology doctoral trainees in a psychodynamic/interpersonal training clinic. *Journal of Counseling Psychology, 62*, 184–201. doi:10.1037/cou0000053

Hilsenroth, M. J., Kivlighan, D. J., & Slavin-Mulford, J. (2015). Structured supervision of graduate clinicians in psychodynamic psychotherapy: Alliance and technique. *Journal of Counseling Psychology, 62*, 173–183. doi:10.1037/cou0000058

Howe, M. J. A. (1999). *Genius explained.* New York, NY: Cambridge University Press.

Hunt, E. (2006). Expertise, talent, and social encouragement. In K. A. Ericsson, N. Charness, P. J. Feltovich, & R. R Hoffman (Eds.), *The Cambridge handbook of expertise and expert performance* (pp. 31–38). Cambridge, UK: Cambridge University Press.

Jennings, L., & Skovholt, T. M. (Eds.). (2016). *Expertise in counseling and psychotherapy: Master therapist studies around the world.* New York, NY: Oxford University Press.

Johansson, F. (2002). *The Medici effect: Breakthrough insights at the intersection of ideas, concepts, and cultures*. Boston, MA: Harvard Business School Press.

Juran, J. M., & De Feo, J. A. (2010). *Juran's quality control handbook: The complete guide to performance excellence* (6th ed.). New York, NY: McGraw-Hill.

Kahneman, D. (2011). *Thinking, fast and slow*. New York, NY: Farrar, Straus and Giroux.

Kanigel, R. (1991). *The man who knew infinity: A life of the genius Ramanujan*. New York, NY: Scribner.

Ladany, N. (2007). Does psychotherapy training matter? Maybe not. *Psychotherapy: Theory, Research, Practice, Training, 44*(4), 392–396. http://dx.doi.org/10.1037/0033-3204.44.4.392

Ladany, N., & Inman, A. G. (2012). Training and supervision. In E. M. Altmeier & J. I. Hanson (Eds.), *Oxford handbook of counseling psychology* (pp. 179–207). New York, NY: Oxford University Press.

Lambert, M. J. (2010). *Prevention of treatment failure: The use of measuring, monitoring, and feedback in clinical practice*. Washington, DC: American Psychological Association.

Larson, E. L., Patel, S. J., Evans, D., & Saiman, L. (2013). Feedback as a strategy to change behaviour: The devil is in the details. *Journal of Evaluation in Clinical Practice, 19*(2), 230–234. doi:10.1111/j.1365-2753.2011.01801.x

Malouff, J. (2012). The need for empirically supported psychology training standards. *Psychotherapy in Australia, 18*(3), 28–32.

Marsella, A. (1998). Toward a "global-community psychology": Meeting the needs of a changing world. *American Psychologist, 53*(12), 1282–1291. doi:10.1037/0003-066X.53.12.1282

Martin, D. J., Garske, J. P., & Davis, M. K. (2000). Relationship of the therapeutic alliance with outcome and other variables: A meta-analytic review. *Journal of Consulting and Clinical Psychology, 68*(3), 438–450. doi:10.1037/0022-006X.68.3.438

McGaghie, W. C., Issenberg, S. B., Barsuk, J. H., & Wayne, D. B. (2014). A critical review of simulation-based mastery learning with translational outcomes. *Medical Education, 48*(4), 375–385. doi:10.1111/medu.12391

Miller, S. D., Hubble, M. A., Chow, D. L., Seidel, J. A. (2013). The outcome of psychotherapy: Yesterday, today, and tomorrow. *Psychotherapy, 50*(1), 88–97. doi: 10.1037/a0031097

Miller, S. D., Hubble, M. A., & Duncan, B. L. (2007). Supershrinks: What's the secret of their success? *Psychotherapy Networker, 31*, 27–35, 56–57.

Miller, S. D., Duncan, B. L., Sorrell, R., & Brown, G. S. (2005). The partners for change outcome management system. *Journal of Clinical Psychology, 61*(2), 199–208. doi:10.1002/jclp.20111

Moss, R. K., & Mousavikizadeh, V. (2017). Implementing feedback-informed treatment: Challenges and solutions. In D. S. Prescott, C. L. Maeschalck, & S. D. Miller (Eds.), *Feedback-informed treatment in clinical practice: Reaching for excellence* (pp. 101–121). Washington, DC: American Psychological Association.

Norcross, J. C. (Ed.). (2011). *Psychotherapy relationships that work: Evidence-based responsiveness* (2nd ed.). New York, NY: Oxford University Press.

O'Hanlon, W. H., & Hexum, A. L. (1990). *An uncommon casebook: The complete clinical work of Milton H. Erickson, M.D*. New York, NY: W. W. Norton.

Orlinsky, D. E., & Rønnestad, M. H. (2005). *How psychotherapists develop: A study of therapeutic work and professional growth*. Washington, DC: American Psychological Association.

Orlinsky, D. E., & Rønnestad, M. H. (2013). Positive and negative cycles of practitioner development: Evidence, concepts, and implications from a collaborative quantitative study of psychotherapists. In M. H. Rønnestad & T. M. Skovholt (Eds.), *The developing practitioner: Growth and stagnation of therapists and counselors* (pp. 265–290). New York, NY: Routledge.

Orlinsky, D. E., & Rønnestad, M. H. (2015). Psychotherapists growing older: A study of senior practitioners. *Journal of Clinical Psychology, 71*(11), 1128–1138. doi:10.1002/jclp.22223

Owen, J., Wampold, B. E., Rousmaniere, T. G., Kopta, M., & Miller, S. (2016). As good as it gets? Therapy outcomes of trainees over time. *Journal of Counseling Psychology, 63*, 12–19. doi:10.1037/cou0000112

Prescott, D. S., Maeschalck, C. L., & Miller, S. D. (Eds.). (2017). *Feedback-informed treatment in clinical practice: Reaching for excellence*. Washington, DC: American Psychological Association.

Railton, P. (2016a). Introduction. In M. E. P. Seligman, P. Railton, R. F. Baumeister, & C. Sripada (Eds.), *Homo prospectus* (pp. 1–31). New York, NY: Oxford University Press.

Railton, P. (2016b). Intuitive guidance: Emotion, information, and experience. In M. E. P Seligman, P. Railton, R. F. Baumeister, & C. Sripada (Eds.), *Homo prospectus* (pp. 33–85). New York, NY: Oxford University Press.

Reese, R. J., Usher, E. L., Bowman, D. C., Norsworthy, L. A., Halstead, J. L., Rowlands, S. R., & Chisholm, R. R. (2009). Using client feedback in psychotherapy training: An analysis of its influence on supervision and counselor self-efficacy. *Training and Education in Professional Psychology, 3*, 157–168. doi:10.1037/a0015673

Rønnestad, M. H., & Orlinsky, D. E. (2005). Therapeutic work and professional development: Main findings and practical implications of a long-term international study. *Psychotherapy Bulletin, 40*, 27–32.

Rousmaniere, T. (2017). *Deliberate practice for psychotherapists: A guide to improving clinical effectiveness.* New York, NY: Routledge.

Rousmaniere, T., Goodyear, R. K., Miller, S. D., & Wampold, B. E. (2017a). Introduction. In T. Rousmaniere, R. K. Goodyear, S. D. Miller, & B. E. Wampold (Eds.), *The cycle of excellence: Using deliberate practice to improve supervision and training* (pp. 3–22). Washington, DC: American Psychological Association.

Rousmaniere, T., Goodyear, R. K., Miller, S. D., & Wampold, B. E. (Eds.). (2017b). *The cycle of excellence: Using deliberate practice to improve supervision and training.* Washington, DC: American Psychological Association.

Rousmaniere, T., Swift, J. K., Babins-Wagner, R., Whipple, J. L., & Berzins, S. (2014). Supervisor variance in psychotherapy outcome in routine practice. *Psychotherapy Research, 26*(2), 196–205. doi:10.1080/10503307.2014.963730

Schuckard, E., Miller, S. D., & Hubble, M. A. (2017). Feedback-informed treatment: Historical and empirical foundations. In D. S. Prescott, C. L. Maeschalck, & S. D. Miller (Eds.), *Feedback-informed treatment in clinical practice: Reaching for excellence* (pp. 13–35). Washington, DC: American Psychological Association.

Seidel, J. A. (2017). Feedback-informed treatment in a private practice setting. Personal advice and professional experience. In D. S. Prescott, C. L. Maeschalck, & S. D. Miller (Eds.), *Feedback-informed treatment in clinical practice: Reaching for excellence* (pp. 125–140). Washington, DC: American Psychological Association.

Seidel, J. A., Miller, S. D., & Chow, D. L. (2013). Effect size calculations for the clinician: Methods and comparability. *Psychotherapy Research, 24*(2), 474–482. doi:10.1080/10503307.2013.840812

Shenk, J. W. (2005). *Lincoln's melancholy: How depression challenged a president and fueled his greatness.* New York, NY: Mariner.

Syed, M. (2010). *Bounce: Mozart, Federer, Picasso, Beckham, and the science of success.* New York, NY: HarperCollins.

Tracey, T. J. G., Wampold, B. E., Goodyear, R. K., & Lichtenberg, J. W. (2015). Improving expertise in psychotherapy. *Psychotherapy Bulletin, 50*(1), 7–13.

Tracey, T. J. G., Wampold, B. E., Lichtenberg, J. W., & Goodyear, R. K. (2014). Expertise in psychotherapy: An elusive goal? *American Psychologist, 69*, 218–229. doi:10.1037/a0035099

Walfish, S., McAlister, B., O'Donnell, P., & Lambert, M. J. (2012). An assessment of self-assessment bias in mental health providers. *Psychological Reports, 110*(2), 639–644. doi:10.2466/02.07.17.PR0.110.2.639-644

Wampold, B. E. (2017). What should we practice? A contextual model for how psychotherapy works. In T. Rousmaniere, R. K. Goodyear, S. D. Miller, & B. E. Wampold (Eds.), *The cycle of excellence: Using deliberate practice to improve supervision and training* (pp. 49–65). Washington, DC: American Psychological Association.

Wampold, B. E., & Brown, G. S. (2005). Estimating variability in outcomes attributable to therapists: A naturalistic study of outcomes in managed care. *Journal of Consulting and Clinical Psychology, 73*(5), 914–923. doi:10.1037/0022-006X.73.5.914

Wampold, B. E., & Imel, Z. E. (2015). *The great psychotherapy debate: The evidence for what makes therapy work* (2nd ed.). New York, NY: Routledge.

Watkins, C. E., Jr. (2011). Does psychotherapy supervision contribute to patient outcomes? Considering thirty years of research. *Clinical Supervisor, 30*(2), 235–256. doi:10.1080/07325223.2011.619417

Whyte, D. (2011). *Keynote Address: Crossing the unknown sea.* 2011 Psychotherapy Networker Symposium, Washington, DC. Retrieved from http://archive.playbacknetworker.com/crossing-the-unknown-sea

APPENDIX

Outcome Measures and Forms

OUTCOME RATING SCALE (ORS)

Name: _____ Age (Yrs): _____ Sex: M/F

Session #: _____ Date: _____

Who is filling out this form? Please check one: Self _____ Other _____

If other, what is your relationship to this person? _____

Looking back over the last week, including today, help us understand how you have been feeling by rating how well you have been doing in the following areas of your life, where marks to the left represent low levels and marks to the right indicate high levels. *If you are filling out this form for another person, please fill out according to how you think he or she is doing.*

Individually
(Personal well-being)

|--|

Interpersonally
(Family, close relationships)

|--|

Socially
(Work, school, friendships)

|--|

Overall
(General sense of well-being)

|--|

International Center for Clinical Excellence

Source: www.centerforclinicalexcellence.com
© 2000 Scott D. Miller & Barry L. Duncan

CHILD OUTCOME RATING SCALE (CORS)

Name: _____ Age (Yrs): _____ Sex: M/F

Session #: _____ Date: _____

Who is filling out this form? Please check one: Child _____ Caretaker_____

If caretaker, what is your relationship to this child? _____

How are you doing? How are things going in your life? Please make a mark on the scale to let us know. The closer to the smiley face, the better things are. The closer to the frowny face, things are not so good. *If you are a caretaker filling out this form, please fill out according to how you think the child is doing.*

Me
(How am I doing?)

☹ |--| ☺

Family
(How are things in my family?)

☹ |--| ☺

School
(How am I doing at school?)

☹ |--| ☺

Everything
(How is everything going?)

☹ |--| ☺

International Center for Clinical Excellence

Source: www.centerforclinicalexcellence.com
© 2003 Barry L. Duncan, Scott D. Miller, & Jacqueline A. Sparks

OUTCOME MEASURES AND FORMS 285

YOUNG CHILD OUTCOME RATING SCALE (YCORS)

Name: _____ Age (Yrs): _____

Sex: M/F_____

Session #: _____ Date: _____

Choose one of the faces that shows how things are going for you. Or, you can draw one below that is just right for you.

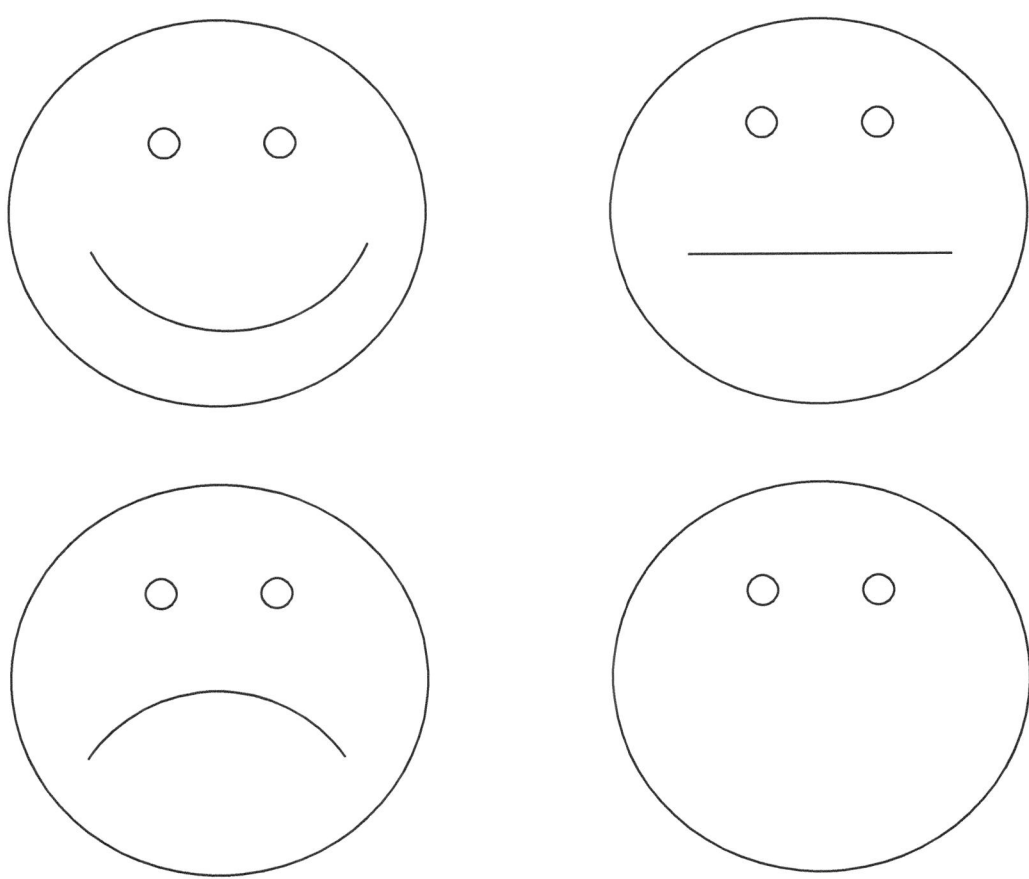

International Center for Clinical Excellence

Source: www.centerforclinicalexcellence.com
© 2003 Barry L. Duncan, Scott D. Miller, Andy Huggins, & Jacqueline A. Sparks

SESSION RATING SCALE (SRS V.3.0)

Name: _____ Age (Yrs): _____ Sex: M/F

Session #: _____ Date: _____

Please rate today's session by placing a mark on the line nearest to the description that best fits your experience.

Relationship

I did not feel heard, understood, and respected. |--| I felt heard, understood, and respected.

Goals and Topics

We did *not* work on or talk about what I wanted to work on and talk about. |--| We worked on and talked about what I wanted to work on and talk about.

Approach or Method

The therapist's approach is not a good fit for me. |--| The therapist's approach is a good fit for me.

Overall

There was something missing in the session today. |--| Overall, today's session was right for me.

International Center for Clinical Excellence

Source: www.centerforclinicalexcellence.com
© 2002 Scott D. Miller, Barry L. Duncan, & Lynn Johnson

CHILD SESSION RATING SCALE (CSRS)

Name: _____ Age (Yrs): _____ Sex: M/F

Session #: _____ Date: _____

How was our time together today? Please put a mark on the following lines to let us know how you feel.

Listening

did not always listen to me. |--| listened to me.

How Important

What we did and talked about was not really that important to me. |--| What we did and talked about were important to me.

What We Did

I did not like what we did today. |--| I liked what we did today.

Overall

I wish we could do something different. |--| I hope we do the same kind of things next time.

International Center for Clinical Excellence

Source: www.centerforclinicalexcellence.com
© 2003 Barry L. Duncan, Scott D. Miller, & Jacqueline A. Sparks

YOUNG CHILD SESSION RATING SCALE (YCSRS)

Name: _____ Age (Yrs): _____

Sex: M/F_____

Session #: _____ Date: _____

Choose one of the faces that shows how it was for you to be here today. Or, you can draw one below that is just right for you.

International Center for Clinical Excellence

Source: www.centerforclinicalexcellence.com
© 2003 Barry L. Duncan, Scott D. Miller, & Jacqueline A. Sparks

GROUP SESSION RATING SCALE (GSRS)

Name: _____ Age (Yrs): _____

ID#: _____ Sex: M/F

Session #: _____ Date: _____

Please rate today's group by placing a hash mark on the line nearest to the description that best fits your experience.

Relationship

I did not feel heard, understood, respected, and/or accepted by the leader and/or the group.

|--|

I felt heard, understood, respected, and accepted by the leader and the group.

Goals and Topics

We did *not* work on or talk about what I wanted to work on and talk about.

|--|

We worked on and talked about what I wanted to work on and talk about.

Approach or Method

The leader and/or the group's approach is not a good fit for me.

|--|

The leader and group's approach is a good fit for me.

Overall

There was something missing in group today—I was not engaged.

|--|

Overall, today's group was right for me—I felt engaged.

International Center for Clinical Excellence

Source: www.centerforclinicalexcellence.com
© 2007 Barry L. Duncan & Scott D. Miller

CLIENT OUTCOMES GRAPH V25

(Ages greater than 19 – Clinical Cutoff = 25)

Client Name: _____ Age: _____

ID: _____

	1	2	3	4	5	6	7	8	9	10	11	12
40												
35												
30												
25												
20												
15												
10												
5												
0												
Session Number	1	2	3	4	5	6	7	8	9	10	11	12

-------------------- SRS Cutoff
————————— ORS Clinical Cutoff

Session #	ORS/CORS	SRS/CSRS/GSRS
_____	_____	_____
_____	_____	_____
_____	_____	_____
_____	_____	_____
_____	_____	_____
_____	_____	_____
_____	_____	_____
_____	_____	_____
_____	_____	_____
_____	_____	_____
_____	_____	_____
_____	_____	_____

CLIENT OUTCOMES GRAPH V28

(Ages 13 to 19 – Clinical Cutoff = 28)

Client Name: _____ Age: _____

ID: _____

40												
35	--	--	--	--	--	--	--	--	--	--	--	--
30												
25												
20												
15												
10												
5												
0												
Session Number	1	2	3	4	5	6	7	8	9	10	11	12

------------------- SRS Cutoff
———————— ORS Clinical Cutoff

Session #	ORS/CORS	SRS/CSRS/GSRS
_____	_____	_____
_____	_____	_____
_____	_____	_____
_____	_____	_____
_____	_____	_____
_____	_____	_____
_____	_____	_____
_____	_____	_____
_____	_____	_____
_____	_____	_____
_____	_____	_____
_____	_____	_____

CLIENT OUTCOMES GRAPH V32

(Ages 12 or younger – Clinical Cutoff = 32)

Client Name: _____ Age: _____

ID: _____

Session Number	1	2	3	4	5	6	7	8	9	10	11	12
40												
35												
30												
25												
20												
15												
10												
5												
0												

-------------------- SRS Cutoff
———————— ORS Clinical Cutoff

Session #	ORS/CORS	SRS/CSRS/GSRS
_____	_____	_____
_____	_____	_____
_____	_____	_____
_____	_____	_____
_____	_____	_____
_____	_____	_____
_____	_____	_____
_____	_____	_____
_____	_____	_____
_____	_____	_____
_____	_____	_____
_____	_____	_____

LEEDS ALLIANCE IN SUPERVISION SCALE (LASS)

Supervisee Name: _____

Date of Supervision Session: _____

INSTRUCTIONS:

Please place a mark on the lines to indicate how you feel about your supervision session.

(Approach)

| This supervision session was not focused. | |---| | This supervision session was focused. |

(Relationship)

| My supervisor and I did not understand each other in this session. | |---| | My supervisor and I understood each other in this session. |

(Meeting My Needs)

| This supervision session was not helpful to me. | |---| | This supervision session was helpful to me. |

International Center for Clinical Excellence

Source: www.scottdmiller.com

© Wainwright, N. A. (2010). *The development of the Leeds Alliance in Supervision Scale (LASS): A brief sessional measure of the supervisory alliance*. Unpublished Doctoral Thesis, University of Leeds, England, UK.

SONAR SESSION FEEDBACK CHECKLIST

S

Start/Setup

O

Outcome Measurement

N

Now

A

Alliance Measurement

R

Respond

Source: Bertolino, B. (2013). The SONAR session feedback checklist (SSFC) (v1.5). Retrieved from https://www.bobbertolino.com/handouts

Index

abilities, focus on, 38
acceptance and commitment therapy (ACT), 197
ACE. *See* active client engagement
acknowledgment, 123, 147–148
   and possibility, 161–163
   and vision for future, 163–166
ACORN. *See* A Collaborative Outcomes Resource Network study
ACT. *See* acceptance and commitment therapy
actionable failure, 250–251
actionable feedback, 276
action and interaction class, 194
action change, 138
action complaints, 138
action praise, 138
action problems, 138
action requests, 138
action stage, 188–189
action-talk, 152–153, 156, 157, 216, 229
   clarifying client concerns, 137–140
   forms of, 138
active client engagement (ACE), 89–129
ADDRESSING acronym, 49
ADHD. *See* attention deficit hyperactivity disorder
adherence, 9
Adler, Alfred, 145–146
Adlerian therapy (individual psychology), 197
advanced skills, 255–257

allegiance effect, 7
alliance, 39, 71
   collaboration keys, 68–86
   outcome correlation, 63–64
alliance, attending, 220–226
   check-ins, 221
   dependence, 223–224
   responding to ruptures, 225–226
   responding to SRS feedback, 221–223
   using subscales, 224–225
ambiguity, 216
ambiguous/vague reports, 137, 216–217
American Journal of Orthopsychiatry, 30
American Orthopsychiatric Society conference, 30
American Psychological Association (APA), 5–6
   defining EBP, 27–30
   Division 29 Task Force standard, 26–27, 123, 187
   Task Force on Evidence-Based Practice, 71
analogies, 159
anecdotes, 159
APA. *See* American Psychological Association
"appreciative allies" concept, 40
apprehension, 204, 239–240
attention deficit hyperactivity disorder (ADHD), 155

295

attribution of change, 229–234
  "blame" client for change, 230–231
  sharing credit for change, 233–234
  speculation, about change, 231–233
attunement, 269–270
awareness, 50
  of verbal and nonverbal language, 119–122

Beatles, The, 248, 257, 261
behavioral rehearsal, 269
behaviorism, 36
behavior therapies, 197
"The Bell Curve: What Happens When Patients Find out How Good Their Doctors Really Are?" (Gawande), 12, 70
Berwick, Don, 12
BFTC. *See* Brief Family Therapy Center
bias, 11–13
bipolar disorder (BPD), 155
blame, 154, 230–231
bleeding pattern, in ORS scores, 209
Bohart, A. C., 44–45
bona fide models, 6, 30, 193–194
BPD. *See* bipolar disorder
Brief Family Therapy Center (BFTC), 145–146
Brown, Laura, 156
Bruce Lee, 257

Campbell, Joseph, 249
CBT. *See* cognitive behavioral therapy
CCH. *See* Cincinnati Children's Hospital
CF. *See* cystic fibrosis
changes
  advantages/disadvantages of, 185
  amplifying, 235
  attribution of, 229–234
  intention to, 186
  optimism about, 185–186
  perceptions and meaning of, 184–186
  preparing for, 90–91
  processes, 32
  and progress, 165–166
  readiness to, 182–190
  sharing credit for, 233–234
  stages of, 186–190
  theory of, 177–182
check-ins, 125–126, 221, 277
children outcome rating scale (CORS), 94
children session rating scale (CSRS), 98
Cincinnati Children's Hospital (CCH), 12, 70, 203
circular questions, 127
classes of intervention (COI), 175, 194–198
  course corrections, 197–198
classes of problems, 194–195
Clement, Paul, 108
client
  characteristics, 29–30, 32, 56
  contributions, 191
  feedback, 107
  outcome patterns, 208–211
  participation, 191
  permission, extending, 157–159
  preferences, accommodation of, 48, 81–86
  progress, monitoring, 55
  strengths and resources, activating, 217–220
  theory of change, 177–182
clinical cutoffs, 203
clinical expertise, 28–29
clinical significance, 203, 205
COE. *See* cycle of excellence
cognition and views class, 194
cognitive behavioral therapy (CBT), 9, 195, 197
cognitive therapy (CT), 172, 196, 197
COI. *See* classes of intervention
collaboration, 102
  creating context of, 89
  with outside entity, 149
collaboration keys, 68–86, 111
  addressing expectations, 76–81
  attending to preferences, 81–86
  creating space, 73–76
  information-gathering processes, 68–70
  routine outcome monitoring (ROM), 70–73

A Collaborative Outcomes Resource Network (ACORN) study, 254
collateral raters, 105–106
common factors, in effective therapy
  evolving from, 34–36
  history and conundrum, 30–34
  and placebo effects, 42
communicate hope and optimism, 56
communicate respect for clients and their cultures, 49–51
communities of practice, 278
competence, 9, 18, 29
concerns/problems
  relationship to, 183–184
  reports of, 213–215
confirmation bias, 261
Confucius, 172
congruence, 47, 123
consensus, 8
constructivism, 37
contemplation stage, 187–188
content questions, 118
contingent linking, 165–166
contradictory feelings, 167
Converging Themes in Psychotherapy (Goldfried and Padawer), 31
conversations, strengths-/pathology-based, 66
Cook County Hospital, 90–91
coping style, 182–183
CORS. *See* children outcome rating scale
cost offset research, 4
counseling, 16
counterevidence, 217
countertransference, 56
couples therapy, 83
creating space, for person in distress, 73–76
crystal balls, 146
Csikszentmihalyi, Mihaly, 37
CSRS. *See* children session rating scale
CT. *See* cognitive therapy
cubism art, 248
cultural competence, 50
cultural curiosity, 74–75
culture
  client's theory of change, 179–182
  of feedback, 104
  influences, 191
  strengths-based questions, 113–114
Cummings, E. E., 251
curiosity, 250
cycle of excellence (COE)
  determining baseline level of effectiveness, 258–260
  engaging in deliberate practice, 262–264
  feedback, 260–262
  framework, 258
cycling, in ORS scores, 210–211
cystic fibrosis (CF), 12, 70

DBT. *See* dialectical behavior therapy
decision-making processes, of clients, 226
"deep domain-specific" knowledge, 263
deliberate practice (DP)
  in context, 270–272
  deep domain-specific knowledge, 263
  engaging in, 262–264
  making plan for, 265
  in psychotherapy, 263–264
  strategies, 253
deliberate questions, 177
dependence, 223–224
depersonalization, 155, 157
de Shazer, Steve, 145
deterioration, 206–208, 220
  failure to identifying, 11–13
  responses to, 211–226
    activating client strengths, 217–220
    attending alliance, 220–226
    reexamining focus of therapy, 212–217
determinism, 154
Diagnostic and Statistical Manual of Mental Disorders (DSM), 26, 155
  DSM-5, 2
diagnostic labeling, 155
dialectical behavior therapy (DBT), 197
difficult material, in therapy, 56
dipping, in ORS scores, 209–210
disempowered populations, 102–103

Division 29 Task Force standard, 26–27, 123, 187
documentation, 69
Dodo bird effect, 7
DP. *See* deliberate practice
dropout, 126, 274
Dr. Seuss, 251
DSM. *See* *Diagnostic and Statistical Manual of Mental Disorders*

early client engagement
   alliance–outcome correlation, 63–64
   strengthening alliance through collaboration keys, 68–86
   strengths-based language and conversations, 64–67
EBP. *See* evidence-based practice
eclectic therapists, 193
Edison, Thomas, 250–251
education/school/vocational training strengths-based questions, 115
effectiveness, baseline level of, 258–260
effective therapy/therapists
   common factors, 30–34
   evidence-based practice, 25–30
   principles and core strategies, 25–57
   qualities and actions of therapists, 54–57
   strengths-based approach, 36–54
   understanding client expectations, 92
effect sizes (ES), 254, 259–260
8-Key Checklist for Method Selection (8-KCMS), 190, 191, 194, 195
80/20 rule, 70, 90–91, 111, 176, 203, 238–239, 276
Einstein, A., 250
electronic medical record (EMR), 106
EMDR. *See* eye movement desensitization and reprocessing
empathy, 47, 123, 255
empirically supported treatments (ESTs), 6, 25, 26, 176
EMR. *See* electronic medical record
endurance, 270
engagement, with clients, 73–76
epiphanies, 202

Erickson, Milton, 36, 51, 120–121, 146, 165
   Milton H. Erickson Foundation, 1
   using utilization concept, 169–171
Ericsson, K. A., 249, 265, 268
error-centric culture, 198, 250–251
ES. *See* effect sizes
ESTs. *See* empirically supported treatments
ETRs. *See* expected treatment responses
evidence-based practice (EBP), 179
   best available research, 28
   clinical expertise, 28–29
   defining, 27–30
   and empirically supported treatments, 25–27
   patient characteristics/culture/preferences, 29–30
evocation of strengths and resources, 89
Evolution of Psychotherapy conference, 1–2, 30
The Evolution of Psychotherapy (Zeig), 2
exception-oriented questions, 112–113
existential therapy, 197
expectancy
   and hope, 191
   and placebo factor, 33, 41–44
expectations, addressing, 76–81
expected treatment responses (ETRs), 106, 260
experiences, normalizing clients, 159–161
experiential and affective class, 194
explanations and treatment plans, 55
exploratory conversations, 116
exploratory questioning, 126–129
externalization, 183
external resources, 44
extratherapeutic factors, 33, 44
eye movement desensitization and reprocessing (EMDR), 197
Eysenck, Hans, 3

facilitative interpersonal skills (FIS) approach, 255, 268–269
failures, learning from, 250–253

family
    social relationships, strengths-based questions, 114
    therapy, 83
feedback, 57, 108–109, 126, 213, 222
    gathering and responding to, 253–254
    maximizing effects of, 276–277
    obtaining, 260–262
    quality/timeliness/usefulness of, 274–276
    tailoring of, 255
feedback-informed treatment (FIT), 29, 92, 109, 111, 201
FIS. *See* facilitative interpersonal skills approach
FIT. *See* feedback-informed treatment
"fit and effect" concept, 30, 35, 193
Fitzgerald, F. Scott, 166
fluctuations, 220
4WH questions, 118, 152, 228–229
Frank, Jerome, 31, 42, 156, 192
Freireich, Emil, 41
Freud, Sigmund, 36, 251
future-focused therapy, 191
future-oriented messages, 64
future-talk, 163–166

Gates, Bill, 248, 251
Gawande, Atul, 12, 41, 70, 277
genuineness. *See* congruence
Gestalt therapy, 197
Gilligan, Steve, 255
Gladwell, Malcolm, 257
global statements, 162
goals
    agreement on meaning/purpose of treatment, 140–147
    identifying progress toward, 151–152
    with multiple clients, 147–151
    and outcomes, revisiting, 237
    turning problem statements into, 164–165
    use of scaling questions, 152–153
Goldman, Lee, 90–91
Gretzky, Wayne, 248
grit and determination, 249–250
group session rating scale (GSRS), 98

growth mindset, 16
GSRS. *See* group session rating scale

Heine, R. W., 31
hobbies/interests, strengths-based questions, 115–116
Hoch, P., 31
hurdles, 277
    and setbacks, as opportunities, 240–244
hypnosis, 197

IHI. *See* Institute for Healthcare Improvement
imitation, 256
impossibility, 47, 154
improvement, 226–235
    amplifying change, 235
    attribution of change, 229–234
    driven mindset, 249, 258
    necessity of, 52
    professional, 29
inclusion, 166–169
individual functioning, 39
individual psychology, 145, 197
information
    acquisition of, 89
    gathering processes, 68–70, 89–129, 191, 229
Institute for Healthcare Improvement (IHI), 12
Institute of Medicine (IOM), 27
internalization, 183
internal strengths, 44
interpersonal functioning, 39
interpersonal skills, 54, 268–269
intervention, 175–198
    classes of problems/classes of intervention, 194–198
    invite, acknowledge, and match (I-AM) approach, 175
    matching, 176–190
        readiness to change, 182–190
        theory of change, 177–182
    model-outcome contradiction, 192–194
    path to models, 190–191

interviewing, 76–77
　for strengths, 92, 110–129
　　strengths-based content-area questioning, 112–116
　　strengths-based exploratory questioning, 116–129
invalidation, 154
　experiences of, 233–234
invite, acknowledge, and match (I-AM) approach, 175
involvement, in meetings, 82
IOM. *See* Institute of Medicine

Jobs, Steve, 249
Johansson, Frans, 262
Jordan, Michael, 251
Joyce, James, 251
Jungian analysis, 197

key competency, 41
Kuhn, Thomas, 27

labeling, 155–156
Lambert, Michael, 16, 32, 33
language
　and interaction, 191
　strengths-based, 64–67
　using to strengthening alliance, 153–172
LASS. *See* Leeds Alliance Supervision Scale
Leeds Alliance Supervision Scale (LASS), 276
Legg, Mike, 256
life changing experience, 202
Lincoln, Abraham, 250
lineal questions, 127
linguistic subtlety, 153
linking process, 147–148

Madsen, W. C., 40
maintenance stage, 189–190
mapping, 175
marginalized populations, 102–103

marital therapy, 238
Martin, George, 261
Maslow, Abraham, 36, 193
matching, 176–190
　client's theory of change, 177–182
　language, 119–129
　readiness to change
　　coping style, 182–183
　　perceptions and meaning of change, 184–186
　　relationship to concerns and problems, 183–184
　　stages of change, 186–190
May, Rollo, 36
The Medici Effect: Breakthrough Insights at the Intersection of Ideas, Concepts, and Cultures (Johansson), 262
mental health labels, 155
mental health professionals, role of, 52
meta-analysis, 3, 9, 28, 44
metaphor, 160
MI. *See* Motivational Interviewing
mindfulness, 65
mindset, 244
miracle question, 145
model and technique factor, 33
model-outcome contradiction, 192–194
monitoring, routine and ongoing, 111
Motivational Interviewing (MI), 111, 185, 197
Mozart, Wolfgang Amadeus, 248, 255
muscles of resilience strategies, 242
myths, about therapist effectiveness, 16

narrative therapy, 197
National Institute of Mental Health (NIMH), 3
National Registry of Evidence-Based Programs and Practices (NREPP), 94
negative emotions, 64
negative experiences, of therapy, 80
neurobiological class, 194
NIMH. *See* National Institute of Mental Health
nonaccountability, 154

nondescriptiveness, 155
NREPP. *See* National Registry of Evidence-Based Programs and Practices

obsessive compulsive disorder (OCD), 155
OCD. *See* obsessive compulsive disorder
O'Hanlon, Bill, 164
OMS. *See* outcomes management systems
open door approach, 240
optimism, 56
organizational cultures, 273
ORS. *See* outcome rating scale
outcome rating scale (ORS), 94–98, 137, 182, 201–202, 251, 252
   clinical cutoff for, 95
   example, 97–98
   feedback message for client, 206, 208
   introducing, 95–96
   scoring, 96–97
   subscales of, 96
   in subsequent sessions, 107–108
outcomes
   and alliance, 39, 71–72
   gathering information about client progress, 274
   goals and, 140, 238
   scores, 243
outcomes management systems (OMS), 106–108, 206, 259
Outliers: The Story of Success (Gladwell), 257
outside helpers, 147–151
overprediction, of client improvement, 11–13, 254
oxymoron, 167

paraphrasing, 123, 136
Pareto principle, 70
partial statements, translating statements into, 162
partners for change outcome management system (PCOMS), 94, 259
   further considerations, 102–108
   outcome rating scale (ORS), 94–98
   routine outcome monitoring (ROM) to, 108–110
   session rating scale (SRS), 94, 98–102
passion, 249–250
past tense, using, 161–162
pathology-based conversations, 64, 65, 66, 155
pathology-based labeling, 155
patient characteristics, 29–30
patient's participation, 47
PBE. *See* practice-based evidence
PCOMS. *See* partners for change outcome management system
perceptual statements, translating statements into, 162
permission
   extending clients, 157–159
   "not to have to" permission, 158
   "to" and "not to have to" permission, 158
   "to" permission, 158
personal characteristics/qualities, strengths-based questions, 113
personal philosophies, 41, 169, 192, 250
person-centered therapy, 197
person-first language, use of, 156
Persuasion and Healing: A Comparative Study of Psychotherapy (Frank), 42
Picasso, Pablo, 198, 248
placebo effects, 42
planned/pre-established interventions, 154
plateauing, in ORS scores, 211
positive emotions, 64
positive regard, 47, 123
posttraumatic growth, 44
practice
   advanced skills, 255–257
   gathering and responding to feedback, 253–254
   mastering basics, 254–255
   putting in time, 257–258
   real-world practice, 257
   settings, 17, 18
practice-based evidence (PBE), 176

precontemplation stage, 187
predictive algorithms, 260
preexisting beliefs, 79
pre-interviews, 76
premature terminations, 274
preparation stage, 188
Prescott, C. L., 108
presupposition, 165
pretreatment/preservices expectancy, 42
previous therapy (behavioral healthcare) experiences
   strengths-based questions, 116
problem/situation, exception-oriented questions, 112–113
problem-specific questions, 177
process questions, 118
prodigies, 256
professional development, 28
   achieving clinical excellence, 247–278
   cycle of excellence
      determining baseline level of effectiveness, 259–260
      engaging in deliberate practice, 262–264
      obtaining systematic, ongoing, formal feedback, 260–262
   deliberate practice
      in context, 270–272
      deep domain-specific knowledge, 263
      engaging in, 262–264
      making plan for, 265
      in psychotherapy, 263–264
      strategies, 253
   further ideas
      attunement, 269–270
      behavioral rehearsal, 269
      endurance, 270
      visual rehearsal, 269
   path to clinical excellence, 277–279
   road to excellence, 248–258
      grit and determination, 249–250
      learning from failures, 250–253
      practice, 253–258
   supervision, 272–277
      maximizing effects of feedback, 276–277
      quality/timeliness/usefulness of feedback, 274–276
      ROM purpose, 272
      supervisees' performance and, 273–274
   therapeutic effectiveness
      strategies for practice to improving, 264–270
      understanding, 247–248
progress in therapy, 235–244
pronouns, use of, 184
psychoanalysis, 36
   and psychodynamic therapies, 197
psychotherapy
   commonalities across models of, 32
   deliberate practice in, 263–264
   effectiveness of various methods and models, 5–8
   evolution in, 2
   "good news, bad news" conundrum, 3–5
   major models of, 197
   training and supervision, 8–10

quality feedback, 276
quality reviews, 69
questionnaires, 111

Railton, P., 270
Ramanujan, Srinivasa, 248–249
randomized controlled trial (RCT), 3, 26, 27, 28
rational-emotive behavior therapy, 197
RCI. *See* reliable change index
RCT. *See* randomized controlled trial
readiness, to change
   coping style, 182–183
   perceptions and meaning of change, 184–186
   relationship to concerns and problems, 183–184
   stages of change, 186–190
reality therapy, 197
real-time feedback, 39, 73
real-world practice, 257
reflective practitioner, 17–19

reflexive questions, 128
Reilly, Brendan, 90–91
relative size (RES), 259
reliable change, 260
reliable change index (RCI), 202–203
reporting, meaning and, 29
RES. *See* relative size
research foundations, 29
Resolution on Recognition of Psychotherapy Effectiveness, 7
Ricks, D., 10–11
ripple effect, 235
risks, to therapist effectiveness and outcomes, 11–13
Rogers, Carl, 36, 47, 159, 161
role-play scenarios, 241, 268
ROM. *See* routine outcome monitoring
Rosenzweig, Saul, 7, 30
Rousmaniere, Tony, 271
routine outcome monitoring (ROM), 11, 12, 28, 39, 53, 68, 70–73, 92, 93–110, 175, 190, 191, 201, 254, 272–273
Rowling, J. K., 251
Rumi, Jalal al-Din, 172
ruptures, responding to, 225–226

safety, 86
SAMHSA. *See* Substance Abuse Mental Health Services Administration
scaling questions, 152–153
Sculley, John, 249
SED. *See* severely emotionally disturbed
seesawing/fluctuating, in ORS scores, 210–211
Seidel, Jason, 277–278
self-actualization, 36
self-assessment bias, 11–13
self-awareness, 50, 277
self-change, 45, 230
self-disclosure, 160
self-reflection, 19
Seligman, Martin, 37
serious and persistent mental illness (SPMI), 155
session rating scale (SRS), 98–102, 186, 201, 251
 cutoff, 98
 examples, 100–102
 introducing, 98–99
 responding to feedback, 221–223
 scoring, 99–100
 subscales, 224
setbacks and hurdles, as opportunities, 240–244
setup, outcome, now, alliance and respond (SONAR), 109–110
Session Feedback Checklist (SSFC), 109–110, 125, 202
severely emotionally disturbed (SED), 155
SFBT. *See* solution-focused brief therapy
sharing credit, for change, 233–234
significant change, 260
simulations
 -based learning, 267
 information obtained from, 274
skill development
 facilitative interpersonal skills (FIS), 268–269
 review video recordings, 266
 simulation-based learning, 267
 video review strategies, 266–267
skills
 advanced, 255–257
 mastering basic, 254–255
 refinement, 265
SOC. *See* stages of change
social relationships, 235
social role functioning, 39
solution-focused brief therapy (SFBT), 146, 197
solution-talk and problem-talk, 67
"Some Implicit Common Factors in Diverse Models of Psychotherapy" (Rosenzweig), 30
SONAR. *See* setup, outcome, now, alliance and respond
speculation, 231–233
splitting, idea of, 168–169
SPMI. *See* serious and persistent mental illness
spreadsheets, 106

SRS. *See* session rating scale
stages of change (SOC), 186–190
    action, 188–189
    contemplation, 187–188
    maintenance, 189–190
    precontemplation, 187
    preparation, 188
standard community care, 6
stigmatizing words, eliminating, 156
stories, 159
strategic and structural family therapies, 197
strategic questions, 128
strengths-based approach, 15, 25, 179, 181, 220
    definition of, 38–39
    evidence to practice, 40–54
    and psychotherapy, 36–40
strengths-based conversation, 64–67
strengths-based information gathering, 92
strengths-based questioning
    content-area questioning, 112–116
    exploratory questioning, 116–129
The Structure of Magic (Bandler and Grinder), 273
Strupp, Hans, 10
Stuart, John T., 250
subscales, SRS, 224–225
Substance Abuse Mental Health Services Administration (SAMHSA), 27, 94
summarizing, 124, 136
supershrinks, 11
supervision, 262, 272–277
    maximizing effects of feedback, 276–277
    quality/timeliness/usefulness of feedback, 274–276
    ROM purpose in, 272–273
    supervisees' performance and, 273–274
supportive services, 223
supportive therapy, 6

TAR. *See* thought, action, and reflection (TAR) process

Task Force on the Promotion and Dissemination of Psychological Procedures (TFPP), 5–6
TAU. *See* treatment as usual
TDCRP. *See* Treatment of Depression Collaborative Research Program
termination, 189, 239
TFPP. *See* Task Force on the Promotion and Dissemination of Psychological Procedures
theory of change, 177–182
therapeutic alliance, 46–49, 54, 220
    accommodation of client's preferences, 48
    agreement on goals, meaning, or purpose of treatment, 47
    agreement on means and methods used in treatment, 47–48
    client's view of relationship, 46–47
therapeutic conversations
    advanced listening and attending skills, 153–172
        acknowledging and validating clients' internal experience, 161–163
        extend clients permission, 157–159
        future-talk, 163–166
        inclusion, 166–169
        normalizing clients experiences, 159–161
        using person-first language, 155–157
        utilization, 169–172
    bringing focus to, 135–153
        action-talk, clarifying client concerns, 137–140
        clarifying problems, goals, and progress through scaling, 152–153
        goal consensus, 140–147
        goal-setting with multiple clients, 147–151
        identifying progress toward goals, 151–152
therapeutic relationship
    with clients, 48–49
    factor, 32, 33
    focus on, 39

therapist
  continuity, 16–17
  effects, 13–19
  exploring performance, 10–13
  influence of, 1–19
  matching client's language, 120–122
  personal philosophy, 14–16
  reflective practitioner, 17–19
  worldview, 14–16
therapist effectiveness, 54–57
  myths about, 16
  and outcomes, 11–13
  strategies for practice to improving
    making a plan for deliberate
      practice, 265
    professional development, 269–270
    skill development, 266–269
    skill refinement, 265
  understanding, 247–248
therapist performance
  gathering information about client
    progress, 274
  information obtained from
    simulations, 274
  observation of, 273
therapist qualities, 32
thought, action, and reflection (TAR)
  process, 19, 68
Tilsen, Julie, 75
timelines, of feedback, 276
time machine, 146–147
Tomm, K., 127
tracking process, 147–148
transition, from therapy, 239–244
transtheoretical model, 186
  of change, 32
treatment
  plan, 55
  structure, 32
treatment as usual (TAU), 238
Treatment of Depression Collaborative
  Research Program (TDCRP), 42
trouble zones, 244

unconditional positive regard, 47
unimprovement, 204–206
  responses to, 211–226
    activating client strengths,
      217–220
    attending alliance, 220–226
    reexamining focus of therapy,
      212–217
utilization, 169–172

vague words, 137, 141
validation, 123, 163
video recordings, reviewing, 266
video-talk, 140
visual, auditory, tactile (kinesthetic),
  gustatory, and olfactory (V/A/T/
  G/O) realms, 194
visual rehearsal, 269

Wampold, Bruce, 34–36, 44, 54, 255
Watson, G., 30–31
well-being, 38
  check-ups, 239
Wenger, Etienne, 278
Whyte, David, 249–250
Wizard of the Desert (Vesely), 51
Wolpe, Joseph, 2
work/employment/career, strengths-
  based questions, 114–115
working alliance, with clients, 46–49,
  54–55

YCORS. *See* young children outcome
  rating scale
YCSRS. *See* young children session
  rating scale
YIN. *See* Youth In Need (YIN), Inc.
young children outcome rating scale
  (YCORS), 95
young children session rating scale
  (YCSRS), 98
Youth In Need (YIN), Inc., 102,
  206, 275

Zeig, Jeff, 1–2